Praise for *Skinny Liver*

"*Skinny Liver* sounds a powerful wake-up call that clearly connects dietary and other lifestyle choices to potentially life-threatening liver disease. More importantly, Kirkpatrick deftly empowers the reader with a scientifically validated, comprehensive, user-friendly plan to prevent and even reverse what has become a major health epidemic."
—David Perlmutter, MD, #1 *New York Times* best-selling author

"Fatty liver disease is a silent epidemic that is affecting 30 percent of all Americans. Grounded in cutting-edge research, Kristin Kirkpatrick's accessible, practical program will help you prevent liver disease and safeguard your overall health."
—Mark Hyman, MD, Director, Cleveland Clinic Center for Functional Medicine, #1 *New York Times* best-selling author

"In today's toxic world, we are bombarded with chemicals in our environment, food supply, water, and personal care products, and our liver takes the brunt of the stress. If your liver becomes overwhelmed, it can lead to fatigue, weight gain, liver disease, autoimmune disease, and even cancer. In *Skinny Liver*, Kristin Kirkpatrick teaches you the secrets on the ideal diet, supplements, and lifestyle to cleanse your liver and take your health to the next level."
—Dr. Josh Axe, author *of Eat Dirt*, founder of DrAxe.com

Regenerative Health

Regenerative Health

DISCOVER YOUR METABOLIC TYPE AND RENEW YOUR LIVER FOR LIFE

Kristin Kirkpatrick, MS, RD, LD,
and Ibrahim Hanouneh, MD

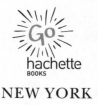

NEW YORK

Copyright © 2024 by Kristin Kirkpatrick and Ibrahim Hanouneh

Illustrations by Tomoko Shibusawa

Cover design by Amanda Kain
Cover copyright © 2024 by Hachette Book Group, Inc.

Hachette Go, an imprint of Hachette Books
Hachette Book Group
1290 Avenue of the Americas
New York, NY 10104
HachetteGo.com
Facebook.com/HachetteGo
Instagram.com/HachetteGo

First Edition: February 2024

Published by Hachette Go, an imprint of Hachette Book Group, Inc. The Hachette Go name and logo is a trademark of the Hachette Book Group.

The Hachette Speakers Bureau provides a wide range of authors for speaking events. To find out more, go to hachettespeakersbureau.com or email HachetteSpeakers@hbgusa.com.

Hachette Go books may be purchased in bulk for business, educational, or promotional use. For information, please contact your local bookseller or Hachette Book Group Special Markets Department at: special.markets@hbgusa.com.

The publisher is not responsible for websites (or their content) that are not owned by the publisher.

Library of Congress Cataloging-in-Publication Data has been applied for.

Library of Congress Control Number: 2023935798

ISBNs: 978-0-306-83015-0 (hardcover); 978-0-306-83017-4 (ebook)

Printed in the United States of America

LSC-C

Printing 1, 2023

To my first and forever best friends,
Dima and Mo—Ibrahim

To my amazing husband, Andy—the cape
actually belongs on you—Kristin

contents

Your Liver or Your Life

S PIDER-MAN HAS MANY impressive talents and skills. He can climb walls. Shoot webs. Sense danger. But perhaps his most crucial superpower is his ability to repair himself, as it's what enables him to continue maintaining the peace.

Your liver is a lot like Spider-Man. It has many skills, performing more than three hundred vital roles in the body. These include metabolizing and deriving energy from your food, removing toxins from the blood, and working in synchrony with all the other major organs, including the heart, brain, and kidneys. What truly sets the liver apart from all other organs, however, is that it can regenerate itself—if someone donates a portion of their liver to a loved one in need of a transplant, the donor's and the recipient's livers will have grown back to original size within just a few weeks. It's truly an incredible feat— like something out of a comic book.

And that's a very good thing because, just like a superhero, your liver regularly endures attacks from multiple angles. (You'll learn more about those assaults and other risk factors for fatty liver in the chapters to come, but they include easily accessible, low-nutrient-dense foods that are higher in calories but lower in nutrients; too little sleep overall or poor-quality sleep; insufficient movement; environmental toxins; type 2 diabetes; and poor metabolic health.)

There is one vital way that your liver is different from Spider-Man: in the movies, Spider-Man may take longer to regenerate after a series of intense challenges, but he eventually bounces back. Your liver, on the other hand, can get to a tipping point where its regenerative abilities are lost and the only option is a liver transplant.

This fact is what inspired us to write our first book, *Skinny Liver: A Proven Program to Prevent and Reverse the New Silent Epidemic— Fatty Liver Disease*, in 2017. We wrote *Skinny Liver* to raise awareness of the growing epidemic of non-alcoholic fatty liver disease (NAFLD) and to share the eating and lifestyle strategies we've used to help our combined thousands of patients slow or even reverse the progression of this silent disease. In NAFLD, healthy liver tissue gets replaced by fat cells not because of drinking too much alcohol but because of eating too many of the wrong types of foods. We call NAFLD *silent* because most people who have fatty liver disease don't know it. As you'll learn, its symptoms are generally vague until the disease is very far along; most people only learn they have it after having their blood drawn at their annual physical and being told that their liver enzyme levels are elevated.

And it's so important that your liver stays healthy. While you may not have been thinking of the liver as the target of your health efforts, it is the hinge that decides which way the gates of your health swing, playing a role in chronic inflammation, heart health, mental health, cognitive health, and metabolic health (including type 2 diabetes). Let's get those gates moving in the right direction.

The good news is that, except for the final stages, thanks to the liver's regenerative properties, fatty liver disease is absolutely treatable, even reversible. We see patients with fatty liver restore their liver health every day. We are a medical doctor (MD—that's Ibrahim) with a specialty in liver disease who previously worked at the Cleveland Clinic and at the Mayo Clinic, and who now sees patients and manages research at MNGI Digestive Health in Minneapolis; and a registered dietitian (RD—that's Kristin) in the Cleveland Clinic Department of Wellness and Preventive Medicine. We believe that our combination of medical and nutritional expertise, as well as our experiences treating patients at some of the top medical centers in the United States and coaching them through making behavioral changes that last, is exactly what's needed to treat a medical disease for which there are no pharmacological or surgical solutions. Together, we offer a full-spectrum approach to health that's too often missing from modern medicine.

Why We Need Regenerative Health Now More Than Ever

We urgently need to raise awareness of liver health because the prevalence of fatty liver disease has gotten significantly worse in the years since we wrote our first book—now, one in four people worldwide has been diagnosed with it, while millions more remain unaware that they are somewhere on the liver disease spectrum. Most alarmingly, this worsening trend is also true for children and young people—and since the longer you have the disease the more likely it is to progress past the reversible stage, this is not good news.

There have been good developments in the last few years, too: as cases of fatty liver have grown, so has our understanding of how to treat it.

What's New in Liver Health: The Four Metabolic Types

As you'll learn in this book, in the past few years there has been a fundamental shift in our knowledge of the causes of non-alcoholic fatty liver disease. After all, medical knowledge, just like health, isn't "set it and forget it." We used to think (and some doctors who haven't been following and processing the latest research still maintain) that obesity was the primary driver of fatty liver disease, and therefore, the sweeping advice was simply to lose weight. Now we know that it's not the numbers on the scale that matter—it's other numbers that reflect your overall metabolic health, such as your blood glucose levels, blood pressure, and waist circumference, that do.

The new approach to treating fatty liver disease is much more individualized. We now understand, for example, that you can be overweight but still be metabolically healthy, and that you can be at what's considered a healthy weight but be metabolically at risk.

In this book, we introduce the four metabolic types—the Preventer (healthy and lean), the Fine-Tuner (healthy and non-lean), the Recalibrator (unhealthy and lean), and the Regenerator (unhealthy and non-lean). And we help you identify which quadrant you fall into and guide you on customizing your eating and lifestyle plan to your particular metabolic profile.

We've also customized our advice to the four specific stages of liver disease and outlined how to prevent fatty liver from settling in in the first place—both for you and for your children. You'll be able to find the eating plan that matches your metabolic profile, your stage of liver disease, your lifestyle, and your goals. And if you have kids and want to help them avoid developing NAFLD now or in the future, we've also included a Family plan that can help you eat healthier as a family without having to focus on losing weight (which can be problematic for multiple reasons that we'll delve into in Chapter 10).

All of our plans are based on the Mediterranean diet—consistently shown to be one of the healthiest eating plans around—with more of a focus on reducing overall consumption of carbs and upgrading the carbs that you do eat in order to make them more nutrient-dense. None of our plans are very low carb—also known as ketogenic—because we design them to be something you can follow for life. We also provide guidance on how to take care of your liver by finding ways to move more, counter the effects of stress, and learn how good it feels when you are giving your liver what it needs to function at its best.

Making Changes That Last

We know how tempting it is to jump in with both feet and completely overhaul your diet and lifestyle—particularly if you've recently been told that you have some form of fatty liver disease and you want to get going. The thing is, fatty liver develops slowly, over time. And so any changes you make to address it also need to last for the long term. Throughout this book, we've included checklists and check-ins to help you be thoughtful about the changes you adopt and track your progress along the way. We suggest you pick up a notebook or journal that you can devote to your Regenerative Health journey—you'll also be able to look back and see how many changes you've made, which will be very helpful in motivating you to keep going.

Your Body Has Superpowers, but It Needs Your Help

Remember, diet and lifestyle modifications are not only the best ways to treat and reverse the disease—they are the *only* ways. This means your liver is counting on you to take care of it so that it can continue taking care of you.

Just as Spider-Man's alter ego, Peter Parker, was told by his uncle, "With great power comes great responsibility," you, too, have a great responsibility to take care of your liver so that it can continue to help you take the assaults of our modern world in stride and retain its power to regenerate itself and your health.

part one

The New Science of Loving Your Liver

chapter 1

Healthy Liver, Healthy You

I MAGINE THAT YOU are flying above a major metropolitan city. You can see the main highway that feeds the majority of traffic into, through, and out of town. You can also see the cloverleaf exits that shunt traffic onto smaller roads that lead to different neighborhoods. If you were on the ground, you might think that the roads you take every day are the most important for the flow of traffic in and around the city, but from thirty thousand feet up, you can see that the net-work of roadways is a cohesive whole that keeps life flowing—in other words, they all matter.

Your health is like a greater metropolitan area. Your vascular system is a lot like those roadways, and your health is reliant on each of those roads flowing easily to the major centers of commerce that are your heart, kidneys, digestive system, bones, and liver. If there's a blockage in that flow at any point, the health of the entire system is in peril.

In this analogy, the liver is like the public utilities department, sweeping the streets of trash (or, in your body's case, toxins), running the buses that help people get where they need to go (the macronutri-ents in your food that need to get to your cells), and dispersing the things the city needs to stay safe, like salting the roads ahead of a snowstorm (in your body's case, distributing vital ingredients like vitamins and minerals). The liver provides the infrastructure that everyone expects to just *work* but nobody gives much thought to until something goes wrong.

You may be thinking, "There's nothing wrong with my liver." But odds are, you're wrong.

The thing is, your liver is the strong and silent type. It doesn't give a lot of clues that it's not doing well. In fact, most people don't dis-cover they have a liver issue until they visit a health care provider who either makes an educated guess that a struggling liver may explain the person's symptoms or orders routine blood tests that come back with eyebrow-raising results.

Chances are, your liver is involved if you are concerned about:

- Chronic inflammation—this common condition, which is associated with nearly every chronic disease, including type 2 diabetes, insulin resistance, dyslipidemia, and cardiovascular disease, can be exacerbated if excess fat cells in the liver burst, triggering an immune response that can lead to inflammation within the liver itself that ripples out to the rest of the bloodstream
- Your heart health—and since cardiovascular disease (for example, heart attack and stroke) is the number one cause of mortality for men and women, this is an appropriate concern
- Your metabolic health, because your doctor has told you that you are prediabetic or you've been diagnosed with type 2 diabetes, as one in three Americans have been
- Your digestive health, because you have inflammatory bowel disease or celiac disease, or simply because you've been noticing your weight creep up
- Your bone health, because you're one of the 12.6 percent of Americans over age fifty who have been diagnosed with osteoporosis (nearly 20 percent for women), or the 43.1 percent of Americans over the age of fifty who have low bone density[1]
- Your reproductive health, particularly if you have been diagnosed with polycystic ovarian syndrome
- Your brain health, because you've noticed some mild forgetfulness, foggy thinking, or changes in cognitive ability
- Your mental health, as fatty liver is significantly correlated with depression and anxiety, particularly in women[2]

Let's take a look at the most important connection, the one between your liver and your heart.

The Liver and the Heart: A (Potentially Tragic) Love Story

Although developing fatty liver disease can be a major blow to your health—one that can even become deadly over time—believe it or not, the liver isn't likely to be the cause of death for the vast majority of people with fatty liver.

Ibrahim often tells his patients that the liver is like a car. It can get dented and beat up through everyday wear and tear. It can even be involved in minor accidents and still get you where you need to go. It may not look pretty, but it remains functional despite a fair amount of adversity. It's only if you keep crashing the car that it won't be able to take you to work anymore. And just as most cars on the road aren't dented beyond recognition, only a small percentage of people with fatty liver develop cirrhosis or liver cancer.

The most common cause of death in patients with fatty liver is cardiovascular disease—most often meaning a heart attack, heart failure, or stroke. That's not just an interesting coincidence; it's because the state of the liver is negatively impacting the health of your cardiovascular system. This is a big deal, because cardiovascular disease is the leading cause of death worldwide.

The liver and the heart are like romantic partners who each have their separate roles but who collaborate to keep the train on the tracks. The liver makes cholesterol, for one. And when fatty liver develops, the liver makes more of a specific type of cholesterol known as very low-density lipoprotein (VLDL). Once VLDL is circulating in the blood, it is vulnerable to being transformed into small, dense, low-density lipoprotein (LDL), the worst kind of the "bad" form of cholesterol. This LDL then begins to build up in arteries and reduce the flow of blood to the heart. In addition, as fat in the liver builds up, there is more inflammation in the liver, and fatty liver disease progresses into the "bad" territory. When this happens, proinflammatory chemicals can get into the blood and contribute to impaired vascular system function. It's like the liver starts spewing out trash that clogs up the roadways used to carry blood and nutrients to and from the heart.

We don't mean to be all doom and gloom. Remember that your liver can regenerate. Unless you are in the later stages of liver disease, it *can* get better. And remember that taking better care of your liver will take better care of your entire being—your heart, your kidneys, your brain, your bones, and your metabolic health. In fact, if you are among the one in three people who are either prediabetic or diabetic, the

---

FUNCTIONS OF YOUR SUPERHERO ORGAN

Filtering toxins out of blood

Transforming those toxins so they can be excreted

Forming bile, which carries toxins out of the body

Making cholesterol

Metabolizing and storing fat, carbohydrates, and proteins

Processing, storing, and secreting glucose

Metabolizing and storing vitamins and minerals, including vitamin A (important for eye health), vitamin K (important for blood clotting), vitamin D (vital for bone health and immunity), and calcium and phosphorous (key components of bone health)

Making and storing proteins that help the blood clot properly

---

liver-friendly plans we share in this book will help to address your metabolic dysfunction, too.[3]

A Crisis for Many

Fatty liver has very few symptoms until the disease is very far along—so unless you're looking for it, you likely won't find it. And the truth is, fatty liver is spreading like wildfire. Three and a half decades ago, between 1988 and 1994, the prevalence of NAFLD was 5.5 percent. Just a few years later, between 1999 and 2004, it jumped to 9.8 percent. Between 2005 and 2008, it ticked up again, to 11 percent.[4] And now, additional studies have put the current prevalence of fatty liver at closer to 40 percent.[5] Some studies have found even higher rates of prevalence, even in asymptomatic people, as high as 46 percent.[6]

The number of Americans with late-stage liver disease—past the point of possible reversal—that was not associated with alcohol more than doubled in the decade between 1999 and 2009.[7] And the number of patients on the waitlist for liver transplant due to a non-alcohol-related case of liver disease has been steadily increasing since 2002 like a roller coaster inching its way up to the highest part of the track.[8]

At this rate, one in two people will have NAFLD worldwide by the time today's kindergartners are in high school. Think about that—every other person in the world!

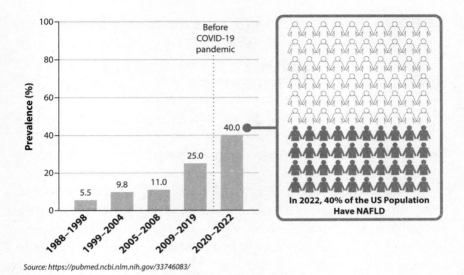

Source: https://pubmed.ncbi.nlm.nih.gov/33746083/

Figure 1.1. Prevalence of NAFLD in the United States

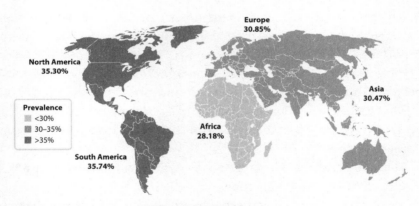

Source: https://www.cghjournal.org/article/S1542-3565(21)01280-5/fulltext

Figure 1.2. Global Prevalence of NAFLD

The First and Second Waves: Obesity and Type 2 Diabetes

As important as it is to quantify how many people are experiencing non-alcoholic fatty liver disease, it's just as vital to understand *why* it's as pervasive as it is.

Since the 1970s, obesity has become significantly more common around the globe. And obesity is regularly mentioned in scientific literature as a cause of non-alcoholic fatty liver disease. In addition, as obesity rates have risen, the prevalence of NAFLD has followed a similar path, like a dog on a leash following its human.

However, just because obesity and non-alcoholic fatty liver disease are correlated, this doesn't necessarily mean obesity *causes* NAFLD. The true root of NAFLD is more nuanced than that (and is something we'll dive into in Chapter 2).

Another condition that closely correlates with NAFLD is diabetes. That one in two people will be diagnosed with NAFLD in the near future is shocking, but it makes sense when you consider how fatty liver is often found in people who have been diagnosed with type 2 diabetes or who are prediabetic. While in the general population, two out of five adults have fatty liver, in people with type 2 diabetes, it's three out of four. That's a difference of 40 percent versus 75 percent. And most of those people have no idea that their livers are in peril.

According to the CDC, one in ten Americans have diabetes, and one in three Americans have prediabetes.[9] Other sources, such as the International Diabetes Foundation (IDF), put this number much higher—the IDF says that one in seven Americans are living with diabetes.[10] Because full-blown diabetes and prediabetes significantly ratchet up your risk of developing fatty liver, and both are on such an upward trajectory, it stands to reason that fatty liver is on the same dramatic rise.

The connection between type 2 diabetes and fatty liver disease is so strong that the American Diabetic Association updated their standards of care in 2019 to state that every patient with type 2 diabetes should be evaluated for the presence of fatty liver. Increasingly, it is reasonable to assume that if you are prediabetic or diabetic, your liver is in danger.

The Third Wave: COVID-19

As bad as these trends are, COVID-19 only made them worse. Part of the reason for this rise is that during the lockdown portion of the pandemic, three things that are harmful to liver health skyrocketed: stress, overeating, and alcohol consumption. In general, we moved a lot less, we ate a lot more processed foods, and we drank more. While we are now past those intense days, their effects can still be felt on our livers—particularly if some of the coping mechanisms we developed during that time solidified into lasting habits. While you were trying to just get through the pandemic, you could have overworked your liver to the point that you developed the early stages of fatty liver disease. Or if you already had it (even if you didn't know it), your fatty liver disease could have progressed without your realizing it.

Beyond that, the COVID-19 virus does directly attack the liver. It is not uncommon to see abnormal liver tests in patients infected with COVID-19, as the virus targets specific receptors on liver cells that then become damaged, and liver enzymes then leak out of those cells, making their levels elevated. After the virus recedes, liver tissue typically will regenerate and chronic or progressive injury won't develop—unless you're one of the approximately 20 percent of people whose COVID symptoms linger, in what's known as long COVID, where symptoms last weeks or even months beyond the initial infection. A 2022 survey conducted by the CDC found that 40 percent of adult Americans had been infected with COVID. Of those, about 20 percent experienced long COVID—that's over 20.5 million people in the United States alone.[11] As the virus continues to infect more people, and more people repeatedly, the number of people with long COVID will only rise, which is concerning not just because of the symptoms' effects on quality of life but also because NAFLD has been found to be highly prevalent in people who have long COVID.

Although the worst days of the pandemic are behind us, COVID is still very much a part of our reality, and with continual risks of recurring infections—which increase the risk of developing long COVID—we now have yet another reason to prioritize our liver health.

In a common example of COVID's lasting effects, one of Kristin's patients had been following our liver health plans and had made some really great advances in swapping out ultra-processed foods, eating fewer carbs, and improving her markers of metabolic health (in her case, her waist size decreased and her blood sugar and triglyceride levels came down). She was enjoying a partial reversal of her NAFLD and on her way to full reversal when COVID hit. She went from working in an office to working from home. The fact that she was always home coupled with the stress and anxiety of the pandemic made emotional eating an easy outlet. This woman has kids, who were now home from school. To feed her hungry kids during the day, she started keeping a lot of snack foods on hand, which are high in refined carbs and sugar, and began eating them herself.

Hers was a perfect storm of conditions that so many of us faced, and she lost all the gains she had made—she was headed toward "the bad" stage of fatty liver disease, and her metabolic profile (particularly her blood sugar and waist size) worsened.

Kristin put her on a moderate-carb plan that was easy to implement, and she is making progress. Her story is a great example of how even the best plan has to take into account your environment and whatever may be happening in your life. New stressors provide all the more reason to have a range of options to choose from so that you can personalize your plan to your body and your life.

The Crest of the Wave: Our Children

Speaking of schoolkids, the most alarming trend in the spread of fatty liver disease is its appearance in children. While most patients are diagnosed with NAFLD in their forties or fifties,[12] fatty liver is becoming more common in children and young adults. This is particularly troubling because liver disease takes time to progress. There are typically one to three years between NAFLD and NASH (non-alcoholic steatohepatitis, when the liver becomes inflamed), and then another three to five years between NASH and fibrosis (when the liver starts to become scarred). Cirrhosis (when scar tissue replaces a significant portion of healthy liver tissue) typically takes from twenty to twenty-five years to develop, and liver cancer comes next. So the longer you have fatty liver, the higher your odds of developing cirrhosis or liver cancer—the two stages of disease for which transplant is the only treatment.

In Ibrahim's practice, he is seeing more and more patients in their mid- to late twenties with the stage of liver disease that you normally see at age fifty or sixty. This is the natural result of becoming metabolically unhealthy in childhood: you can end up being twenty years into liver disease before you're thirty.

Just as with adults, COVID-19 did not help the health of our children. As they quarantined indoors and took classes virtually, their sedentarism and screen time rose exponentially, and for many, their metabolism suffered as a result. Parents who were trying to complete work while also taking care of their kids, or who had to report to work and leave their kids at home, faced a number of difficult situations and decisions during those days. Too often (but understandably), parents had to rely on packaged convenience foods to make mealtimes easier— but these are the very foods that contribute to liver disease.

Whitney Houston sang it, and it's true—the children are our future. If we continue on the current trend of metabolic challenges in childhood, we will see a significant increase in cirrhosis and liver cancer in the not-too-distant future that will only add to the trends already rising in the current adult population. And as you'll learn, when the liver is impaired, other diseases follow. Research has confirmed that children and young adults with biopsy-confirmed early stage liver disease have significantly higher rates of mortality overall, including from cancer and heart disease.[13]

We realize this is a hard truth to hear, but we also know that oftentimes adults are motivated to change their eating and lifestyle habits when they understand the impact those habits have on their family members—which is exactly why we've created a family-friendly plan to help all members of your household take better care of their livers.

There Is Still Time to Flatten the Curve

The writing on the wall couldn't be clearer: our livers, and thus our whole-body health, are in peril, and everyone, even if you are lean and metabolically healthy, needs to take better care of their liver. Quite frankly, unless you are super healthy and make it a point to eat mostly unprocessed foods with only a moderate intake of foods that spike your blood sugar, the chance of your having fatty liver to some extent is pretty low. But if you're experiencing insulin resistance, prediabetes, or full-blown type 2 diabetes—or a combination of other metabolic dysfunctions, such as high cholesterol, high blood pressure, or high triglycerides—that chance is high. And if you care for one or more children who eats a typical American diet of fast and processed foods with few fruits and vegetables, and you're thinking it's OK for them to eat these high-calorie/low-nutrient foods because they're young and resilient and have a high metabolism, the time to rethink that choice is now.

All of this may seem like bad news, but simply by realizing the extent of how prevalent fatty liver is and what risks it exposes you to, you are already miles ahead of the general population.

Most of Kristin's patients don't come to her for help addressing their liver problems. They want her perspective as a dietitian to help them address the weight that they can't seem to lose as well as their lack of energy. Mainly, they want some guidance on how to clean up their diet.

She always checks in on their liver health, because it is such a common companion to metabolic dysregulation. And nine times out of ten, she discovers that their liver is somewhere on the fatty liver disease spectrum.

We know no one wants to hear that their liver is struggling, but both of us have noticed in our practices that when patients realize their liver is in jeopardy, they get motivated to take better care of themselves, and they do it quickly. Perhaps the reason for their acceptance and willingness to change is the knowledge that, eventually, their livers can get past the point of no return, when only a transplant can save them. Or perhaps they want to avoid the stigma of liver disease because of its association in most people's minds with alcohol or drug use. Some of them take it as an overall wake-up call to attune to their own health in general. Whatever the reason, we'll take it! We know that motivation can pay off in across-the-board health improvements—for your liver, yes, but also for all the other organs and systems connected by the roadways of your body. And the sooner you start making changes, the more fully your liver can recover and your fatty liver disease can reverse.

Liver Disease: The Good, the Bad, and the Ugly

Some fat in the liver is healthy—fat comprises about 5 percent of a normal liver. Problems typically start to arise when you consume too many nutrient-poor calories that consist primarily of added sugars or simple carbs: think of your basic, standard American diet, with lots of bread, pasta, cookies, chips, fries, ice cream, flavored yogurts, and sweetened beverages (including sweetened coffee drinks, sodas, and energy drinks), along with few vegetables and little fiber.

Your liver is charged with processing all that sugar. Every time it does so, it uses up a lot of adenosine triphosphate (ATP), the primary molecule of energy used by your cells to metabolize sugar as well as fat. Consuming too many carbs depletes your ATP, and you have less of it to process fat, which means you have more fat on hand. Because the liver can't break the fat down so that it can be burned for fuel, it stores it. It's kind of like how your house can get overrun with clutter and you just keep sticking items in the basement.

Once you get to the point where fat makes up more than 5 to 10 percent of your liver—and you aren't a heavy user of alcohol or drugs—you reach the threshold of having non-alcoholic fatty liver disease (NAFLD). While people typically understand the threat to the liver that abusing alcohol and drugs poses, they are less likely to be aware that diet and toxin exposure can be just as threatening. Sugar is as bad as alcohol for your liver. As Ibrahim likes to say, sugar is "alcohol without the buzz."

When the fat in the liver is joined by inflammation, it's called non-alcoholic steatohepatitis (NASH). NAFLD and the early stages of NASH are what Ibrahim calls "the good" stage of liver disease, because these stages can be reversed (which is exactly what this book will show you how to do), and in reversing them, you can prevent cardiovascular disease.

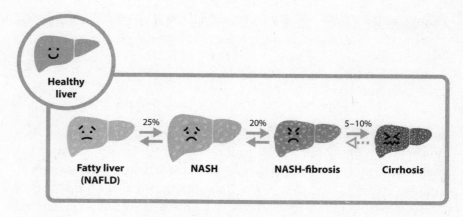

Figure 1.3. The Stages of Fatty Liver Disease

To continue the cluttered house analogy, as your liver becomes more fatty and inflamed, at some point you can't really use the basement anymore because there's no place left to walk, and it becomes a fire hazard because it's so packed with stuff. There is a big opportunity to clean out that basement, but that opportunity will go away the more crowded it gets down there.

When the fat and inflammation of NASH leads to pervasive scarring, you reach "the bad"—a stage of liver disease called NASH-fibrosis. At this point, you have to pay close attention to your diet and lifestyle and intervene as soon as possible to slow progression and possibly reverse the damage that has happened. And "the ugly" stages are cirrhosis—when so much of the liver tissue has been replaced by scar tissue that it can no longer function—and liver cancer—when malignant cells take root in the liver and potentially spread to other parts of the body. For "the ugly" phase, liver transplant might be necessary.

Even though only a small percentage of people with NAFLD will progress to "the bad" or "the ugly" stages of liver disease, a small percentage of a big number is still a lot of people. Assuming a total US population of 329.5 million people, that's 6.59 million Americans with fibrosis, and 1.3 to 2.6 million American with cirrhosis. That's simply too many.

THE STAGES OF FATTY LIVER DISEASE

The Good

NAFLD. Mostly asymptomatic, although some people with NAFLD may experience fatigue, a general malaise, or mild abdominal pain on the right side. A physical exam may reveal that the liver has become enlarged, although less than a third of NAFLD patients have an enlarged liver. NAFLD is discovered or confirmed by elevated levels of liver enzymes on a blood test, or thanks to an ultrasound, CT scan, or MRI that reveals a significant presence of fat in the liver.

NASH. The only definitive way to differentiate between NAFLD and NASH—in other words, to determine if there is inflammation present in the liver in addition to excess fat—is to do a liver biopsy. Although there is a research-backed algorithm that uses the results of a few simple blood tests and your age to gauge how far your liver disease has progressed (which we tell you about on page 50), we believe a biopsy is still the best method. Of people with NAFLD, 25 percent will go on to develop NASH.

The Bad

NASH-fibrosis. This stage of liver disease is identified by the presence of inflammation and scarring. Of all people with NASH, 20 percent will go on to develop NASH-fibrosis.

The Ugly

Cirrhosis. This is the stage of liver disease where too much of the liver tissue has been replaced by scar tissue.

Of people with NASH-fibrosis, 5 to 10 percent will go on to develop cirrhosis. It generally takes twenty to twenty-five years from the first development of fatty liver to progress to cirrhosis.

Liver Cancer. Of people with cirrhosis that develops as a result of fatty liver, 1 to 2 percent will develop liver cancer each year. Even though the risks are low, because liver cancer is much more treatable in its early stages, individuals with cirrhosis should get a liver ultrasound every six months to promote early detection.

How Happy Is Your Liver?

While we will share more specific diagnostic tools in Chapter 2 to help you determine your metabolic profile, this assessment can help you start to objectively assess which risk factors for fatty liver you may have. After all, typically, we're not motivated to change our behaviors until we start to realize that a specific health condition actually pertains to us and to understand how our daily habits may be fostering that health condition.

Health Risk Assessment

It's hard to get a clear picture of how your daily choices may be impacting your health. Truthfully, we all tend to think we're doing a little better at making healthy choices than we actually are, and we minimize any unhealthy choices we make. When new patients come to see us, they'll often tell us they "eat pretty well," but when we drill down, we discover that there is almost always room for significant improvement—maybe they're drinking soda every day, or smoking cigarettes, or not eating very many vegetables at all. We designed this assessment to help you raise your awareness of your own habits—to identify the habits that warrant your attention, and to also give yourself credit for the healthy choices that you are making. We hope that gaining some objectivity on your current habits will help motivate you to start making healthier choices.

To use it, first resolve to be honest and brave. Then, place a checkmark near every item in each column that pertains to you. This is not a diagnostic tool—in order to truly determine which metabolic profile fits you best, you'll need some actual measurements, which we walk you through in Chapter 3. For now, the more checkmarks you have in Column A, the higher your risk for some form of non-alcoholic fatty liver disease—as well as other chronic diseases, such as type 2 diabetes and cardiovascular disease—and the more likely you are to fit the Regenerator or Recalibrator metabolic profiles. From there, Columns B, C, and D show a continuum, with Column D being the most protective of liver health; the more you have in Column D, the better for your liver and the more likely you are to be a Preventer or a Fine-Tuner.

We'll include this assessment again at the end of the book so that you can visually assess the progress you've made by seeing fewer checkmarks in Columns A and B and more in Columns C and D. Just remember that the ultimate goal isn't necessarily to have every single answer in Column D. As you will learn throughout this book, our plans are for the long haul, and we know that small changes add up—and are definitely more doable. Every answer that you move from the left to the right between now and the end of this book is a big win. Think about it: while it might be faster to try to jump ten feet over a roaring river, the more certain way is to go step by step over rocks in the stream.

Liver Health Risk Assessment

	Column A	Column B	Column C	Column D
Diet				
I eat red meat (beef or pork) or red processed meat (sausages, hot dogs, pepperoni, etc.)	Pretty much every day _____	A few times a week _____	Once a week or so _____	Rarely _____
I eat more than 25 grams of added sugar in a day (the amount in 1/2 a can of soda, 1–2 scoops of ice cream, 2 cookies, or a slice of cake)	Pretty much every day _____	A few times a week _____	Once a week or so _____	Rarely _____
I eat more than 50 grams of low-fiber carbs in a day (from an assortment of white bread, wraps/tortillas, pasta, white rice, crackers, pretzels, standard breakfast cereals)	Pretty much every day _____	A few times a week _____	Once a week or so _____	Rarely _____
I eat fast food	Pretty much every day _____	A few times a week _____	Once a week or so _____	Rarely _____
I eat at least three servings of fruits and vegetables of different colors	Rarely _____	Once a week or so _____	A few days per week _____	Every day _____
I have a total of at least seven servings of fruits and/or vegetables in a day (a serving equals a large handful of fruit and colorful vegetables and two handfuls of fresh raw greens)	Rarely _____	Once a week or so _____	A few days per week _____	Every day _____

	Column A	Column B	Column C	Column D
I eat at least 20 grams of fiber in a day (for example, from a blend of beans, oats, vegetables, nuts, seeds, berries, avocados, quinoa)	Rarely	Once a week or so	A few days per week	Every day
	____	____	____	____
Exercise				
The average number of hours I spend sitting in a day are	10 or more	8–10	5–8	Less than 5
	____	____	____	____
I get some light exercise—such as an easy walk, light yoga, or anything that doesn't make me out of breath, for at least 30 minutes	Rarely	Once a week or so	A few times a week	Most days
	____	____	____	____
I work out to the point of being able to notice my breathing	Rarely	Once a week or so	A few times a week	Most days
	____	____	____	____
In general, I spend this much of my day either standing or moving around (i.e., not sitting)	An hour or less	1–2 hours	3–4 hours	4 hours or more
	____	____	____	____
Alcohol				
I drink alcohol	5 or more days per week	3–4 days per week	1–2 days per week	Less than once per week
	____	____	____	____
When I drink alcohol, I have this many servings (one serving equals one drink—5 ounces of wine or 1 ounce of hard alcohol—for women, or two drinks for men)	4 or more	3–4	2–3	1
	____	____	____	____
Smoking or Vaping				
My relationship with smoking or vaping is	I currently smoke cigarettes or vape multiple times per day	I currently smoke cigarettes or vape 1–2 times per day	I used to smoke cigarettes or vape, and I quit less than five years ago	I used to smoke cigarettes or vape, and I quit more than five years ago, or I have never smoked or vaped
	____	____	____	____

	Column A	Column B	Column C	Column D
Coffee				
I drink unsweetened coffee	Rarely or never	Once or twice a week	2 or more cups per day	1–2 cups per day
	_____	_____	_____	_____
Sleep				
Most nights I sleep	Less than 5 hours	5–6 hours	6–7 hours	7 hours or more
	_____	_____	_____	_____
I have been diagnosed with sleep apnea	I have been diagnosed with sleep apnea and I am not treating it	I don't know if I have sleep apnea but am told I snore loudly with periods of not breathing	I have sleep apnea and I am treating it	I do not have sleep apnea
	_____	_____	_____	_____
Stress Management				
I practice something to reduce my experience of stress (for example, meditate, stretch, garden, journal, talk to a counselor, do yoga)	Rarely	Once a week or so	A couple of times per week	Most days
	_____	_____	_____	_____
Waist Size The circumference of my waist is (see page 45 for measuring instructions)	40 or higher (for men) or 35 or higher (for women)			39 or lower (for men) or 34 or lower (for women)
	_____			_____
Type 2 Diabetes	I have been diagnosed with type 2 diabetes	My doctor has told me I'm prediabetic	I have not consulted with a doctor about my blood sugar levels	I've had my blood sugar levels tested and my doctor tells me they are in a healthy range
	_____	_____	_____	_____

For a deeper understanding of how the things you eat and drink, how much you move or exercise, and how your stress and your sleep all influence your liver health, keep reading. We'll also dive into what has long been considered a primary risk factor for fatty liver disease—obesity—and how it's not really the number on the scale that drives fatty liver but your metabolic profile. This is where we get to start customizing your approach to preventing, reversing, or managing fatty liver, and where things start getting exciting.

chapter 2

What's Weight Got to Do with It—or Not

F OR MANY YEARS, obesity has been presumed to be a primary risk factor for fatty liver disease. And it is true that losing weight is often accompanied by a slowing, reducing, or even reversal of fatty liver disease.

But in recent years we've learned that pointing the finger at obesity is too simplistic. It's not weight classification, or even body mass index (BMI, which factors in height in addition to weight) that contributes to fatty liver disease. (Because many doctors still use BMI, and therefore you may know your own BMI number, we will occasionally refer to it in this book; however, we don't use it as a guideline in determining your metabolic health.)

After all, not every person who fits the medical definition of obese or severely obese will develop fatty liver disease. And just because you're what's considered to be a healthy weight according to the medical tables, there is no guarantee that you're immune to developing fatty liver disease.

Much more important to the state of your liver than the number of pounds that you weigh is the state of your metabolic health; metabolic health is, specifically, your blood sugar and insulin levels, your levels of lipids (both kinds of cholesterol and triglycerides), your waist size, and whether or not you have type 2 diabetes. While fatty liver disease has a broad array of risk factors—which we'll cover in this chapter—it is metabolic health that matters the most. Luckily, it is also the most changeable (unlike, say, your age, or what your mother ate when she was pregnant with you).

WHAT'S IN A NAME?

Metabolic health is such a crucial component of liver health that there is a movement to change the names of non-alcoholic fatty liver disease (NAFLD) and non-alcoholic steatohepatitis (NASH) to metabolic-associated fatty liver disease (MAFLD) and metabolic-associated steatohepatitis (MASH). This name change would shift the definition from what it's *not* caused by (alcohol) to what it *is* caused by—metabolic health. It would also help patients, health care providers, and researchers to focus on this true root cause, which can improve outcomes.

The medical community isn't the only group rethinking obesity. Throughout our society, there's been a backlash to the diet industry and a movement to embrace bodies of all shapes and sizes as normal and healthy. For all these reasons, we've fine-tuned our approach to treating fatty liver disease. Rather than focusing just on weight loss, we've shifted our aim to improving metabolic health—and if you're already metabolically pretty healthy, to taking steps to stay that way.

There are four basic categories of metabolic health. Knowing which one you fall into—or which two you straddle—will help you tailor your efforts to improve your liver health to your unique body.

We'll walk you through those four metabolic profiles—and help you determine which profile fits you best—at the end of this chapter. But first, let's look at how the medical approach to obesity has changed.

Our Evolving Understanding of Obesity

For decades now, doctors, nutritionists, dietitians, researchers, and the general public have believed that weight gain is the direct result of overeating—an "eat less, weigh less" idea that's known in the scientific literature as the energy balance model (EBM).

In many ways, EBM makes sense. After all, the number of available calories worldwide has risen right alongside the prevalence of obesity over the last several decades.[1]

And if fat is simply the result of eating more calories than you burn, then it stands to reason that having more calories available—especially in a processed, shelf-stable, convenient, and, frankly, addictive form—would cause rates of obesity to rise around the world, which they have.

But we've come to realize that weight gain isn't as simple as how many calories we're consuming. This shift in our understanding of what truly leads to weight gain and rising obesity rates is known as the carbohydrate-insulin model (CIM). This framework suggests that it's not the sheer volume of calories consumed that triggers weight gain; it's the *type* of calories that matters.

The Direct Link Between Sugar Consumption and Fatty Liver

The term "fatty liver" is a little misleading—many people think that it's eating fat that contributes to it, when it's really excess carbohydrates, particularly simple carbs like sugar and refined, fiber-stripped grains, that are primary food sources of fatty liver.

This is bad news because, in the United States, we eat double the amount of sugar per day compared to people in any other country in the world.[2] According to data from market research firm Euromonitor, the average American eats 30 teaspoons, or just over a half cup, of sugar every day.

We now know that a diet high in added sugars and refined, low-fiber carbs such as white flour (which the liver converts into glucose, making it essentially the same as eating sugar), causes a rise in blood sugar that kicks off a problematic cascade.

First, it increases the release of insulin (the hormone used to direct sugar into the cells and out of the blood) and suppresses glucagon (a hormone that cues the release of stored glucose when blood levels are too low). The result? The insulin tells your liver to store the extra calories from all that glucose as fat, and the dip in glucagon means your liver rarely gets the cue to release any of that stored fat.

As you can see in Figure 2.1, The High-Carb Metabolic Health Spiral, over time, a diet high in refined sugar and carbs can produce so much insulin that your insulin receptors get desensitized to the messages that insulin is sending, resulting in what's known as insulin resistance. When that happens, the pancreas will keep producing more and more insulin in an attempt to get blood glucose levels down. When insulin levels are high, your brain detects that there isn't enough energy circulating in the blood, so it sends a chemical signal to do two things: eat more, and conserve energy by slowing your metabolism.

It's a quadruple whammy, but it doesn't stop there.

As your stomach empties, your gut sends hormonal signals to the brain, where a network of neurons becomes engaged and creates the state of being that many people call "hangry"—unpleasant hunger accompanied by cranky mood and a high drive to find food quickly. And if you're trying to diet by restricting your calories, this neuronal network stays active for longer.[3] So, not only are you hungry, you're in the grip of a hormonal storm that makes you feel the need

INSULIN RESISTANCE AND YOUR LIVER

Insulin is the hormone that regulates the amount of blood sugar in circulation. When you eat carbs, the pancreas releases insulin to reduce your glucose levels. But when you eat too many carbs too often, there's so much insulin floating around that the receptors for it get overworked and stop getting its messages. As a result, there's a lot of insulin in your bloodstream with nowhere to go.

Because insulin is also a fat-storage hormone, when your insulin levels are high, it tells the body to hold on to every calorie and tuck it away as fat. Too much insulin also stimulates the liver to make more glucose in a process known as *gluconeogenesis*.

When the insulin receptors in your muscles are burned out, they don't get the message to take up glucose out of the blood. So now you have really high glucose, which stimulates the pancreas to make more insulin, driving your insulin levels even higher.

Insulin resistance is like a merry-go-round, and the only way off is to reduce the number of carbs you eat, give your liver a break and stop cueing it to make more glucose and store more fat, and allow your insulin receptors to regain their sensitivity.

Insulin resistance is a step on the path to type 2 diabetes, but just like the earlier stages of fatty liver disease, it is reversible. And the Renew Your Liver plans can help you do it.

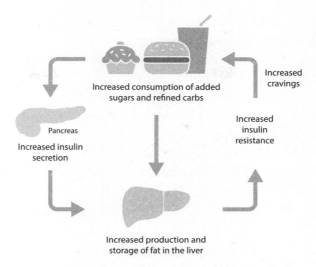

Increased consumption of added
sugars and refined carbs

Increased
cravings

Pancreas
Increased insulin
secretion

Increased
insulin
resistance

Increased production and
storage of fat in the liver

Figure 2.1. The High-Carb Metabolic Health Spiral

to find that food *now*—making it more likely that you'll reach for something convenient, processed, and likely to increase your blood sugar level.

Beyond contributing to insulin resistance and intense cravings, processing all that sugar is exhausting to the liver, and a direct cause of an increased storage of fat within the liver. Why is a high-carb, low-fiber diet so tiring to the liver? Breaking down sugar is an energy-intensive process, and the lack of fiber in processed carbs makes it worse. Without fiber, glucose gets dumped into your bloodstream more quickly than it would if fiber were present to slow down the digestion process. For every molecule of sugar that you eat, the liver uses two molecules of adenosine triphosphate (ATP) to metabolize it. Remember, ATP is the form of energy that is created by your mito-chondria (organelles located within your cells) and that fuels the vast majority of processes that are happening throughout your body at any given moment. The more sugar and the less fiber you eat, the lower the ATP stores in your liver and the less energy it will have on hand to do its work. And so, instead of metabolizing sugar, your liver will store it as fat—the same way that you might be tempted to tidy your kitchen by sticking all the dirty dishes in the oven instead of taking the time and energy to wash and put away each one.

Insulin resistance makes it even harder for the liver to replenish the ATP that it uses. As a result, even more of the sugar that you consume will be stashed away as fat. The cycle of fat storage, increased cravings, and slower metabolism speeds up. In other words, you have a dietary recipe for disaster.

And the biggest problem is that those foods that raise your blood sugar and kick off this negative spiral are everywhere. They are seemingly impossible to avoid and just as difficult to resist.

The Rise of Un-put-down-able Foods

Ultra-processed foods—whether they're chips, frozen meals, cookies, breakfast cereals, or hot dogs—have become the source of the vast majority of our daily calories, and our reliance on them is only growing. A 2021 study found that American adults got 57 percent of their daily calories from ultra-processed foods in 2017-2018, up from 51.5 percent in 2001-2002.[4] For children, it's even worse: ultra-processed foods were the source of 67 percent of the daily energy consumption for American kids in 2018, up from 61.4 percent in 1999.[5]

Yet these foods aren't really made from what you would recognize as, well, food. They're made from things that have been extracted from foods, like starches, fat, and fillers. Sure, they may provide calories, but they don't necessarily provide nutrition. Beyond that, they've been modified with chemical flavorings, salt, and sugar so that they appeal to your taste buds so strongly that you really can't eat just one (if you're old enough to remember that slogan for Lay's potato chips). Ultra-processed foods have been stripped of vitamins, minerals, and the fiber that helps you feel full—it's hard not to eat the whole bagful. If you tried to eat as much broccoli as would fit inside a bag of potato chips, you'd never be able to finish it because you'd get full about a third of the way through. There's even a fancy new term for these ultra-processed foods: they're called *hyperpalatable.*

Hyperpalatable foods are so tasty and convenient that they're crowding out the healthier foods on our plates. According to the CDC, only one in ten American adults is eating the recommended servings of fruits and vegetables per day.[6]

Studies show that hyperpalatable foods are a disaster for the liver. The fact that they are highly refined—and therefore stripped of most of their fiber, which slows down digestion—means that they cause blood sugar levels to jump quickly, which, remember, causes the liver to store more fat. Another way of saying that a food causes a spike in blood sugar is saying that it is high-glycemic (*glyc-* is a prefix that means sugar or glucose in medical terms). Both animal and human studies have shown that foods that are high-glycemic increase the accumulation of fat in liver cells, which leads to fatty liver disease.[7] And hyperpalatable foods also contribute to the other metabolic roots of fatty liver disease—namely, insulin resistance and type 2 diabetes.[8]

A HELPFUL TOOL FOR CHOOSING CARBS WISELY: GLYCEMIC LOAD

You've probably heard of the glycemic index, which ranks how quickly and how severely a specific food can cause your blood sugar to rise. The glycemic index goes from 0 to 100, and 100 represents the spike that 100 grams of pure sugar (glucose) elicits. Foods that are higher on the glycemic index tend to be more refined, meaning they have less fiber, which slows digestion and the impact on blood sugar.

The glycemic index has been a very helpful tool in helping people understand which foods are more likely to cause a blood sugar spike and subsequent crash. The problem is that the glycemic index doesn't take into account how much of a food you actually typically eat, so it can't measure the impact on blood sugar of a real-world serving of that food.

Glycemic load is another measure of a food's impact on blood sugar that does factor in serving size. The formula for determining a food's glycemic load is to start with that food's glycemic index, multiply that by the number of carbs in a serving of the food, and then divide it by 100. The result is a much lower scale of numbers that gives a more accurate view of just how much, and how quickly, a food will raise your blood sugar levels.

For example, watermelon is a high-glycemic index food (it has a glyce-mic index of 80) because it doesn't have a lot of fiber to slow the absorp-tion of its natural sugars. But when you look at how many carbs are in an actual serving of watermelon, it's so low that it won't have a very big impact on your blood sugar—its glycemic load score is only 5.

Glycemic load is the measure we used to develop each of the eating plans in this book. But we're not saying you can never ever have a high-glycemic-load food again—just that you should reserve these foods for rare occasions and not let any of them be one of your go-to everyday foods. We specifically selected the foods that are a mainstay of the eating plans that we'll outline starting in Chapter 6 for a number of reasons—their accessibility, their palatability, because they are on the lower end of the glycemic load scale, and for their nutrient density. Note that although there is no specific definition from the USDA on what "nutrient-dense" means, we define it as:

- high vitamin and mineral content in relation to its caloric content and volume
- a good source of fiber, whether soluble or insoluble
- either a whole food or made with whole-food ingredients you can pronounce and recognize
- a source of healthy fats and/or protein

If you've gotten hooked on the hyperpalatable stuff, and your weight and/or your metabolic health has been negatively impacted as a result, know that it's not because of some personal failing. The food industry knows how to hook your taste buds and keep you eating what they want.

On top of all this, we are living in an environment where hyperpal-atable food is both everywhere and ridiculously accessible. You don't even have to talk to someone to place your order for takeout anymore—you can order it on an app and have it brought to your doorstep 24/7. Even the old adage to shop the perimeter of the grocery store—where the fresh produce and meats are—doesn't apply anymore, because so many of us are ordering our groceries online.

The truth is, we have to accept that we live in a world that is set up to disrupt our metabolic health—and that our bodies are wired in such a way that once we experience this disruption, it's hard to break the physiological cycle of eat food–hold on to fat–get hungry–get hangry–eat more hyperpalatable food.

Impaired metabolic health is by no means an individual failing–it's a structural failing of our food systems. It is better to shift your focus away from losing weight, which can feel overwhelming if not impossible, and toward what you do have control over: improving your metabolic health.

MAKING BETTER HEALTH YOUR GOAL INSTEAD OF WEIGHT LOSS

Kristin knows firsthand how daunting losing weight can feel. She says:

Before I became a dietitian who helps patients, I *was* the patient. Starting when I was about fourteen, I was an overweight kid. Not just overweight—obese. I spent my adolescent years ping-ponging between dieting and overeating. I always wanted to lose weight, because I wanted a flat belly like my friends had. I'd gear up every New Year's for a whole new way of eating, only to be back to the same old habits by March. It wasn't until one annual checkup when my pediatrician realized I was only a few numbers away from a diabetes diagnosis that I was sent to a dietitian.

She told me to eat less overall and increase my intake of fruits and vegetables—not exactly anything I didn't already know. Plus, I hated those foods at that time. I walked out of that office with a paper outlining a 1,200-calorie diet that had nothing to do with who I was, my particular health challenges, or the environment I lived in (in my Polish-Dominican household, we existed on white rice and pierogies).

I spent the next ten years figuring out that when I focused on dieting, counting calories, and carefully measuring my portion sizes, I only felt more deprived, and what successes I did have came with a lot of misery. But when I instead focused on eating more nutrient-dense versions of the foods that I loved instead of trying to eat only "healthy foods," I not only enjoyed the process, I actually got healthier. I also learned that I didn't have to completely give up the foods I love—such as those pierogies, and also, bacon!—so long as I only had them occasionally. That also helped me not feel deprived and to see what I was doing not so much as dieting but as revamping my eating habits in a way that helped me feel my best. This is exactly the same approach that I offer to my patients—to put their health first and let their weight take care of itself.

Fat Itself Is a Major Player

We've learned more about fat—or, technically, adipose tissue—too. We used to think fat was inert, basically a storage unit for extra calories. But, depending on where it is located, it can exert an influence on bodily processes. Fat that is stored in the belly, close to the liver, can release inflammatory molecules known as cytokines that, when present in small amounts, are helpful messenger molecules of the immune system. But when they are present in big numbers—a so-called cytokine storm—the inflammation they produce triggers an even bigger inflammatory response that can be more damaging to the body than the original offender. Even at more moderate levels, the cytokines emitted by fat can contribute to systemic inflammation, which is a cofactor in nearly every chronic disease.

Another factor that makes belly fat more dangerous than fat that is stored around the hips and thighs is that the portal vein, which brings about 80 percent of the blood into the liver, runs through the belly fat and will carry triglycerides from that belly fat directly into the liver.

In essence, gaining weight in your belly can trap you in a cycle of gaining more fat in your liver.

The Kind of Fat That Helps You Lose Belly Fat

There is one type of fat, or adipose tissue, in your body that is beneficial, and that is known as brown fat. As opposed to white fat, which stores excess energy in the form of triglycerides (which are harmful to cardiovascular health), brown fat helps release stored energy by producing heat. Higher quantities of brown fat are associated with a lower body weight.

Sadly, the amount of brown fat lessens naturally with age—which may explain why you tend to put on weight and even to develop fatty liver disease as you grow older. However, it appears that it's possible to stimulate the production of brown fat, even in older adults, by eating certain nutrients—many of which are regular parts of the Mediterranean diet (and thus are in all of the food plans contained in this book). The nutrients that produce brown fat include the antioxidant resveratrol, which is found in the skins of grapes, berries, cocoa, and red wine; curcumin, which is the active component of turmeric; and omega-3 fatty acids, which are found in fatty fish such as salmon as well as walnuts and flaxseeds. Increasing levels of brown fat means the body gets more efficient at burning fat for energy.

Why Bariatric Surgery Isn't a Cure-All

If belly fat is a primary cause of fatty liver disease, and losing belly fat a potent way to treat and even reverse it, wouldn't bariatric surgery be a reasonable approach to losing weight and reversing fatty liver disease? This stomach-reducing surgery does have some evidence to support its effectiveness—a 2021 Cleveland Clinic study found that, among people with both obesity and NASH, those who had the surgery had a significantly lower risk of developing further complications. They had an 88 percent lower risk of developing cirrhosis and a 70 percent lower risk of experiencing a severe cardiac event such as heart attack or stroke.[9]

While it's true that bariatric surgery can have positive outcomes, it doesn't address the underlying problem, which truly isn't weight, or even waist circumference—it's addiction to high-carb, high-glycemic, low-nutrient foods and the negative impact those foods have on your metabolic health. It also generally results in rapid weight loss, which can actually make fatty liver worse because as the body breaks down fat into fatty acids, the liver becomes flooded. If you already have fatty liver (which is likely if you had impaired metabolic health in addition to having a lot of excess weight), then your liver is already compromised. Those fatty acids can create inflammatory molecules known as reactive oxygen species, which may correspond to further liver damage. Further, because rapid weight loss is typically the result of a state of malnutrition (you're eating significantly less, so your body isn't getting all the nutrients it needs), there are fewer antioxidants on hand to help protect you from the inflammatory effects of break-down of that stored fat.

Not only that, but surgery is not required. As we'll cover more deeply in just a moment, making significant improvements to even "the ugly" stages of fatty liver only requires the loss of 10 percent of your body weight.

Furthermore, studies show that some bariatric patients have a greater risk of developing an alcohol addiction. A large review of more than forty thousand bariatric surgery patients found a link between bariatric surgery and certain substance use disorders, including alcohol abuse.[10] In another study, researchers followed more than two thousand patients who had bariatric surgery at ten different hospitals across the country. Nearly 21 percent of those studied developed an alcohol use disorder.[11]

It's likely that some bariatric surgery patients are unknowingly swapping a food addiction for an addiction to alcohol. Neuroscientists have found a correlation between alcoholism and a genetic deficiency in the brain's dopamine-binding receptors that they suggest could lead patients who have this deficiency to turn to alcohol once the ability to binge eat is removed.[12] This all implies that we should look at the myriad factors for disease rather than treating obesity itself.

Although most people think, "I'll get the surgery and be thin!" they don't realize that you *can* become overweight again, and quickly. In both of our practices, we've seen plenty of bariatric surgery patients gain back the weight they lost. Kristin has seen people close to her who have opted for stomach reduction surgery and put all the weight back on within two years.

Beyond that, the surgery isn't without its own risks. In that same Cleveland Clinic study, four of the surgery group died from complications of the surgery within the first year.

Many people simply don't have access to bariatric surgery as an option. They may not weigh enough—Kristin has actually had patients joke that they need to put on some weight in order to be eligible. Most programs require passing a psychological assessment in order to be eligible, and insurance companies use their own criteria when deciding whether or not they will cover it. Getting that approval can be a very complex process, and unless you are in a position to pay out of pocket, it can be financially inaccessible, as the average cost of weight-loss surgery is between $17,000 and $26,000.[13]

Honestly, although you may feel that weight-loss surgery is the surest path to better health, you are actually holding in your hands a more realistic, safer, more affordable, and effective plan to get you there right now. And with the guidance you'll receive on how to customize your eating plan to both your stage of fatty liver disease and your metabolic profile, you won't have to subject yourself to a drastic, one-size-fits-all surgical option. You'll be able to hand-tailor your food and lifestyle choices to precisely what your unique body needs to be its healthiest.

And yet, if you do meet the classification of obese or severely obese and go to your doctor about any symptom or medical issue you may be experiencing, it's all too likely that they will suggest bariatric surgery as a catch-all treatment. Even though the medical understanding of obesity is changing, it's still very much the case that doctors will make it the scapegoat for everything you're experiencing. That's what happened to Jon.

Jon's Story: The Dangers of Focusing Exclusively on Obesity

Jon had been overweight since he was a kid. By the time he was forty, he weighed 350 pounds. One Sunday afternoon in January 2020, Jon felt a sharp pain in the center of his abdomen that seemed to be moving to the right. Fearing appendicitis, he went to the ER, where he got a CT scan, some fluids, and an all-clear before they sent him home. Although he didn't receive a diagnosis at that visit, the incident was scary enough to motivate Jon to change his diet—eating fewer carbs and more greens. He started losing weight, but then COVID-19 happened, and those healthy new habits went out the window.

During lockdown, Jon gained another twenty-five pounds. By that summer, he started noticing something hard and palpable in his abdomen, in the region of his stomach. While not a doctor, Jon works in health care, so he knew enough to recognize that he likely had a hernia.

Jon went to see his primary care doctor, who said it wasn't a hernia—Jon just needed to lose weight. He asked Jon if he had ever considered bariatric surgery to help with weight loss. Knowing that bariatric surgery might help him lose weight, but wouldn't do anything to help change the habits that had led to the extra weight, Jon declined. But he did ask for a referral to a surgeon because he felt strongly that something was amiss, whether it was a hernia or not, and he wanted to find out what it was.

Because the pandemic disrupted medical care, it took months for Jon's appointment with the surgeon to come up. In the meantime, he got through the pandemic the best he could on his own—which is to say, like so many people, he ate whatever was convenient and tasted good, including a lot of fast food and soda.

When he finally got in to see the surgeon, it was March 2021. At that appointment, the surgeon asked Jon if he was there to address his hernias—plural. This doctor was looking at that original CT scan from the ER where two hernias were evident, despite what the hospital and primary care doctors had said. "It was such a frustrating moment for me, because it meant my primary care doctor had looked at me and only seen my obesity and not my actual medical condition," Jon says. The surgeon set a goal weight of three hundred pounds for Jon, and at that point, he could have surgery to repair his hernias.

Having a goal weight got Jon back in touch with his motivation to get healthy, and he started a new eating plan. He cut out all refined carbs and soda and started having one meal a day, at lunch time. If he was hungry at night, he'd have an apple and some almonds or string cheese. After a month, he added in walking a mile a day, a distance that he gradually increased over time. By July 2021, he had reached his goal weight, and he had surgery to repair his hernias later that summer.

Around the time of his surgery, Jon received an email that a new lab had been posted to his medical portal. Turns out it wasn't actually new—it was the same CT scan from that first visit to the ER in January 2020 (his doctor's office was merging with another practice and consolidating their files). It showed that Jon had an enlarged liver due to fatty liver disease, a fact that no care provider had mentioned in the multiple appointments Jon had had in the nearly eighteen months since. Jon knows how serious fatty liver disease is. The fact that he had been in the first stage of fatty liver disease without knowing it fueled Jon to keep up his efforts to stay healthy, because now he had an even deeper goal than simply losing weight. At the time of this writing, Jon has lost 137 pounds. His labs are all normal. A follow-up scan shows that his liver is normal-sized and healthy looking. And he's normalized his healthier approach to eating and exercising into his everyday lifestyle, realizing that he can occasionally have pizza or bread or another meal in the evening and not backslide.

Some of the major perks Jon has enjoyed are shopping for clothes at Target (and not having to visit a store for "big and tall" men) and realizing that he actually loves many foods he had always thought he didn't like, such as avocados, tomatoes, and mushrooms. But the biggest benefit has been a significant uptick in his mood. "My personality has changed—I realize that I had been overindulging to numb. Now I can appreciate the good things in my life that I just didn't truly see before—the people around me and my career. I'm even putting myself out there and trying to meet someone, something I never considered as a possibility before."

It's Not the Amount That Counts

Another problem with the obesity narrative and the push for bariatric surgery is that it can make you think that any excess weight is problematic and that to be healthy you need to have a dramatic transformation into a super-lean person, like something off of a *People* magazine cover or an episode of *The Biggest Loser*.

There are two major problems with this thinking:

1. It can convince you that your goal is so big that it's paralyzing—if you think you need to lose fifty, sixty, or more pounds, it's common to feel like you don't even know where to begin.
2. It's false. You can greatly improve, and in some cases even reverse, fatty liver disease with diet and lifestyle changes that improve your health greatly irrespective of weight loss.

Research shows you can reverse NAFLD with a weight loss of only 5 percent of your body weight. That means if you weigh 250 pounds, you only need to lose 12.5 pounds. If you have NASH, losing 7 percent of your body weight is all it takes for significant reduction. And if you have fibrosis or cirrhosis (in other words, scarring of the liver), even a 10 percent weight loss will help significantly.[14]

You don't need to lose a lot of weight, and you also don't need to do it quickly. As we've covered, losing too much weight too quickly can only make your fatty liver worse. That's because quick weight loss is often the result of being undernourished—and your liver needs access to ample nutrients in order to function well. Also, rapid weight loss just isn't sustainable. And what your liver truly needs is a lasting pivot in your eating and lifestyle habits away from foods that spike your blood sugar levels to ones that provide longer-lasting energy and fullness. (Which is not to say that you have to eat perfectly healthy every day for the rest of your life—we promise, you can still have your favorite foods occasionally!)

It's much healthier for the liver—and more sustainable from a behavior change perspective—to aim to lose the percentage of body weight that your stage of liver disease requires over a minimum of three months.

When Kristin shares these fairly low and slow weight-loss goals with her patients, they don't believe her. They've been conditioned—as so many of us have—to think that the only way to be truly healthy is to be super trim, and the only kind of good weight loss is dramatic weight loss.

It's time to walk away from using weight as a barometer of overall health and to look to metabolic health instead. Let's look at the four profiles of metabolic health so that you can determine which one you fall into and, therefore, what you need to prioritize in terms of supporting your metabolic health in general and your liver health in particular.

chapter 3

The Four Metabolic Types

S INCE WE NOW know that obesity itself is the result of a metabolic imbalance, we also know that we can seek to address those imbalances, and when we do, we'll improve all conditions that are metabolically related—including fatty liver, type 2 diabetes, and cardiovascular disease. As a bonus, excess weight can come off too, if needed, but weight loss isn't the primary goal.

To address your particular metabolic imbalances, you first have to know what they are. As we mentioned in the introduction, there are four basic profiles of metabolic health:

- The Preventer (healthy and lean)
- The Fine-tuner (healthy and non-lean)
- The Recalibrator (unhealthy and lean)
- The Regenerator (unhealthy and non-lean)

Determining which one of these profiles you fit best will also determine which dietary and lifestyle approach will best meet your needs.

Before you go through the process of figuring out your profile, remember that they aren't set in stone. You can progress from unhealthy and non-lean to healthy and non-lean, or to healthy and lean. Of course, it is possible to travel in the other direction, too, from healthy and lean to any of the other profiles—but by following the plans we share in this book, you'll be significantly reducing the odds of that happening.

To determine which profile you fall into, you'll need to know some specifics about your indicators of metabolic health. Some of them, like waist circumference, you can gather on your own, while for others you'll need a blood test (to determine your cholesterol levels) or access to a blood pressure cuff (to measure your blood pressure, which can be done at home if you have the device, or at a pharmacy, or at your doctor's office). They are all part of a standard physical, however, so you may already have this information in your medical portal (also known as "My Chart") from your last checkup. If you don't, you can obtain them with one simple appointment.

Indicators of Metabolic Health

In order to figure out which metabolic profile fits you best, you'll need to know which of the following metabolic risk factors you do or do not have.

Your waist circumference. Studies have shown over and over that waist circumference is more indicative of overall health than weight or BMI, and there is a very strong relation between abdominal fat—what's known as central obesity in the scientific literature—and fatty liver disease.

That's because the fat that accumulates in the abdomen is more inflammatory—and therefore, harmful—than the fat that settles around the hips, butt, and thighs. And the fat that accumulates within the abdominal cavity among your abdominal organs, known as visceral fat, is more dangerous than fat that collects just beneath the surface of the skin, known as subcutaneous fat. Part of why visceral fat is a problem is because it is closer to your abdominal organs, and the blood vessels that supply and wash visceral fat drain directly into the internal organs in the abdomen. The lack of space means you have less room for healthy tissue, and that can impair organ function. And you want every organ in the abdominal cavity to be working at its best.

Visceral fat is more physiologically active than lower-body fat—but not in a good way. Studies have found that visceral fat produces a potent inflammatory molecule known as interleukin-6 (Il-6) that enters the bloodstream and contributes to systemic inflammation. The more visceral fat you have, the more chronic, systemic inflammation you will experience, the more out of whack your insulin levels will be, and the more likely it is that your liver will be storing fat.

THE BEST WAY TO MEASURE WAIST CIRCUMFERENCE

To determine your waist circumference, use a flexible measuring tape—if you don't have one, you can order one online for about $5 (search for "body measuring tape").

First, place your hands on your hips and use your fingers to feel for the top of your hip bones, technically known as your *iliac crests*. Then wrap the tape around your torso so that it touches the skin just above the tip of your iliac crests, making sure that the tape is horizontal all the way around and not riding up too high in front or low in the back. Pull the tape so that it's snug but not making an indent in your skin, and take your measurement at the end of a normal exhale.

Periodically remeasuring your waist circumference is a great way to track your progress toward better metabolic health without having to step on a scale.

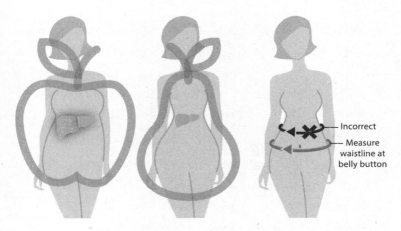

Figure 3.1. Body Types and How to Measure Waist Circumference

Type 2 diabetes or prediabetes. As we covered in Chapter 1, type 2 diabetes is a close companion of fatty liver. If you have been diagnosed with type 2 diabetes, your risk of having some stage of fatty liver disease is 75 percent, and if you've been told by your health care provider that you are prediabetic, your risk is somewhere between the 40 percent chance that the general population has and the 75 percent of people who have developed type 2 diabetes.

High blood pressure. High blood pressure is defined as being equal to or greater than 130 mm/hg systolic (the first number) and 85 mm/hg diastolic (the second number). It is one of the conditions that make up metabolic syndrome, which is a constellation of risk factors for type 2 diabetes, heart attack and stroke, and fatty liver.

Imbalanced blood lipids. Because there are different types of cholesterol that range from good to not bad to downright harmful, determining whether you have imbalanced blood lipids (fats) is not as simple as looking at your total cholesterol number. You want your HDL cholesterol (the good kind that protects you from heart disease) to be at least 40 mg/dl if you're male and 50 mg/dl if you're female, and your triglycerides (a different form of fat that is considered to be a building block of cholesterol) to be less than 150 mg/dl.

Metabolic Profile #1: The Preventer (Healthy and Lean)

While we may still uphold an ideal of being thin, it's important to understand that only about one in ten Americans fits this profile.[1] Even if you are one of them, it's still vital that you take steps to stay metabolically healthy—Chapter 7 contains a preventative plan designed to do just that.

Percentage of the population: 12 percent
Waist circumference:

    Men: 40 inches or less
    Women: 35 inches or less

Two or fewer of the following risk factors:

- Type 2 diabetes or prediabetes
- High blood pressure (equal to or greater than 130/85)
- Low HDL cholesterol (less than 40 mg/dl for men and 50 mg/dl for women)
- High triglycerides (150 mg/dl or higher)

Focus: Preventing metabolic dysfunction

Metabolic Profile #2: The Fine-Tuner (Healthy and Non-lean)

This category often includes pear-shaped individuals who carry most of their excess weight in their hips, butt, and thighs. It can also include those who have a high level of muscle mass that makes them heavier but not necessarily less healthy. If you fit this profile, you may have a nutrient-dense diet but also indulge in processed foods from time to time and may engage in physical activity that builds muscle.

Percentage of the population: 32 percent[2]

Waist circumference:

     Men: 40 inches or higher

     Women: 35 inches or higher

Plus no more than *one* of the following risk factors:

- Type 2 diabetes
- High blood pressure (equal to or greater than 130/85)
- Low HDL cholesterol (less than 40 mg/dl for men and 50 mg/dl for women)
- High triglycerides (150 mg/dl or higher)

Focus: Reducing carbs and increasing nutrient density in a sustainable way

Metabolic Profile #3: The Recalibrator (Unhealthy and Lean)

Most of Kristin's patients who are not overweight but are metabolically unhealthy are sugar addicts—they just don't eat enough calories to put on weight, and/or they may be so physically active that they remain thin.

Percentage of the population: 18 percent[3]

Waist circumference:

     Men: 40 inches or less

     Women: 35 inches or less

Three or more of the following risk factors:

- Type 2 diabetes
- High blood pressure (equal to or greater than 130/85)

- Low HDL cholesterol (less than 40 mg/dl for men and 50 mg/dl for women)
- High triglycerides (150 mg/dl or higher)

Focus: Reducing your sugar intake and increasing your consumption of nutrient-dense foods

Metabolic Profile #4: The Regenerator (Unhealthy and Non-lean)

The majority of our patients fall under this category and already have NAFLD or may have even progressed to NASH or NASH-fibrosis.

Percentage of the population: 38 percent

Waist circumference:

  Men: 40 inches or higher

  Women: 35 inches or higher

Two or more of the following risk factors:

- Type 2 diabetes
- High blood pressure (equal to or greater than 130/85)
- Low HDL cholesterol (less than 40 mg/dl for men and 50 mg/dl for women)
- High triglycerides (150 mg/dl or higher)

Focus: Reducing carbs to stabilize metabolic health, getting more active, and reducing waist size

Prevalence of the Four Metabolic Profiles

Looking at the breakout of the prevalence of the four metabolic profiles reveals a fascinating portrait of who is healthy and our evolving attitudes about weight. This is further evidence that it's not as simple as saying that if you're overweight or obese you are automatically unhealthy.

A Flow Chart for Determining Your Metabolic Profile

Figure 3.3 provides a simple schematic that can help you identify which metabolic profile you fall into. If you don't know your blood

Distribution of the Metabolic Profiles

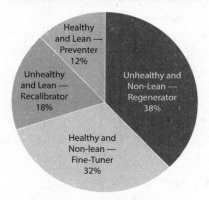

Sources: https://www.cell.com/cell-metabolism/fulltext/S1550-4131(17)30429-1;
https://www.liebertpub.com/doi/10.1089/met.2018.0105; https://www.jci.org/articles/view/129186

Figure 3.2. Distribution of the Metabolic Profiles

How to Determine Your Metabolic Health Profile

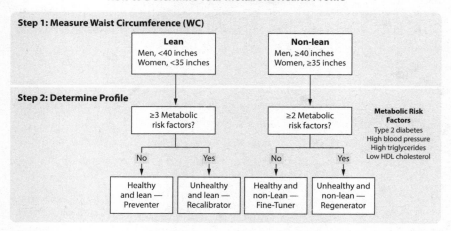

Figure 3.3. How to Determine Your Metabolic Health Profile

pressure, triglyceride levels, and HDL levels, they are part of the blood work your physician orders at your annual physical—if your physical was more than six months ago, make your appointment now so that you can use current results to help you choose the right plan for you.

As a reminder, here are the definitions of markers of metabolic health:

- High blood pressure: equal to or greater than 130/85
- High triglycerides: equal to or greater than 150 mg/dl
- Low LDL cholesterol: below 40 mg/dl for men or 50 mg/dl for women

The Other Piece of the Personalization Equation

In addition to knowing your metabolic profile, you also want to factor in whether or not you already have non-alcoholic fatty liver disease and, if so, which stage you are in.

While liver biopsy is the only true way to assess the extent of scarring in the liver, researchers have developed a formula called the FIB-4 score, which assesses your state of liver disease noninvasively. To learn your FIB-4 score, you can use an online calculator that asks for your age and a few basic blood test results, including levels of two liver enzymes—alanine transaminase (ALT) and aspartate transaminase (AST)—and your platelet count. It's accessible at gihep.com/calculators/hepatology/fibrosis-4-score/.

FIB-4 Scores
Here's how your FIB-4 score relates to the stage of fatty liver disease:
"The good," or NAFLD: less than 1.3
"The bad," or NASH-fibrosis: 1.3-2.67
"The ugly," or cirrhosis: greater than 2.67

Next Stop: Boosting Your Liver Health

Now that you have a good idea of your metabolic profile and the state of your liver health, it's *almost* time to start learning about diet and lifestyle plans to help you renew your liver. First, though, in Part 2, we're going to cover the tools and strategies that everyone needs to start taking better care of their liver. Some are easy swaps and quick fixes that will help you get a jump start, and others are behavioral strategies and mindset shifts that will motivate you to get going on implementing any changes you need to make and maintaining them over the long term.

We know you're probably itching to dive into finding the right plan for you, and we promise—it's coming soon! Just as we wouldn't send you off on a cross-country road trip without a full tank of gas, a map, food, and water, we won't send you off into a new eating plan without the things you need to make it to your ultimate destination—which, in this case, is a much happier liver.

part two

Regenerating Your Health

chapter 4

Reduce Your Risks

W HEN WE MEET people socially and tell them what we do for a living, many of them think—or say out loud—something to the effect of, "Oh, that's nice, but it doesn't pertain to me because I don't have liver disease."

Because of the already high and ever-increasing prevalence of non-alcoholic fatty liver disease, that line of thinking all too often just simply isn't valid.

Regardless of whether you have been diagnosed with a form of NAFLD, there are certain strategies and practices that your liver is begging for you to adopt. We'll share those things that apply to everyone, regardless of your metabolic profile or stage of fatty liver disease, in this chapter. But first, we'll help you paint a clearer picture of your unique risk factors.

The Fatty Liver Risk Factors Beyond Your Control

As we've established, non-alcoholic fatty liver disease is as prevalent as it is for some global, systemic reasons. That being said, there are also risk factors that are more personal to you—some of them you had no say in, and some that you do have direct influence over. Let's look at the ones that aren't something that you can control but that you can take steps to overcome nonetheless by following the guidance in this book.

Your Age
Fatty liver doesn't blow in like a hurricane. It grows like a tree. The older you are, the more years the tree has had to grow. This is not to say that if you're in your twenties or thirties you have nothing to

worry about: Ibrahim treats plenty of twenty- and thirty-year-olds with NASH-fibrosis and even cirrhosis. Remember, this is why the rising prevalence of NAFLD in children is so concerning—because the longer you have fatty liver, the more time your disease has to progress.

Your Hormones

Another reason age is a risk factor is that as we get older, our reproductive hormones decline. The technical term for this is hypogonadism; if you're a woman, you think of it as perimenopause (the transition to the cessation of your period) or menopause (when you have not had a period for at least a year). But men also experience a drop in reproductive hormones (perhaps you've heard the term "manopause"—a funny name for a real phenomenon). While both men and women experience a decrease in testosterone over time, hypogonadism is a bigger risk factor for women because estrogen helps to clear insulin. As you get closer to and beyond menopause, you have less and less estrogen on hand to regulate your insulin, and thus your blood sugar levels are likely to be higher and your liver is more likely to store glucose as fat. The good news here is that the eating plans we outline in this book will all work toward lessening the impact of age-related hormone fluctuations on your metabolic health.

Length of Time Your Metabolic Health Has Suffered

Because fatty liver disease progresses over time, the longer your markers of metabolic health have been compromised, the longer your liver has had to move along the path from "the good" toward "the ugly." If you were metabolically healthy for most of your life but then gained weight around your waist at midlife, your liver hasn't had as much time to accumulate fat as it would have if you had had a large waist circumference since you were younger.

What Your Mother Ate When You Were In Utero

Here's something you *really* have no control over—your mother's diet and liver health when she was pregnant with you. Women with fatty liver are very likely to have a child with fatty liver. What's worse, if you take that newborn and put them on an eating plan that should fight fatty liver, it doesn't reverse quickly. Researchers theorize that the cytokine storm that happened during pregnancy in those affected by NAFLD impairs the child's liver's ability to regenerate. There is also a link between gestational diabetes and fatty liver in the mother and the baby.

While you can't go back in time and change what your mother ate when she was pregnant with you, if you are a woman who is hoping to have a child or children, you have quite a lot of influence over your own liver health, and thus your children's liver health. Following the plan in this book that makes the most sense for you will help you exert that influence.

Genetics

Genetics is also a factor in who is more likely to develop fatty liver and who isn't.

Some conditions that are associated with fatty liver tend to run in families, like dyslipidemia, which is an imbalance of fats, including cholesterol and triglycerides, that increases the risk of cardiovascular disease and fatty liver. Fatty liver itself has been found to be more likely in siblings, or among parents and children, who also have some form of the disease.[1]

There are also specific genes that are associated with a higher risk of fatty liver disease: people with a variant in the patatin-like phospholipase domain-containing protein 3 gene (PNPLA3) were shown to be twice as likely to have a fatty liver as those who don't. Genetic variations aren't always bad—a different variant in this same gene is thought to play a protective role in people who have it.[2]

There are other genetic variations on specific genes that have been identified as playing a role in a propensity toward fatty liver disease. Among them are variants of the HSD17B13 gene,[3] TM6SF2 (which regulates the metabolism of fat in the liver), E165K (a variant of which impairs the secretion of very low-density lipoprotein [VLDL] and triggers the storage of liver fat),[4] and GKRP (which increases how much glucose the liver uptakes),[5] and that's just for starters. Now that these genetic variants have been identified, it opens up new possibilities for identifying risk and, potentially, for developing new treatments. Although genetic tests that identify the genes associated with fatty liver disease aren't widely available yet, even for clinicians, they could become a powerful way to assess predisposition to developing fatty liver disease and help identify those patients who need to take extra care with their metabolic health.[6]

KEEPING YOUR GENETICS IN PERSPECTIVE

It's easy to tell yourself things like, "Fatty liver is just in my genes," especially if you have a family member who has it or if you've gotten a genetic testing report that shows you have increased risk of developing it.

But our understanding of genetics has evolved to the point where we know that it's not the presence of a specific gene variant that dictates your health outcome—it's whether that gene is turned on or turned off. And that is dictated by epigenetics. "Epi" means above, and "epigenetics" refers to the material that sits on top of your genetic material and influences whether your genes are expressed (turned on) or not (turned off). And epigenetics can be influenced, both positively and negatively, by your diet, how much you exercise, your sleep, your stress, and your environment. For this reason, if you have variants that increase your risk, it doesn't mean that they are determinative.[7]

Again, genetic variants can also work in your favor and make your efforts to change your diet and lifestyle more impactful.[8] Thanks to epigenetics, you have so much power to positively influence your health and reduce your risk of all manner of diseases, including fatty liver disease. Let this knowledge empower you to do the things we outline in this book to support your metabolic health, and know that you are making changes that can benefit you all the way down to the level of your DNA.

The Risk Factors You Can Control

Let's talk about the things you can do something about—these are things you can immediately start doing differently, even before you figure out exactly which eating plan is best for you based on your metabolic profile and stage of fatty liver disease.

Your Alcohol Consumption

Although we're talking about non-alcoholic fatty liver disease—and not the liver disease that develops as a direct result of drinking excessively over the long term—drinking taxes the liver because it is responsible for metabolizing the ethanol in alcoholic beverages. Alcoholic beverages are a source of sugar, carbs, and calories as well, three things that an overworked liver is likely to store as fat. The more often you drink, and the more you drink, the more liver fat you tend to have.

Ibrahim explains alcohol consumption to his patients this way—it's not the use of a bad thing, it's the overuse of a good thing. And it's really easy to overuse alcohol. The current dietary guidelines for Americans from the National Institutes of Health (NIH) allow for two drinks per day for males and one drink per day for females, but there's a lot of debate among medical professionals and researchers about whether even that small amount is excessive. Additionally, even if you are following these guidelines, you are probably a little off. Kristin has her patients first pour as much wine as they typically drink into the glass they normally drink from and then pour the wine into a measuring cup. Many realize that what they thought was five ounces (which is the serving size of wine as defined by the NIH) actually measures out to seven ounces or more.

The truth is, if you have non-alcoholic fatty liver disease—particularly at advanced stages ("the bad" or "the ugly")—or fit into either of the metabolically unhealthy profiles, you should not drink any amount of alcohol every day. If you are among the low percentage of people who are metabolically healthy, most people argue that moderate drinking is OK. Just remember that moderate drinking is no more than two drinks in a day for men and one for women. Kristin says, "Moms who drink a couple glasses of wine every night with dinner or after the kids are asleep, I am looking at you! Many of my mom clients admit to having as many as three glasses at night. Gradually working to reduce that to two, one, or no glasses per night (perhaps only having a glass on weekend nights, or alternating nights) will not only help your liver regenerate itself; it can help you cut carbs, sugar, and calories, and shed some excess weight." This step-down approach is especially important for women, because research shows that women are at greater risk for alcohol-associated liver disease at lower levels of consumption than men, and that risk starts to increase substantially in women who consume more than one drink a day.[9]

ARE LOW-CARB ALCOHOLIC BEVERAGES A BETTER CHOICE?

There are so many different types of alcohol being marketed to carb-conscious consumers, it can definitely be confusing!

"Low carb" does not always mean low alcohol. In fact, many wines and beers marketed as being low in sugar or low in carbs will have just as much alcohol as their higher-sugar counterparts. Bottom line, if you are in the market for a "healthier" form of alcohol, focus on options that are lower in both sugar *and* alcohol. We also suggest keeping your portion size and frequency lower, especially if you are in the later stages of liver disease, or cut out alcoholic beverages altogether.

In general, you want to stick with red wine when possible because it is a traditional part of the Mediterranean diet, which, as we have mentioned, has a library of research to support its overall healthfulness and its ability to support liver health in particular. It's the antioxidant content of red wine—thanks to the fact that it includes the skins of the grapes, which is where the deeply hued polyphenols are—that makes it an acceptable part of the plan. (In white wine the grape skins are removed, and so are the majority of antioxidants.) Additionally, enjoying a meal over a glass of wine with people helps foster a communal atmosphere that is also beneficial for health.

It's still important to keep your red wine intake moderate, though, not just because of the carb content but also because of the alcohol content. Even though red wine does have some health benefits, alcohol is, after all, a neurotoxin. When you drink it, your body will prioritize getting that alcohol out of your system over metabolizing glucose and fat; studies have even found that alcohol causes a spike in insulin during the four hours after consumption.[10]

Here are some other things to keep in mind regarding your alcohol intake:

- **Think about your stage of liver disease:** If you have NAFLD or NASH, a little alcohol is OK so long as you stick to the recommended guidelines. Once you get into fibrosis or cirrhosis, it's better for your liver if you skip alcohol as much as possible.

- **Consider the carb/sugar content:** Different types of alcoholic beverages have different amounts of sugar. While all wine is made from grapes, and grapes are rich in natural sugars, not all wines have the same sugar content. The longer a wine is fermented, the more the natural sugars are depleted by the fermentation process, and the drier the wine is as a result. The types of red wine that tend to be on the drier side include cabernet sauvignon, malbec, merlot, pinot noir, sangiovese, syrah, and tempranillo. Sweeter red wines typically include port, zinfandel, sherry, and marsala. A typical beer contains twelve to fourteen grams of carbs, whereas most light beers have somewhere between three and six—all per twelve-ounce serving. Most hard seltzers have one or two grams of carbs per twelve-ounce serving.

- **Familiarize yourself with a proper portion size:** Remember, a serving of red wine is five ounces, not "a glass," so make sure your "glass" of wine is actually five ounces and not larger (pour it first into a measuring cup and then into a glass so you can learn what a true portion looks like). A serving of beer or hard seltzer is twelve ounces—not a pint, which is sixteen ounces.

- **Look for a lower alcohol content:** The lower the alcohol content of your wine or other alcoholic beverage, the better. Why? More alcohol means more calories. It also means less metabolism of the carbohydrates in the drink (as well as the carbs, protein, and fat in your meal that accompanies that glass of alcohol) as your body will focus on detoxing the alcohol first. Most labels will show a beverage's alcohol by volume (ABV) as a number followed by a % sign. The average wine is 11–13 percent alcohol, but it can go as low as 5 percent and as high as 20 percent. Beer and hard seltzer are in the 4–5 percent ABV range.

If you prefer hard liquor, gin, rum, tequila, vodka, and whiskey are all carb-free. Of course, liquor is also higher in ABV than wine, which is why a recommended daily serving of hard alcohol is one ounce for women and two ounces for men. Use a shot glass to be sure of your portion size. Also, be mindful of your mixers. If you don't enjoy hard liquor neat or on the rocks, choose a low-carb mixer such as seltzer, water, or sugar-free tonic, then add flavor with a squeeze of lemon or lime or a dash of bitters.

Your Gut Health

Many patients with fatty liver disease also experience challenges to their gut health. One such challenge is increased intestinal permeability, also known as leaky gut, when the lining of the intestines becomes damaged and porous, allowing food and bacteria to leak out of the digestive tract into the bloodstream. Another is bacterial overgrowth in the small intestine (a.k.a. small intestinal bacterial overgrowth, or SIBO).

Patients with fatty liver disease also have significant alteration of the gut microbiome. Research has shown that patients with NAFLD experience a decrease of the abundance of good bacteria and an increase of the abundance of bad bacteria.[11] In other words, studies have found differences in the gut microbiomes of people with NAFLD and healthy individuals.

The overgrowth of unfriendly bacteria can increase the formation of fat in the liver by metabolizing fructose into acetate, which promotes the creation of fat.[12] It can also produce ethanol (otherwise known as alcohol, meaning it's like your bad gut bugs are going to the bar and overindulging even if you never drink)[13] and contribute to leaky gut (which can then tax the liver by requiring it to filter the harmful compounds released into the bloodstream). These findings suggest that improving the health of the microbiome will become an important tool in fighting fatty liver disease.

In addition, stress, any trauma you have experienced, and your environment can adversely affect your microbiome. (If you have any gastro-intestinal challenges, such as bloating, constipation, or diarrhea, or have been diagnosed with irritable bowel syndrome, you know these symptoms tend to intensify with stress.) We continue to find more things that impact the microbiome and more areas of health that the microbiome influences. We simply can't ignore taking good care of our gut.

Luckily, there are many steps you can take to boost your good gut bacteria—eating fermented foods such as sauerkraut, kefir, yogurt, miso, and tempeh; eating more fiber-rich foods such as whole grains, legumes, and low-glycemic-load fruits and vegetables; and reducing your consumption of refined sugars and grains, which feed unfriendly bacteria. All of the Renew Your Liver plans will help you adopt these strategies, which can greatly benefit your gut health.

In addition, researchers are already looking to identify signatures of gut microbiomes in advanced stages of fatty liver in order to make detection easier and able to be done earlier.[14]

There are some emerging therapies designed to improve gut health that may sound out-there but can be effective ways to repopulate the bacterial population, including fecal transplant, where the fecal matter of one individual is implanted in another individual. Indeed, a landmark 2006 paper published in *Nature* showed that fecal transplantation from obese mice to regular-sized mice led to increased fat mass.[15] Fecal transplant is still experimental for the treatment of metabolic syndrome and fatty liver disease. Although it's not ready for prime time yet, there is early evidence that fecal transplantation from a healthy donor to a patient with NAFLD could improve inflammation in the liver[16] and intestinal permeability.[17]

While we wait for more evidence to support the safety and efficacy of fecal transplant as a treatment for NAFLD, you may want to consider supplementing with probiotics, or gut-friendly bacteria. Ibrahim's take is that they don't cause harm and may cause good (refer to the Supplements for Overall Health [and Liver] Support section of this chapter for guidance on choosing and taking a probiotic supplement). A 2019 review of randomized clinical trials in humans observed the following benefits of taking probiotics: improved levels of liver enzymes, lower levels of triglycerides, decreased inflammation in the liver, reduction of liver fat, and reduced body weight.[18]

Your Daily Servings of Fruits and Vegetables

Fresh produce is typically high in fiber and nutrients and low in calories. Eating it regularly—at least three servings a day—crowds out room on your plate and in your belly for food that is more processed and nutrient-poor. Also, people who eat a lot of fresh produce tend to have other healthy habits, including not smoking, drinking less, and exercising more. To be clear, while increasing your veg intake is the goal, we'd like you to emphasize greens, such as collards, spinach, and kale, as well as cauliflower, broccoli, and so on, but less so the high-glycemic-load vegetables such as potatoes and corn. When setting up your plate, we recommend making fresh produce the main attraction, with lean protein, healthy fats, and whole grains as accessories.

Sleep Apnea

This sleep disorder, in which a person will stop breathing for anywhere from a few seconds to thirty seconds repeatedly throughout the night, is strongly associated with inflammation, insulin resistance, increased LDL (the harmful form of cholesterol), and fatty liver. Studies have also found that people with sleep apnea have higher levels of the liver enzymes ALT (alanine aminotransferase) and AST (aspartate aminotransferase), and a 500 percent higher risk of developing liver disease than those who don't have it.[19] If you haven't been diagnosed with sleep apnea but you (or your partner, who hears your ragged breathing at night) suspect that you may have it, it's worth speaking with your doctor about it. Your liver (and your partner) will thank you!

Hormonal Health

Nothing in the body works in isolation. Disruptions in your hormones—chemical messengers of your endocrine system that influence the function of your organs, among other things—can also influence your liver health. Polycystic ovarian syndrome (PCOS), for example, is a condition that affects one in ten women in the United States. It is associated with elevated levels of sex hormones (known as androgens) and can result in ovarian cysts, missed periods, and infertility. Women who have PCOS are about four times as likely as women without it to develop type 2 diabetes, which is also strongly associated with fatty liver disease. To up the stakes even further, fatty liver disease tends to progress quickly if you have PCOS.

Hypothyroidism is a common condition (more than three million cases are reported in the United States every year) where the thyroid gland doesn't make enough thyroid hormone. Since the thyroid rules metabolism in the body, hypothyroidism can feel like your gas tank is running on empty: fatigue, weight gain, and an intolerance to cold are typical symptoms. Thyroid hormones are also vital for healthy liver function. As evidence, there are two places in the body with thyroid receptors—the thyroid gland and the liver. It makes sense because thyroid hormone helps with metabolism, and the liver has the job of metabolizing fats and other nutrients. If your thyroid hormone is low, it makes sense that your liver may be struggling to break down fat and will have to resort to storing it instead of moving it along.

Ibrahim has found hypothyroidism to be common in his fatty liver patients. As a result, when he gives talks to medical schools, he tells them to screen fatty liver patients for hypothyroidism.

The good news here is that both PCOS and hypothyroid are treatable—for PCOS, your doctor may suggest going on birth control pills to regulate your hormone levels, and for hypothyroidism your doctor may prescribe a synthetic thyroid hormone. There are also efforts under way to research and develop drugs that selectively stimulate the thyroid receptor in the liver, which could lead to the increased metabolism and breakdown of fat. In addition, the dietary programs that we include in this book can all help normalize your hormonal imbalances, particularly by reducing your insulin levels.

FOUR HEALTHY HABITS TO REDUCE ALL HEALTH RISKS

In a 2012 study, researchers from the Medical University of South Carolina examined the health records of nearly twelve thousand adult men and women of all ages and weights in an effort to gauge the effect of four specific healthy habits on mortality.[20] These habits were as follows:

- Eating at least five servings of fruits and vegetables per day
- Not exceeding two alcoholic drinks per day (for men) or one per day (for women)
- Exercising regularly (more than twelve times per month)
- Not smoking

Perhaps not surprisingly, their analysis found that each one of these healthy habits offered protection against early death and that reduction in risk rose with each additional habit—meaning, those who engaged in all four of the habits were less likely to die early than those who only engaged in three, and so on.

What *was* surprising was that people in all weight categories—regular weight, overweight, and obese—experienced a reduction in risk of death, not just those who were obese or overweight. This furthers our argument that even if you are classified as having a "normal" weight, and even if your metabolic markers look good, you still stand to benefit greatly from adopting an eating and lifestyle plan aimed at prevention of fatty liver disease.

Another interesting finding from this study was that it didn't matter how long people engaged in physical activity, only how frequently. This suggests that you don't need to aim for fewer, longer workouts (like jogging for forty-five minutes), as shorter, more frequent types of movement (like simply walking more in your daily life, or doing workouts that are only ten or so minutes long a couple of times a week) offer plenty of benefit. Since you don't necessarily have to find big chunks of time for exercise, this can help you make movement more of a regular habit.

Unfriendly Companions: The Conditions That Often Accompany Fatty Liver

Fatty liver disease is called a silent disease because it presents so few telltale symptoms. Some people do experience itchy or sensitive skin, darker urine and paler stools, a tendency to bruise easily, unexplained weight loss, mild pain in their upper right abdomen, nausea, and/or fluid retention in the legs, ankles, and feet. For the most part, however, symptoms only present themselves when the liver disease has progressed very far along—and then it can show up as persistent fatigue, muscle weakness, mental fog, and memory loss. If only something as definitive as jaundice—when the whites of your eyes and even skin can take on a yellow cast—happened in every instance and stage of fatty liver disease! (Jaundice is caused by an excess of bilirubin, a reddish-orange pigment that's released when red blood cells are broken down. Your liver breaks down bilirubin so that it can be excreted via bile, but when the liver isn't working well, the bilirubin builds up in your bloodstream.) Although jaundice can occur in hepatitis, cirrhosis, and liver cancer, it doesn't typically occur in the first three stages of fatty liver disease.

The experience of having fatty liver disease isn't typically marked by uncomfortable symptoms, but there are some conditions that can accompany fatty liver disease. While they may not be useful in alerting you to the presence of the disease, or which stage you are in, you can expect to experience improvement in the following areas as your liver recovers:

- **Poor sleep.** While impaired sleep is more likely to contribute to fatty liver disease than be caused by it, it is true that people with NAFLD tend to have disordered sleep. One Japanese study found fatty liver disease is most likely to occur in people who sleep either six or fewer hours per night or more than eight hours per night. (It was lowest in the group that slept between six and seven hours per night.)[21] When your liver issues begin to resolve, your sleep issues can, too.
- **Higher risk of cancer.** Even more serious is that fatty liver is associated with a greater risk of developing all cancers, not just liver cancer. A study published in the *Journal of Hepatology* found that men with fatty liver had a higher risk of developing colorectal cancer than men with healthy livers, and women with fatty liver disease were more likely to develop breast cancer. These risks got higher as the severity of the fatty liver disease increased.[22]

    The greater risk of cancer is true not just for adults but also, tragically, for children with fatty liver, too: an important Swedish study compared children and young adults who had biopsy-confirmed NAFLD and NASH with their peers who did not have fatty liver disease. Over the course of fifteen years, the youth with NAFLD and NASH had a significantly higher risk of dying from all forms of cancer than their healthy peers—a risk of 7.7 percent, as compared to a 1.1 percent risk in the population with healthy livers. They also had higher rates of mortality from liver-related disease and cardiovascular disease, although cancer presented the highest risk.[23]
- **Lower quality of life.** Some fatty liver patients can experience loss of appetite, nausea, and even vomiting, particularly in later

stages of the disease. They can also feel some amount of pain or tenderness in the upper right side of their abdomen. These low-lying symptoms are the type of thing that can decrease quality of life, which is a serious loss in and of itself.

- **Fatigue.** This vague and pervasive condition is difficult to attribute to any one particular source. With our always-on lives, it is completely understandable if we feel mildly to moderately run down most of the time. But fatigue has been linked in the literature to fatty liver disease, and in both of our practices, when patients' fatty liver gets better, so do their energy levels.

In some ways, it's a blessing that fatty liver doesn't produce a lot of unpleasant symptoms, because who wants to live with unpleasant symptoms? On the other hand, it can also be hard to find the motivation to change your habits if you are relatively comfortable. We hope that by learning how much regeneration is possible when it comes to the liver, and how likely it is that fatty liver disease will progress and expose you to other risks if you don't take steps to remedy it, you will be inspired to make changes.

Start by Moving—Even Ten Minutes a Day!

Many people think of exercising primarily as a way to burn calories and, therefore, to lose weight. But science suggests that exercise isn't actually all that effective in helping you to lose weight—dietary changes provide most of that benefit. One way that moderate exercise of the type and duration we're about to suggest *does* shine is in improving insulin sensitivity and in helping to keep weight from creeping on or back on—both of which aid in reducing your risk of developing fatty liver or helping you reverse fatty liver if you are already on the NAFLD spectrum. Exercise also improves mood and produces pain-reducing chemicals, making it easier and more doable to make the other lifestyle changes that will keep your health moving in an upward spiral.

Because exercise is so good at keeping fatty liver at bay, it shouldn't be a surprise that the majority of NAFLD patients (between 50 and 60 percent) report getting minimal levels of physical activity. If you fit this profile, it is very important that you start to change this, as of today. As you'll see, it really doesn't take much movement to do a lot of good for your liver.

If you have a general lack of movement in your life, or even if you do workouts fairly regularly but spend most of the day seated, you are experiencing a major risk factor for metabolic syndrome and fatty liver. Inactivity is associated with insulin resistance and increased systemic inflammation as well as increased risk of cancer and heart disease. In fact, a 2018 study by the Centers for Disease Control (CDC) attributed more than 8 percent of all annual deaths in the United States to "inadequate levels of activity."[24] However, that doesn't mean you need to become a gym rat, marathoner, or CrossFit devotee to reap the benefits of exercise. It takes a lot less time and effort than you think.

In fact, one study examined data gathered between 2003 and 2006 as part of the National Health and Nutrition Examination Survey. The data the researchers selected came from a group of five thousand Americans aged forty to eighty-five who had worn an activity tracker for at least seven days. The researchers grouped these people according to how many minutes of physical activity they logged each day and then jumped ahead in time to 2015 to analyze the death rates and determine the risk of mortality experienced by each group. And then they ran various scenarios—if everyone moved for ten additional minutes, how many fewer people would die compared with the original mortality rate? They found that moving around for a mere ten extra minutes a day would prevent 110,000 unnecessary deaths each year.[25]

More specific to liver health, one 2017 review found that an increase in activity of at least sixty minutes per week—which is just 8.5 minutes per day—still helped reduce liver fat and levels of the liver enzymes ALT and AST, which are sometimes used to gauge the presence of fatty liver disease.[26]

This makes sense when you look at the blue zones—parts of the world where people live longer, better lives (places that include Okinawa, Japan; Sardinia, Italy; Nicoya, Costa Rica; Ikaria, Greece; and Loma Linda, California). For the most part, those folks are not making a conscious effort to exercise. They're working in the garden, in the home, or in the community, not setting goals to walk a certain number of steps.

The bottom line? Doing something is much better than doing nothing.

It really doesn't seem to matter what type of exercise you do or even how vigorous it is. The most important qualification of the movement you do is that you can actually do it—whether that's because it's so convenient that you don't have an excuse not to or because you enjoy it or both.

That said, there has been plenty of interesting research on what the different types of exercise do for the liver.

- *Aerobic exercise:* What you might think of as "cardio" (including running, walking, biking, dancing, swimming, pickleball, and using the cardio machines at the gym) activates fat burning. The intensity of aerobic exercise doesn't seem to make much difference.[27]
- *Resistance exercise:* Also known as strength training, resistance training builds muscle fibers and activates enzymes that play an important role in the metabolism of fat in the liver. Like aerobic exercise, resistance exercise does improve liver fat. However,

THE BENEFITS OF MOVEMENT

Aids in digestion

Gives a short-term boost to metabolism

Cues the body to take glucose from the bloodstream and put it into the tissues, where it can be used for fuel

Makes tissues more sensitive to insulin

Prevents stiffness

Strengthens muscles, bones, and joints

Releases endorphins, which reduce the perception of pain

Boosts mood

Promotes more restful sleep

Is associated with an increase in HDL (the good kind of) cholesterol studies lean toward a greater benefit to fatty liver with aerobic exercise or at least a combination of aerobic and resistance exercise. In other words, resistance training alone is not as effective in reducing liver fat.

The CDC recommends either 150 minutes of moderate exercise or 75 minutes of vigorous exercise per week or an equivalent combination of the two. These numbers are what we recommend to our patients—and to you—too. As high as the numbers may sound, when you divide them by seven (the number of days in a week), that's just a hair over twenty minutes per day for moderate exercise—which includes all the daily motions listed in the "Everyday Actions Count as Movement" sidebar—and just over ten minutes per day for vigorous exercise. Those twenty minutes can be a few minutes here and there in the morning, afternoon, and evening. And again, if you can't do twenty minutes, even ten minutes of moderate-intensity movement will still provide a lot of benefit.

NEAT—OR, EVERYDAY ACTIONS COUNT AS MOVEMENT

You don't have to put on exercise clothes or break a sweat in order to get movement going that benefits your health. Any movements you make during the day can add up, thanks to something called non-exercise activity thermogenesis (NEAT)—or the energy that we expend during daily living, basically any time we're not sleeping, eating, or exercising. While we're not too concerned about burning calories because we're not focused on weight loss, things like doing the dishes or walking to the kitchen and making a cup of coffee can add up to significant amounts of expended energy throughout the day. In fact, you can burn five hundred to six hundred calories on all the activities involved in cleaning and maintaining your home during one day, versus the twenty-seven calories you'll burn watching TV for three hours. So moving more means less need for your liver to store those excess calories.

In addition, NEAT has been shown to improve markers of metabolic health, including decreasing insulin sensitivity and blood pressure and increasing high-density lipoprotein (the good kind of cholesterol). It also decreases the risk of dying from cardiovascular disease, as well as dying for any reason, even if you don't regularly get more formal exercise (although we still want you to exercise, too!).[28]

When you feel you don't have the time or energy to exercise, do plenty of the activities listed below, or really anything that gets you up out of the chair and moving around. The same goes for your children. If they won't go do something active, put them to work sweeping!

Standing
Getting up to walk across the room
Going up and down the stairs in your house
Going to get the mail or the newspaper from your mailbox or front step
Folding laundry
Doing dishes
Sweeping and vacuuming
Dusting
Cooking
Showering
Stretching
Returning shopping carts to the corral
Walking the aisles at the big box store
Weeding or watering the garden
Walking your pet (patients who have dogs are less likely to have fatty liver)
Running errands on foot

If you have a disability or physical condition that makes moving painful or uncomfortable, you can start slow and stick to low-impact forms of movement, such as chair yoga, walking, riding a recumbent bike, or swimming. If what you can do on a given day is park farther away from the grocery store, that is absolutely fine. Just try to keep in mind that not moving is a recipe for creating more stiffness and pain, and movement can produce natural pain-relieving and mood-boosting neurochemicals. It's worth it to consult with a physical therapist or physical trainer to develop a routine that gets you moving without aggravating your painful parts so that you and your liver can reap the many benefits of movement. The more you move, the more you'll build up endurance, enjoy mental health benefits, and feel better—all of which will naturally help you want to get more movement.

If your disability or mobility challenges mean that moving more is really not feasible, know that dietary changes have a tremendous beneficial impact on liver health, even without exercise, and you can still do a ton of good by following one of our Renew Your Liver eating plans.

Make Space for Better Sleep

A good night's sleep can make everything seem better—you have more energy, your thinking is clearer, your mood tends to be sunnier, and that's just what you can notice on the surface. Inside your body, how well you slept the night before kicks off a whole host of hormonal reactions, many of which exert direct influences on your metabolism, appetite, and fat storage, and thus on your liver health.

While sleeping too little isn't necessarily associated with fatty liver, it *is* associated with insulin resistance, which ultimately leads to changes in insulin blood levels. This sets the stage for craving quick-burning comfort foods (low-fiber carbs) and gaining belly fat, which certainly does put you on the path to fatty liver.

Lack of sleep alters the function of your digestive enzymes—they never turn off, which means you never get the message that you're full. It also messes with your levels of ghrelin (an appetite stimulant) and leptin (an appetite suppressor), which can lead to your thinking that you're hungry when your body doesn't actually need food and to overeating. And what are you going to crave? Carbs. Think about those days when you stayed up all night in college: you wanted to eat nonstop the next day, and you didn't want to eat broccoli. You wanted pizza.

If you aren't sleeping well, you are probably stressed. If you are relying too much on alcohol to take the edge off, then that will also negatively impact your sleep. Because alcohol is a depressant, once you've metabolized the alcohol (thanks, liver!), you will be comparatively stimulated and wake up. Alcohol also hinders the quality of your sleep, and you don't just want enough sleep, you want it to be solid.

If you sacrifice sleep during the week and try to catch up on the weekend, studies show that your efforts likely aren't helping to prevent the metabolic dysregulation that inadequate sleep triggers.[29]

The good news is that sleeping more can have quick positive effects on your appetite and metabolism. One randomized clinical trial of adults who habitually slept less than six and a half hours per night found that when they increased their sleep duration by just over an hour a night for two weeks, they subconsciously ate less during the day with no specific instructions to do so. This suggests that it doesn't take much additional sleep—or very many days of a little more sleep—to interrupt the hormonal cascade triggered by too little sleep that can increase appetite and cravings for low-fiber carbs.[30] If cravings are a problem for you, try going to bed earlier!

You want to aim for at least seven hours a night—less than that is associated with a disruption in the hormones ghrelin and leptin.[31] According to a National Sleep Foundation survey, just over 35 percent of all adult Americans get less than this amount. And if you're a single parent, active-duty service member, or factory worker, you're even more likely to be getting less than seven hours a night.[32]

It's true that the demands of work, parenting, family, and community involvement can make it seem like you don't have time to sleep, but in reality you don't have time *not* to. Convincing yourself that you're fine on six hours of sleep is all too likely to result in too high of a toll on your metabolic health. If you know you need more sleep but are having trouble getting it, refer to the sleep-related tips in Your Checklist for Change at the end of this chapter. And if you've been diagnosed with sleep apnea, or a partner or person you live with has suggested that your snoring sounds as if you are gasping for air, consult with your doctor about addressing it, as sleep apnea is a confirmed risk factor for fatty liver. In fact, even if you believe you are only a light snorer, talk to your doctor about it and ask for a sleep study in order to rule out sleep apnea. While not everyone who snores is experiencing the periods of low oxygen that are the hallmarks of sleep apnea, it is worth it to make sure that you don't have it and to get treated for it if you do.

Find Ways to Dial Down Stress

You already know that stress isn't good for your health. At its essence, stress is inflammatory.

The two major players in the stress response are the hypothalamus-pituitary-adrenal axis (the HPA axis) and your sympathetic nervous system (SNS). The HPA axis is responsible for activating the SNS—the branch of the autonomic nervous system that rules the "fight or flight" reactions of your body—during a stressful event, and for bringing you back to homeostasis afterward.

Your hypothalamus gland is located in your brain and is always on the lookout for stressors. As soon as it perceives one—whether it's something real like a car that narrowly misses hitting your car or something intangible like a deadline—it sends a hormonal message to the pituitary gland, which is the master regulator of your hormonal system and is located next to the hypothalamus in your brain. The pituitary then releases hormones that signal your adrenal glands to produce pro-inflammatory cytokines and a category of hormones known as glucocorticoids, the most well known of which is cortisol. A lot of steps happen quickly; when they happen continuously, the HPA axis can have a harder time bringing you back to homeostasis and you can get stuck in an inflammatory state.

Stress has been linked to multiple cofactors of fatty liver, including cardiovascular disease and metabolic syndrome. And of course, when you're stressed, it's that much easier to skimp on sleep, drink an extra glass or two of alcohol, smoke cigarettes, or indulge in emotional eating.

A 2020 study was the first of its kind to find a connection between perceived stress and NAFLD itself: Korean researchers assessed the livers of over 171,000 adults using ultrasonography and found that 27.8 percent overall had NAFLD. They also asked the participants to complete a questionnaire that scored their perceived level of stress, and the higher those scores were, the higher the rates of NAFLD prevalence climbed. The increase was even more pronounced for men than for women and for metabolically unhealthy individuals than for metabolically healthy individuals.[33]

While there aren't yet studies that evaluate the effectiveness of stress-reduction practices such as meditation and mindfulness on fatty liver disease in particular, studies have found that these relaxation practices, even when performed in a workplace setting, can reduce cortisol production and quiet the sympathetic nervous system so that the autonomic nervous system can come back to balance.[34]

RELAXATION APPS

Although our smartphones can certainly be a source of stress, they can also provide relief by giving us easy access to guided meditations and other relaxation exercises through the use of apps. Here are some that we recommend to our patients and clients:

- Headspace
- Calm
- Insight Timer
- Healthy Minds Program (free)

Guided visualizations can also be wonderfully relaxing—you simply listen along as someone talks you through a relaxing script. Good sources include the following:

- ImagesofWellness.com
- HealthJourney.com
- Countless videos on YouTube (free)

What all this means is that actively seeking to reduce your stress is a crucial piece of your liver-protecting plan. You can do that in a variety of ways: by saying no to or delegating tasks you don't have the bandwidth for; making time for a formal practice like meditation, breathing, yoga, or tai chi; and/or making it a point to savor the good parts of your life so that your focus is less trained on your worries.

Other parts of your Renew Your Liver plan will also help you counteract stress. Moving more is a great way to burn off angst and clear your mind. And our approach to the act of eating itself—we advocate mindful eating, which we cover in Chapter 5, and intuitive eating, which we cover in Chapter 6—can help you shift out of stress eating. And perhaps just knowing that stress only makes things harder for your liver will give you added incentive to seek ways to reduce it.

Detoxify Your Life—Keeping the Bad Actors Out

So far, we've compared the liver to Spider-Man (for its regenerative properties) and the public works department (for its vital role in keeping all the pathways of your body working). Now we have another analogy for you. Your liver is also like a TSA agent—the person at the airport who is responsible for stopping any bad actors from getting through security and onto an airplane, causing trouble for the rest of the travelers and airport and airline staff. Except, instead of screening for explosives or weapons, your liver is scanning for toxins, whether that's chemicals that come from food or water stored in plastic containers, pesticides on foods or used in your yard, or heavy metals such as lead (from old water pipes or paint) and mercury (from old silver fillings).

Your liver is responsible for filtering these harmful substances out of the blood and either sending them off to be excreted through your urine, sweat, or stool, or tucking them away in your fat cells where they can't harm your organs (most toxins are fat-soluble, which means they get stored within the fat cells). Normally, your liver does a great job of removing any toxins from circulation. But there are toxins coming at us from so many directions that the liver can get overloaded, particularly if it's also busy processing a lot of sugar and losing healthy tissue to fat deposits or even scarring. The more toxins you can keep from entering your body in the first place, the easier you'll make things for the liver.

Toxins are so potently disruptive to liver health that there is a form of fatty liver disease caused by toxin exposure that scientists have named toxicant-associated fatty liver disease (TAFLD). Workers with chemical exposure as part of their job, particularly workers in vinyl chloride factories, most often experience TAFLD and TASH (toxicant-associated steatohepatitis).

Even if you have your garden-variety NAFLD, because your liver is already struggling to some degree, it means that more of the toxins that are coming in every day are not getting out of the body, causing an additional risk to your liver. That's why it's really important that you do what you can to reduce your toxin exposure. This doesn't mean you have to live in a hermetically sealed, perfectly organic environment—little changes really do create important results. To that end, refer to the list of little things that pertain to toxins in the Checklist for Change at the end of this chapter to see what you can start implementing today—whether that's washing your produce to reduce pesticide content, reducing your use of everyday chemicals to clean your home or treat your lawn, or swapping your plastic food storage containers for stainless steel or glass. Every step you take will give your hardworking TSA agent of a liver a break.

The Most Important Thing You Can Do to Protect Your Liver: Reduce High-Glycemic Carbs

Truly, though, unless you work in a chemical plant, the most dangerous toxin to your liver is sugar. It's easy to get nervous about all the toxins out there in the world, but it's much more important to realize that you could potentially be damaging your liver every time you eat.

As we noted earlier, the term "fatty liver," while accurate, is also a little misleading. Many people think that fatty liver must come from eating too much fat, but it's really from eating too many low-fiber, nutrient-poor carbohydrates.

As we covered in Chapter 2, the medical research establishment has started to move away from the "calories in, calories out" model of weight gain and toward the carbohydrate insulin model (CIM). According to CIM, the most important variables for improving metabolic health and preventing or reversing obesity as well as fatty liver disease are reducing hunger and controlling insulin. And the way you achieve both of those aims is by eating fewer carbs.

When you reduce your carb intake, you limit the amount of insulin and modulate its impact—as well as the impact of the other metabolic hormones, glucagon and leptin. These reductions naturally help curb your appetite. Also, protein and fat are more filling than carbs, so you will be less likely to overeat because you're heeding the call of hunger signals. And when you feel famished, your brain is cueing you to eat anything you can get your hands on—it's a survival mechanism intended to prevent death. When you reduce the carbs, you reduce hunger, and best of all, you can do it without focusing on reducing calories. That is a very good thing, because if the last five decades of the diet industry has taught us anything, it's that a focus on cutting calories doesn't help to make lasting improvements to metabolic health, including liver health.

Thanks to the popularity of the ketogenic diet, we now have a lot of studies to show that low-carb diets lessen appetite as well as the responses of insulin, glucagon, and leptin. Lowering carb consumption to less than 50 grams per day (officially known as "low carb") also has been found to be a sustainable approach to weight loss and an effective dietary pattern for type 2 diabetes. Low-carb consumption is the basis of the eating plan we recommend for the "bad" and "ugly" phases of fatty liver disease (NASH, fibrosis, cirrhosis, and liver cancer). As a comparison, the Dietary Guidelines for Americans recommends between 225 and 325 grams of carbohydrates per day!

Lowering your carb intake provides quick results that can help improve your liver health. But for most people, low-carb eating isn't easy to maintain over the long term. We don't want you to feel you have to continue it indefinitely. If you are at either the "bad" or "ugly" stages of NAFLD, after losing 7 to 10 percent of your body weight, you can loosen up the reins a little and shift to either the more moderate-carb approach that we've designed to reverse the first stage of fatty liver disease (NAFLD) or the preventive approach with a Mediterranean diet that has been tweaked to reduce the amount of whole grains included.

A more moderate-carb approach isn't just more doable—it might make you live longer. A 2018 study by Dr. Sara B. Seidelmann in *The Lancet Public Health* looked at a moderate-carb approach, which they defined as 50–55 percent of total daily caloric consumption, and found this relatively easy strategy appeared to reduce the risk of all-cause mortality more than either a low-carb diet (defined as 40 percent or less of caloric intake from carbs) or high-carb (more than 70 percent of daily calories).[35]

To be clear, none of our plans fit the definition of a keto diet—which is technically a *very* low-carb, high-fat diet designed to nudge your metabolism away from burning sugar as its primary source of fuel and toward using fat for energy (what is known as ketosis). You may have tried keto and seen a lot of benefit, or you may be on it now. That's OK.

We just believe in the benefits of more moderate approaches and don't want people to feel that they have to completely transform their diet in order to get healthier. We also don't recommend staying on keto over the long term, and here's why: A 2021 meta-analysis of more than one hundred peer-reviewed studies found that people who follow the keto-genic diet over the long term have significantly increased risk of heart disease, Alzheimer's, type 2 diabetes, and cancer.[36] And really, it's no wonder, as many ketogenic diet followers load up on red meat, pro-cessed meats, and dairy and avoid nutrient-dense foods such as fruit, squashes, root vegetables, and legumes. While our eating plans are lower in carbs than what you're probably used to, their secondary focus is on being nutrient-dense and not necessarily high in fat. For that reason, we advise eating plenty of deeply hued fruits and vegeta-bles and some well-chosen whole grains, beans, and legumes, even if you start with our Low-Carb plan. (These are things that really don't have a place in a ketogenic diet thanks to their carb counts.)

There are a few upsides to the ketogenic diet craze, however—first, it provided a lot of research on the benefits of moderate- and low-carb approaches on liver health, and it made a lot more lower-carb food products available. Now there are all kinds of lower-carb, higher-fiber foods available, such as grain-free buns made primarily out of broc-coli or cauliflower, right in the frozen foods section.

The goal of the Renew Your Liver eating plans isn't to get you into ketosis (but if ketosis is something you *are* interested in, there are some huge benefits to being in this state as well—it's just that we don't recommend it as a long-term strategy). The primary aim of all our plans is to get your insulin and blood sugar levels into an acceptable range. The way to do that is to reduce the amount of food you eat that has a significant impact on your blood sugar. In other words, you want to eat foods that have a lower glycemic load.

Eat More Fiber to Reduce Your Overall Carb Intake

Dietary fiber is a form of carbohydrate. But it's not one that your body can break down. So whenever you eat a food with carbs in it, you can subtract the number of grams of fiber it has from the total carbs. This quick math will give you the total of what's called *net carbs*—or the total number of carbs that your body needs to process.

In addition, fiber slows down the digestion of that food—meaning that if you eat something carb-rich that also has a lot of fiber in it, like an apple with the peel still on it, you won't experience as much of a blood sugar spike as if you had consumed a low-fiber version of that food, such as apple juice (where all the fiber has been removed).

Some companies have started listing "net carbs" on their food packages, although some labels use the terms "active carbs" or "digestible carbs" instead.

So if you're reading a product label and it says there are twenty grams total carbs in the product, with ten grams of fiber, the net carbs—the amount of carbs that counts toward the total digestible carbs—is ten grams.

This is the formula: total carbs − grams of fiber = net carbs.

Net carbs are yet another reason we suggest eating plenty of richly hued vegetables and fruits, whole grains, and beans and legumes—they are all rich in fiber and will naturally help you reduce blood sugar levels.

Carbs Versus Fat—Which Is the Real Villain?

The problem with saturated fat isn't really the fat itself; it's the foods that it comes packaged in, such as processed meats and red meat. Processed meats, such as hot dogs, bacon, and sausages, are problematic

THE RENEW YOUR LIVER EATING PLANS

These plans are:

Plant-based
Nutrient-dense
Low to moderate in carbs
Low to moderate glycemic load
Gut health friendly
Enjoyable
Uncomplicated (ingredients that are easy to find)
Sustainable (keeping the environment in mind)

because they are often preserved with nitrates that, when heated, turn into nitrosamines, which are associated with an increased risk of colorectal cancers. Red meat is associated with heart disease, and remember, the number one cause of death in fatty liver patients is cardiovascular disease.

Research out of the Cleveland Clinic suggests that a direct reason why eating red meat can promote risk of heart disease is through a gut bacteria by-product known as TMAO (trimethylamine N-oxide), which is produced when gut bacteria digest nutrients found in red meat. High levels of TMAO are linked to atherosclerosis and other complications of heart disease, such as blood clots that can break off and lead to stroke or heart attack. Cleveland Clinic researchers have found that people who eat a diet high in red meat have significantly higher levels of TMAO than people whose main sources of protein are white meat or nonmeat food.[37]

Shoring up your gut bacteria population could potentially help you produce less TMAO, which could mean less damage to your vascular system. Luckily, the Renew Your Liver eating plans are also designed to improve gut health and foster beneficial gut bacteria thanks to their being high-fiber (which feeds good bacteria) and low in glycemic load (which means they deprive bad bacteria of their favorite food source—sugar).

Kristin's patients will often come to her and say, "I've got a little bit of fatty liver but I'm really here because I don't want to have a heart attack," or they're worried about brain health. No matter what their primary health concern is, she will remind them that the liver is a key player in the vascular system. Remember when we compared the body to a highway system in Chapter 1? Doing things to take care of the liver ends up taking care of every organ and organ system throughout the body.

If you love a BOGO (buy-one-get-one sale) at the shoe store or grocery store, then you'll love the eating plans in this book, as they each can help to remedy fatty liver while also addressing type 2 diabetes, heart health, brain health, kidney health, and vascular health. It's more like a buy-one-get-the-whole-store deal.

Each of the four Renew Your Liver eating plans helps address the following things:

- Fatty liver
- Type 2 diabetes
- Cardiovascular disease
- Gut health
- Brain/cognitive health

How Renew Your Liver Eating Plans Are Different from Other Popular Diets

Eating Plan	Similarities	Differences
Keto	Shares a primary aim of reducing carb intake and lowering levels of blood sugar and insulin.	Our Renew Your Liver plans include more high-fiber, nutrient-dense carbs, such as richly hued fruits and vegetables and legumes. They also include less red meat, processed meat, and full-fat dairy than is typically part of a keto eating strategy.
The Mediterranean Diet	Both share an emphasis on nutrient-dense foods, healthy fats (especially extra virgin olive oil), and limited red meat, dairy, and sweets.	Our plans include fewer grains than the Mediterranean diet. We also don't advocate for a glass of red wine every day—although it is OK, the less alcohol you drink, the happier your liver will be.
Paleo	Both encourage eating primarily nutrient-dense, whole foods.	Renew Your Liver plans allow for some whole grains, dairy, and legumes—all of which are excluded from the Paleo approach. Our plans also advocate for eating much less red meat than Paleo.
The DASH Diet	This popular diet is also based on the Mediterranean diet, with a distinct goal of reducing blood pressure.	The Renew Your Liver plans rely less on grains (the DASH recommends 6–8 servings per day) and generally include fewer carbs overall than the DASH diet.
The MIND Diet	This combination of the Mediterranean and DASH diets is designed to bolster cognitive health. Like our Renew Your Liver plans, the MIND diet aims to support one organ (in this case, the brain) by upping vegetable intake and moderating carbs.	The MIND diet places much more emphasis on eating green leafy vegetables than we do—we just want you to eat more vegetables of all colors. It also encourages one glass of red wine per day; we recommend drinking as little as possible—no more than one alcoholic beverage for women and two for men per day, but ideally you would have alcohol infrequently or not at all.

Eating Plan	Similarities	Differences
The Nordic Diet	Similar to the Mediterranean diet but with an emphasis on foods from the Nordic regions (such as Sweden and Denmark).	The Renew Your Liver plans have a greater emphasis on extra virgin olive oil and include fewer grains than the Nordic diet (especially our Moderate-Carb and Low-Carb plans).
The Longevity Diet	Created by fasting expert Valter Longo, this diet is similar to the Mediterranean plan with an emphasis on eating like your ancestors, including lots of plants. It also includes following a fasting-mimicking eating plan a few times a year (eating a small number of calories per day for five days in order to reap the benefits of fasting without actually having to forgo all food).	Renew Your Liver plans are somewhat higher in protein than the Longevity diet. A daily intermittent fast is the only type of fast included in the Renew Your Liver plans.
Vegetarian	Both eating styles share an emphasis on plant-based foods.	Many vegetarians replace those calories from animal products with carb-heavy foods such as bread, pasta, and pizza. The Renew Your Liver plans will have you upgrading those carbs to have more fiber and nutrient density, as well as reducing overall carb intake.

Supplements for Overall Health (and Liver) Support

Vitamin D

There is a well-established connection between low levels of vitamin D and fatty liver disease, and although a deficiency isn't the cause of NAFLD, it can accelerate progression of the disease.

The good news is that vitamin D supplements are inexpensive, easy to find, and easy to take (they are typically small capsules, although vitamin D can come in liquid form, too). Also, getting your vitamin D levels up can provide multiple benefits, such as a reduced risk of osteoporosis in both men and women over age fifty, if your levels are at least 50 nmol/L, and a lower risk of developing depression.[38]

There's no one-size-fits-all dosage. How much vitamin D you need depends on your current levels, which can only be assessed with a blood test. It also depends on your current level of sun exposure—you will typically need more during the winter unless you live in a very warm and sunny place, like the American Southwest or Florida—as well as the darkness of your skin, as people with darker skin need more sun exposure to manufacture vitamin D than a lighter-skinned person. For this reason, dosage is a bit of a moving target and one that's best determined by working with your health care practitioners. The dosage is generally somewhere between 1,000 and 5,000 IUs per day.

Omega-3s

Omega-3 fatty acids, particularly DHA and EPA, which are found in fatty fish such as salmon as well as in the tiny shrimp-like creatures known as krill, have been shown to reduce levels of triglycerides. Remember, high levels of triglycerides are a risk factor for fatty liver disease. While studies haven't shown a significant benefit for omega-3 supplementation on fatty liver disease, there is a trend toward benefit. In other words, omega-3s have been found to be effective at achieving lower liver fat and blood levels of triglycerides in NAFLD patients, although outcomes are mixed when it comes to improving markers of more severe NAFLD, such as inflammation and fibrosis.[39] So you are definitely reducing a risk factor and potentially helping to treat existing fatty liver by taking omega-3s.

There is also a plant-based form of omega-3 known as ALA, which is found in algae, flaxseeds, and walnuts. However, the body has to convert ALA into the more active DHA and EPA forms, and that conversion process isn't particularly efficient. You would have to consume a lot of ALA to get the DHA and EPA you'd get from a much smaller amount of fish or fish oil.

For all supplements, you want to purchase those verified by a third party to actually contain what the label says they contain and to not be contaminated with heavy metals, pesticides, or other contaminants— all of which have to be filtered out by your liver and can potentially damage your liver. The top two companies that provide this verification are Consumer Lab (consumerlab.com) and US Pharmacopeia (usp.org). Look for the USP verified mark and/or the CL Seal of

Approval on the label of the supplement you're considering buying—and put it back on the shelf if you don't see it.

Probiotics

Introducing good gut bacteria to your microbiome through the use of supplements is like taking out an umbrella insurance policy on your health. In general, getting a diverse population of different strains of friendly bacteria is one of the most important aspects of having healthy gut microbiota.

When it comes to probiotics, here are some things to look for when shopping:

- *You tend to get what you pay for.* Higher-end brands tend to have higher-quality products. Probiotics need to be treated with care, especially since they are essentially living bacteria.
- *Research the brands.* Instead of just walking into the supplement aisle at your local drugstore or big box store, take a look at the brands they offer, read the labels, and even check out the websites of these brands. High-quality brands will offer high-quality service. Some even offer a free call to help you choose the right product or will send you data that you can review.
- *Take care of your supplements.* Because the bacteria in your probiotic supplement are alive, it means they can die. You can prevent that from happening—or at least forestall it—by storing them away from light, heat, and moisture. The best place to keep them is in the fridge.
- *Follow the dosage instructions.* Read the label carefully and follow its instructions. You could start with a lower dose and work up to the dosage on the label, but don't take more—more is not always better.
- *Expect symptoms early on.* Your microbiome may not be in a great place if you've been eating a lot of sugar for a long time or have taken multiple rounds of antibiotics—two examples of things that can wipe out good bacteria and foster the growth of bad bacteria. If this is the case, once you introduce probiotics, you are likely to experience some bloating, gas, and other mild

digestive issues. While unpleasant, these are actually signs that the probiotic is working. It could take two to four weeks for your body to acclimate.

· *Keep switching it up.* Every probiotic supplement has a different mix of bacterial strains. Because the diversification of healthy microbes is key, you want to switch up your supplement every three to six months.

· *Don't over-rely on your good gut bugs.* Despite the many powerful things probiotics can do for your metabolic and liver health, you can't supplement your way out of a bad diet. You still need to eat well.

It's Not Just What You Eat, It's When You Eat It

Intermittent fasting, a form of time-restricted eating (TRE), is a more recent eating trend that has a lot of research to support its effectiveness.

Intermittent fasting means that you restrict your food intake to a condensed amount of time, or eating window. The benefit of intermittent fasting is that it gives your body, and liver, a break from the work of digesting and gives your blood glucose levels a chance to become depleted, which also lowers insulin levels and improves insulin sensitivity. In addition, intermittent fasting has been found to upregulate (activate) pathways that reduce oxidative stress and repair or remove damaged molecules, which reduces inflammation. Intermittent fasting also promotes the loss of abdominal fat and improves cognitive function. The health benefits of intermittent fasting are so important that a 2019 review published in the *New England Journal of Medicine* went so far as to suggest that physicians and dietitians actually write a prescription for their patients for intermittent fasting![40] It's powerful medicine that is also free.

Perhaps the best part of intermittent fasting is that it is intermittent. You don't have to adapt to long-term caloric restriction or follow a ketogenic diet full time—two other dietary approaches that have been shown to have similar benefits, albeit with a much higher level of difficulty to maintain and potential pitfalls of their own.

If changing your diet is intimidating, know that you can start to help your liver—and your insulin, your inflammation levels, your abdominal fat, and your brain—by starting to change not *what* you eat (we'll get there!) but *when* you eat. When you go at least twelve hours without eating (say, from 8:00 p.m. at night to 8:00 a.m. the next morning), you give your liver a break from metabolizing and your insulin levels a chance to lessen. As amazing as it is, the liver is not meant to process foods *all* day long. Fasting gives it the break it so deserves.

As you become more comfortable with going longer between your last meal of one day and your first meal of the next, you can make the window when you don't eat bigger by postponing your breakfast and moving up your dinnertime. A 2018 study published in the *Journal of Nutritional Science* had one group of participants delay their breakfast by ninety minutes and have dinner ninety minutes earlier than they typically did, resulting in an eating window that was shortened by three hours total. The other group kept up their normal eating habits. After ten weeks, researchers found that the TRE group ate fewer calories, lost fat, and had significantly lower fasting glucose than the control group.[41]

You can start to improve your insulin sensitivity with even a moderate twelve-hour fast every day, which simply means not eating anything after 8:00 p.m. and before 8:00 a.m. the next morning. This way, you'll be asleep for most of your fast. If you've been eating late at night and/or first thing in the morning, this is a great place to start. And if every day is too much of a challenge, aim to do it for the five weekdays and then loosen things up on the weekend.

As with every change we recommend making in this book, the best choice for you is the one you will actually do. If a twelve-hour window without eating is a stretch, there is no shame in starting with a ten-hour window (finishing dinner by 8:00 p.m. and having breakfast at 6:00 a.m. the next morning, for example) and adding one extra hour of fasting a day every week or so. We both have made intermittent fasting a regular part of our lives: Kristin has breakfast at 11:00 a.m. and finishes dinner by 7:00 p.m. most days while Ibrahim keeps a twelve-hour eating window between 7:30 p.m. and 7:30 a.m.

INTERMITTENT FASTING FOR SHIFT WORKERS

Studies have shown that shift workers are at an increased risk of developing belly fat, type 2 diabetes, and cardiovascular disease—in other words, all of fatty liver disease's sidekicks—due to eating out of sync with a typical circadian rhythm.

Results of various studies prove that intermittent fasting for at least two out of five days a week limits consumption, promotes weight loss, and improves metabolic health markers that occur in the body due to shift work.

What does intermittent fasting while on shift work look like?

Example 1:
5:00 p.m.: Wake up and begin your eating window.
7:00 p.m.: Have dinner.
1:00 a.m.: End your eating window.
1:00 a.m.–5:00 p.m.: Fast.

Example 2:
12:00 a.m.–2:00 a.m.: Start of eating window.
8:00 a.m.–10:00 a.m.: End of eating window.
8:00 a.m.–5:00 p.m.: Sleeping and fasting.
5:00 p.m.–12:00 a.m. (the next day): Skip breakfast and continue fasting.
12:00 a.m.–1:00 a.m.: Start of eating window.

Your Checklist for Change

While you're gearing up to adopt a new eating plan that suits your life, your liver, and your metabolic profile—we'll get to those starting in Chapter 6—there are small changes you can begin to make now that will help you start reaping benefits. We call them little things. Because the truth is, if you can't make small changes, bigger changes are that much harder. Getting some smaller successes under your belt now will help you gain momentum for adopting a new eating plan a few weeks from now.

The little things really do matter. Get one or two of these working in your favor and you will have more energy and more motivation to keep going down the little things list and/or to follow one of the four eating plans we outline in Part 3 of this book. You could absolutely decide to stick with making smaller changes from this list for a few weeks or more before you move on to adopting one of the Renew Your Liver eating plans, and you could still make important progress toward your goals by doing so. If you've been drinking every night of the week, cutting back to every other night would absolutely make an important difference in your liver and whole body health. Same with replacing the soda you drink regularly with water or seltzer water. Or booking a doctor's appointment to see if you actually have sleep apnea, particularly if you snore at sleep time. Starting with one thing is absolutely helpful and important to do, even if that's all you can manage for now.

Use this list of little things both as inspiration for small steps you can take each day to protect your liver and as a checklist to track the things you're doing regularly. Once you've made that step a habit, you can check it off, which will help you see your progress.

Of course, you needn't tackle all of these things at once. In fact, please don't! If you only do one of these at a time, it will be *plenty*. Then, whenever you feel ready to add in something new, you'll be able to look at this list and choose something that has a lot of benefit for your liver and your overall health. By the time you get to the eating plan section of the book, you'll already be feeling energized and empowered to keep going.

The items with an asterisk (*) after them are the most important things you can do. If you're not already doing these things, choose one of these to start with. Whatever you choose, write down your answers to the following prompts in your Regenerative Health notebook, a journal or planner, the Notes feature on your phone, or wherever you remind yourself of your goals and to-dos.

I'm committing to adopting the following little things:
When I feel solid in that, this is the next little step I'll add in:

Movement
☐ **Set a standing goal:** Try every hour to stand for at least five minutes during most waking hours, and get extra benefit if you move

around, walk in place, or stretch. Set a timer to remind you to break the sitting spell and get up out of your chair regularly (this is also a feature on Apple watches; you can also ask Alexa to remind you to stand each hour whenever you are at home). If you use a wheelchair or standing is difficult, incorporate chair yoga or other stretches suggested below.

☐ **Stretch:** Add time to your day for a full-body stretch, perhaps when you first wake up or just before bed. Kristin loves to start the day with a cobra stretch on the floor before her cup of coffee.

☐ **Take a short walk after meals:** A lap around the block, the office, or even down the driveway and back after a meal can help promote digestion and move glucose out of your bloodstream and into your tissues, requiring your body to produce less insulin.

☐ **Bump it up just one notch:*** If you mostly sit all day, start building up to twenty minutes of moving around each day (it can be a little here and a little there). If you already move a fair amount during the day, try adding in short bursts of more strenuous exercise three times a week. An Australian study found that performing a ten-minute workout that contained three twenty-second bursts of maximal effort three times a week for twelve weeks did more to improve insulin sensitivity than a forty-five-minute, moderate-intensity cardio workout![42]

Food

☐ **Organize the fridge:** Think about how often you eat with your eyes; then set up your fridge and pantry to accommodate that, keeping nutrient-dense foods in view and at eye level in the fridge to make them easier to choose when you open the fridge for a snack. Additionally, consider glass containers for healthy foods and opaque containers for foods you should have less often.

☐ **Prepare your produce:** Instead of placing fresh produce right into the fridge after shopping, wash and chop and place them in produce-friendly containers. Make eating fresh produce even more convenient by creating single-serving containers of your cut-up fruit and veggies.

☐ **Assess your hunger:** When you head to the kitchen to grab a snack, ask yourself if you are truly hungry. You might be feeling something else—bored, frustrated, tired—and using food to cope. Determine what emotion is driving this action. Becoming an expert in this will take away any need for portion control and willpower—two things that have not been found to work with dietary change.

☐ **Introduce more color:** Aim to have foods of at least two different colors in every meal. For example, add matchstick carrots to your salad, mixed berries to your yogurt or oatmeal, or tomatoes and spinach to your scrambled eggs. Seven colors a day is a good goal to aim for—and it helps you figure out what to select from the produce section on your trips to the grocery store.

☐ **Remember to hydrate:** Set reminders throughout your day to drink more water, which helps your liver perform its detoxifying duties more efficiently.

☐ **Swap white for whole grain:** Remove refined, processed, low-fiber, high-glycemic-load grains from your diet and replace them with grains that are whole. For example, swap in brown rice or quinoa for white rice and whole-grain sprouted breads for white breads.

☐ **Upgrade your carbohydrate choices:** Use bean-based pasta or zucchini noodles instead of regular pasta. Choose quinoa, cauliflower rice, or brown rice over white rice, and start using sprouted whole wheat bread (such as Ezekiel) instead of standard white bread and almond flour or chickpea flour tortillas over white flour tortillas. Upgrading your carbs often means swapping out some of the carbs for more nutrients.

☐ **Replace sugary beverages:*** If you typically drink regular or diet soda, energy drinks, fruit juice, or lemonade, replace them with water or seltzer. If you drink sweetened coffee drinks, such as sea salt caramel or pumpkin spice lattes, try a latte made with unsweetened almond or oat milk and sprinkle cinnamon on top to give a sweet taste without added sugar.

☐ **Feed your gut:** Have something fermented each day, choosing from organic tempeh, organic miso, sauerkraut, kefir, kombucha, kimchi, and olives.

☐ **Cut down on drinking:** Now is the time to start drinking less. If you've been having alcohol every day, cut down to every other day or perhaps just on weekends, and don't exceed more than two drinks per day (if you're a man) or one drink per day (if you're a woman). If you have to do this gradually, that's OK, but keep going.

☐ **Chew more:** Focus on chewing each bite slowly and completely, which has been shown to prevent weight gain, promote satiety, and even boost your metabolism higher after eating than if you ate quickly.[43] If you have an unconscious habit of wolfing your food down, put your fork down after each bite to invite yourself to spend more time with each mouthful of food.

Meal Timing

☐ **Close the kitchen:*** Avoid eating at night, keeping your eating window to twelve hours or less (and if you are a shift worker, refer back to the Intermittent Fasting for Shift Workers sidebar that appears earlier in this chapter). If late-night eating is a habit, tell yourself the kitchen is closed until tomorrow morning, and brush your teeth after dinner so you are less likely to indulge in late-night eating.

☐ **Eat less as the day goes on:** Give yourself—and your liver—more time to metabolize your food by consuming more of your calories earlier in the day (so that your body can focus on detoxing and rejuvenating while you sleep instead of on digesting). A good rule of thumb is to eat breakfast like a king, lunch like a prince, and dinner like a pauper—meaning break your fast with a larger morning meal, have a smaller lunch, and make dinner your smallest meal of the day (think more appetizer and salad than full entrée).

Stress Management

☐ **Prioritize rest:*** Sleep is how your mind resets and when your body regenerates. Be in bed for at least seven and a half hours before you need to wake up, which will help you get a solid seven hours of sleep.

☐ **Pause:** Set aside a few times a day to check in with how you are feeling. Do you need a glass of water? A walk around the block to clear your head? A nap? A hug? A few minutes to stare out the window?

☐ **Prepare:** Take five minutes after your alarm goes off to breathe deeply (in other words, don't immediately pick up your phone and start scrolling your feeds or checking your email). Consider going a step further by deciding on your intention for the day.

☐ **Protect:** Give yourself more time in your day for the things that matter by saying no to unnecessary requests.

☐ **Lighten your load:** Delegate at least one thing this week that doesn't need to be done by you.

☐ **Practice:** Meditation, breathing exercises, yoga, tai chi, and even chores like weeding or sweeping, or crafts such as knitting or drawing, can all help you get into a relaxed mental state. Aim to practice one of these mindfulness-inducing activities for at least ten minutes a day.

Reducing Toxin Exposure

☐ **Swap out food storage containers:** Replace plastic food storage containers with glass, stainless steel, or ceramic versions, and plastic baggies with reusable bags made out of silicon, waxed canvas, or other nontoxic materials.

☐ **Bathe your produce:** Wash all fresh produce in a bath of water and baking soda before eating (use one teaspoon of baking soda for every four cups of water; swirl produce in the baking soda bath for at least thirty seconds, then rinse under cold water).[44]

☐ **Get organic savvy:** Buy organic versions of the "Dirty Dozen" (the twelve most contaminated fruits and vegetables according to the Environmental Working Group—see the latest list at ewg.org), and/or eat more of the "Clean 15" (the fifteen least contaminated).

☐ **Air out your dirty laundry:** Take the plastic off your dry-cleaned clothes and let them air out outside before bringing them in your home, or use a cleaning service that uses greener methods, such as wet cleaning or carbon dioxide cleaning.

☐ **Cut down on chemicals:** Stop or dramatically reduce your use of pesticides and herbicides in your home and yard, and switch to nontoxic household cleaning products.

☐ **Be a natural beauty:** Opt for fragrance-free personal care products that only use ingredients you can pronounce.

Now that you know what types of little lifestyle changes are going to have a big impact on your liver health, you are ready to start looking at more details regarding how you will be eating differently. Your eating plan will be customized for you, but to choose the right one, you'll want to understand the underlying ideas for each plan and have some strategies for more easily adopting a new way of eating.

chapter 5

Feed Your Liver

J UST AS YOU wouldn't set out on a cross-country road trip without plotting a basic route, filling the car with gas, downloading some podcasts or audiobooks to keep you entertained, and packing some water and snacks, you don't want to embark on a new liver-friendly diet and lifestyle without doing a little prep.

In this chapter, we'll cover the steps that too many people skip over when they decide to start eating differently and that are crucial for creating change that lasts. We know you may be in a hurry to get going—perhaps your doctor put the fear of God into you by saying you need to lose a lot of weight, and quickly—but taking the time to integrate the things we cover in this chapter will help you go further and then stay longer.

First, we'll focus on two foundational concepts:

1. Surrounding yourself with healthy foods
2. Resetting your appetite

With that information in hand, at the end of this chapter, you will:

- be better able to understand your hunger and your cravings;
- have healthier foods within arm's reach (and fewer unhealthy foods around);
- have an array of tools to help you manage your portions, painlessly; and
- be armed with strategies to address any negative effects of times you may have tried to "diet" in the past.

We'll also talk you through how to decide if you are indeed ready to adopt a new eating plan. After all, we're giving you a lot in this chapter, and depending on what's going on in your life, now may *not* be the time to dive into an entirely new way of eating. It might be better for you to strengthen some of the skills you'll learn in this chapter and continue working your way through Your Checklist for Change we listed at the end of Chapter 4 so that you aren't tempted to make a bunch of diet and lifestyle changes that aren't sustainable. Honestly, sustainability is the single most important piece of any of the eating plans or information we share in this book. Fatty liver doesn't develop in a day, and it won't resolve in a week or even a month. It's truly best to take things one step at a time, so let's cover the steps that will best set you up for success.

Surround Yourself with Healthy Foods

An important step that will help you recalibrate your appetite and become accustomed to naturally and painlessly eating well is making sure that you are surrounded with healthy foods. That way, you won't have to use your willpower to make different eating choices, which is good, because willpower is a finite resource that burns quickly, like newspaper in a campfire. It's a lot easier to eat well when you don't have a bunch of unhealthy foods in your pantry and refrigerator. There are two parts to surrounding yourself with healthy foods: (1) setting up a liver-friendly kitchen, and (2) making better choices at the grocery store. Let's start with the first part.

Make Your Kitchen Liver Friendly

It's a simple truth that we eat with our eyes first. That's why food manufacturers pay big money to have their products displayed at eye level in the grocery store—what you see, you'll be more likely to grab. That's why you want to set up your pantry and fridge so that they are a constant reminder of healthy eating.

The first piece of this is to get rid of, or to greatly, greatly reduce the amount of, liver-unfriendly food you have in your home. You do get 15 percent to play with—15 percent of your food can be not so liver friendly—but know that if something is in your house, it's going to be very hard to resist eating it.

These are the things you should aim to winnow out of your kitchen:

- *Any product that lists sugar in the first three ingredients.* Of course, the label may not actually say "sugar"—check the list of thirty sneaky names for sugar to the right. Look for sugar on every label, even things you would never imagine could have it! One of Kristin's clients was cleaning out her pantry and was surprised to learn that sugar was the second ingredient in the breadcrumbs her Italian American husband used to make chicken cutlets. (Now she uses a blend of finely ground coconut flakes and almond flour.)
- *Products that consist primarily of refined grains.* These are your basic crackers, traditional pasta, white rice, white flour, and white breads.
- *Hyperpalatable foods.* Get rid of any foods you have that are difficult to stop eating. These generally include things like chips, store-bought cookies, doughnuts, fast food, frozen snacks like pizza rolls, and French fries. If you can't have chips without eating the whole bag, get rid of them or put them on the top shelf, way in the back.

Once you've created some space in your cupboards and refrigerator, put your nutrient-dense, liver-friendly foods front and center—ideally in clear containers so that you can see them and start tantalizing your taste buds with them. This may mean going against the way you've always done things. For example, sticking your vegetables and fruit in the produce drawers means they're out of sight, out of mind and more likely to be "out of" your belly. Instead, store your meat and cheeses in the produce drawer and put your veggies and fruit on the shelves that are at eye level. Give yourself bonus points for prewashing and cutting your produce so that it is that much easier to grab in a moment of hunger.

In the pantry, store your nuts and seeds in glass jars right up front. (If you stocked up on big or multiple bags of nuts and seeds at Costco or Trader Joe's, keep whatever doesn't fit in the jar in the freezer so that it will stay fresher, longer, as the oils in nuts and seeds are prone to rancidity.)

For any of the manufactured food or sweet treats you still have—that 15 percent of food we talked about in the previous section—store them out of sight—on a high shelf, behind other things, or in an opaque

THIRTY SNEAKY NAMES FOR SUGAR

Agave nectar/syrup
Barley malt
Blackstrap molasses
Brown rice syrup
Cane juice syrup
Cane syrup
Carob syrup
Corn syrup
Demerara
Dextrose
Diatase
Evaporated cane juice
Florida crystals
Fructose
Fruit juice concentrate
Galactose
Glucose
Golden syrup
High-fructose corn syrup
Maltodextrin
Maltose
Maple syrup
Molasses
Muscovado
Rapadura
Rice syrup
Sorghum syrup
Sucrose
Treacle
Turbinado

container. If you're living in a house with cookies, putting them toward the back of a cabinet in a stainless-steel canister means you're not seeing them, which means you'll think about them less, and as a result, you'll reach for them less.

You can even keep a healthy snack out on the kitchen counter so that you don't have to go rummaging for something to eat and

LIVER-FRIENDLY KITCHEN TOOLS

Even though you don't need to make elaborate meals to eat a liver-friendly diet, it really helps to have a few tools in your kitchen to make food prep easier and more enjoyable and your food even tastier.

To be clear, you don't *have* to purchase everything on this list if you don't already have them. You can add these things over time—or even put them on your wish list for occasions when loved ones are wondering what you'd like to receive as a gift.

- Chef's knife: Use this building block of the kitchen to cut, peel, slice, and chop any food you might be working with on a daily basis. A chef's knife will help with every kitchen creation, so invest in a quality knife (carbon steel) and blade sharpener to keep your tool in its best condition.

- Immersion blender: This extremely versatile tool can help with pureeing sauces, soups, dips, or smoothies. You can even use it to beat eggs, mix salad dressing, or finely mash sweet potatoes.

- Drip coffee maker: As you'll learn in just a bit, coffee is a liver superfood with a major body of research to support its benefits! A drip coffee maker is perfect for daily coffee drinkers and much more cost-effective (and environmentally friendly) than pod coffee makers. A good coffee maker will ensure each cup of coffee tastes great.

- Coffee bean grinder: Grinding your own coffee beans for each batch of coffee gives you control over the flavor profile. The second the beans are ground, they begin to lose freshness and flavor, so to avoid this and keep your coffee at its best, avoid preground coffee and coffee pods and invest in a grinder of your own.

- Cutting boards: As with a good knife, a cutting board is a building block of the kitchen. If you're just starting out, get a board that can be easily cleaned and won't damage or dull your knife. As you continue outfitting your kitchen, you'll want to consider investing in multiple prep/cutting boards, and one board should be designated for each category of food: one for meats, one for dairy, one for grains and bread, and one for fruits and vegetables. This helps to avoid cross-contamination and keeps the kitchen organized. Designating a color for each category can be helpful as well.

- Cast-iron skillet: Use a cast-iron skillet for essentially anything—making bread, searing meat, sautéing vegetables, reheating leftovers, or even scrambling an egg. It works equally well on the stove top or in the oven, and it is practically indestructible. This is a pan you'll have for years. Kristin has also been using carbon steel pans, which she is loving.

- Food processor: Whether you need to mix, chop, or puree, a food processor does the work for you in a flash. You could spend a little or a lot—a Dash food processor can be $25, while some models go up to $500—but you don't really need to do too much research; you just need something strong enough to mix things together. With a food processor, you can make salsa, pesto, gazpacho, nut butters, and (almond-flour) dough in minutes.

- Air fryer: We know that fried foods—with their high fat content and their hyperpalatability—aren't great for the liver. An air fryer gives you a similar crunch without the added oil. Sweet potato fries, chicken tenders, tofu cubes, zucchini chips, and more all crisp up beautifully without putting your liver at risk.

- Thermapen: This digital meat thermometer helps you cook animal protein—such as chicken breasts, salmon, and turkey burgers—to the perfect temperature, without either under- or overcooking. Kristin doesn't cook meat without it!

perhaps come across that container of cookies. Kristin often has a bowl of roasted chickpeas or cashews that she roasts with a little cinnamon and sea salt on her kitchen island so that she, her husband, or her kids always have something nutrient-dense within reach. Of course, if it's out you might overeat it, but better to overeat something low carb and nutrient-dense than what you might uncover when you are mindlessly looking in the pantry.

Revise Your Shopping Habits

What you eat every day has its roots in what you buy at the grocery store. If you want to change your eating habits, you've also got to change your shopping habits.

First, before heading out, make sure that you've had a nutrient-dense meal within the last couple of hours, because if you grocery shop when you're hungry, you're more likely to buy those hyperpalatable foods.

Once you're at the market, look at your cart and see that it has at least 85 percent whole food. You can still have your 15 percent of old favorites, but if you think about your typical grocery cart, that means the main compartment is filled with whole food, and the section up front where you might park a toddler is all the space available for the ultra-processed stuff.

These are the foods you want to prioritize buying:

- *Colorful whole foods.* In every aspect of the plant world—and thus the whole foods realm—there are ranges in color. A good rule of thumb is that anything with a deeper hue is more nutritious (with the exclusion of highly processed foods—blue Doritos are not what we're talking about here!). So, while of course this includes fruits and vegetables, aiming to eat colorful foods extends beyond the produce drawer to your spice drawer and your pantry. Spices such as turmeric, curry, paprika, red pepper, cinnamon, and black pepper all bring nutrition and color in addition to flavor. In the pantry, think black or brown rice instead of white rice. Buy tricolor quinoa, black beans, red lentils, green lentils, and pasta made with differently hued beans, and rich green extra virgin olive oil instead of pale canola oils. You will naturally increase the nutrient density of your food when you prioritize buying foods in a range of colors.
- *Intact grains.* You've heard of whole grains. We take this idea one step further by encouraging you to look for intact grains, which simply means grains that are as close as possible to the form that they were in when they were still growing. Take oatmeal, for example. While rolled oats are technically a whole grain, they are

steamed and rolled flat, which causes them to lose a little bit of their nutrients and essentially predigests them. Steel-cut oats, on the other hand, are oat groats that have been cut (not steamed and flattened). They are more intact than rolled oats. Other intact grains include popcorn, quinoa, wild rice, and millet. Intact grains are more nutrient-dense—particularly in their fiber content— than typical or even whole grains, so just swapping them out for your typical grains will help improve the nutritional density of your diet.

COLORFUL FOODS AT A GLANCE

How many colorful foods can you work into one meal?

Black	Blue	Purple	Green	Red	Orange	Yellow
Black beans, black olives, black lentils, coffee, cacao	Blueberries, blackberries	Eggplant, purple cauliflower, radicchio, red onion, purple grapes	Lettuce, spinach, kale, collards, broccoli, Brussels sprouts, green peppers, jalapeños, poblanos, green olives, kiwi, edamame	Red peppers, tomatoes, tomato sauce, red lentils, red grapefruit, strawberries, raspberries	Carrots, pumpkin, clementines, butternut squash, sweet potatoes, oranges	Chickpeas, grapefruit, lemons (zest or juice)

- *Lean meats and fatty fish that are as close to nature as possible.* Think bison or grass-finished beef, organic and pastured chicken and eggs, and wild-caught fatty fish. (See more on the animal protein we recommend on pages 115–116.)
- *Ready-to-go dinner foods.* We've all had those nights where you're already hungry, can't find anything to eat in the house, and reach for your phone to order a pizza. You always want to have a few foods that you can use to pull together a meal in ten minutes or less. A lot of these quick foods are frozen. Kristin recommends having a bag of frozen broccoli, a bag of organic frozen chicken

breasts, and a bag of frozen quinoa, brown rice, or cauliflower rice on hand at all times. You can even find cubes of smashed garlic and pureed herbs in the freezer section. The refrigerator case in the produce section is also a great source of these grab-and-go foods—you can find pre-cooked lentils and beets there. Sautéing a few of these foods in one pan with a little extra virgin olive oil, salt, and pepper can help you have a healthy and tasty meal ready even before the pizza delivery guy could show up, and for less money, too. Your go-to meals don't need to come from recipes or be chef-worthy.

- *Fast snacks.* For those times when your hunger sets in and it's not a formal mealtime, it's great to have some nutrient-dense snacks on hand. Nuts and seeds—our favorites are walnuts, almonds, macadamia nuts, sunflower seeds, and pumpkin seeds—are great. You might also like kale chips, roasted seaweed, and whole-grain pretzels and crackers (for a lower-carb version, get nut-based crackers).

- *Skip the sweets.* Avoid buying cookies, ice cream, and other treats. But if you do, buy them in the smallest portion you can find—the pint of ice cream instead of the half gallon, one brownie from the bakery counter instead of a prepackaged box. You also want to check the ingredient list and make sure it contains as few ingredients as possible and that you recognize each item on that list. You can also buy chocolate chips (especially those from brands like Lily's, which are sweetened with stevia, meaning it won't impact your blood sugar) and sprinkle a few into a small ramekin of sunflower and/or pumpkin seeds—this can satisfy your sweet tooth while also providing a good dose of fiber and healthy fats from the seeds. Kristin once had a patient with type 2 diabetes and high blood pressure who really struggled with portion control. He developed what she thought was a brilliant workaround: he used a seven-day pill organizer box to portion out his daily chocolate chip allotment. It worked for him; and when it comes to keeping your old foods to 15 percent of what you eat, there's a solution that will work for you, too.

The Twelve Liver-Friendly Foods to Always Have on Hand

It's really helpful to have your go-to foods available in your fridge or pantry. Here are a dozen of our top foods that benefit your liver and are a part of each of our four Renew Your Liver eating plans.

1. **Coffee.** While technically a beverage, coffee, as it turns out, is essentially a superfood with more than a thousand compounds, the most powerfully beneficial of which are polyphenols (which can slow the growth of cancer cells and reduce the risk of type 2 diabetes) and antioxidants (which are anti-inflammatory and protective against both cancer and heart disease).

   Thanks to how popular it is in so many cultures, coffee is likely the single greatest source of antioxidants in the human diet worldwide. It's also an appetite suppressant, which can help you stave off hunger and cravings, especially when you're changing your palate from hyperpalatable foods to more whole foods.

   Numerous studies have established a link between drinking coffee and reduced risk of a range of common diseases and health issues, including depression, gallstones, heart disease, melanoma, prostate cancer, suicide, and type 2 diabetes. One study, which followed more than two hundred thousand participants for up to thirty years, found that those who had three to five cups of either regular or decaffeinated coffee a day were 15 percent less likely to die early than those who did not drink coffee. The biggest reduction in risk was in suicide—coffee drinkers were 50 percent less likely to die of suicide than those who didn't drink it. Why? Possibly because coffee triggers the production of brain chemicals with antidepressant effects.[1]

   And coffee is great for your liver in particular. A 2017 Dutch study found an association between the regular consumption of coffee and herbal tea and lower likelihood of stiffness in the liver—a hallmark of cirrhosis.[2] Other studies have found that coffee drinkers have a lower risk of cirrhosis and liver cancer and that coffee consumption appears to be protective against the prevalence of NAFLD and is helpful in reducing the inflammation that can happen with NASH and NASH-fibrosis.[3] Coffee also appears to help you not develop liver disease in the first place: researchers assessed the coffee consumption of nearly twenty-eight thousand Americans from 1999 to 2010 and found that those who had three cups a day—whether caffeinated or decaffeinated—had a 25 percent lower risk of having abnormal liver tests than those who had never drank coffee.[4] So love your liver a latte, and drink up!

> *How to drink it:* Of course, you'll want to skip adding sugar and avoid the premixed and presweetened flavored coffees, like most pumpkin spice lattes. (A sixteen-ounce Starbucks Mocha Frappuccino packs fifty-one grams of sugar and fifteen grams of fat—ten of them saturated.) A few drops of liquid stevia or monkfruit—natural sweeteners derived from plants that don't impact blood sugar—can add some of that sweetness back, and it's fine to add a little cream, half-and-half, milk, or your favorite nut milk. And it's better to make your coffee with a paper filter, as it will trap the oily chemicals known as diterpenes that are in coffee beans and that can raise LDL (bad) cholesterol. Most studies show that benefit can be derived with just small quantities but that three cups is probably the sweet spot. However, if you are someone who is a slow metabolizer of caffeine (a nutrigenomics test, which we discuss at the end of Chapter 6, can help you determine this), or if you are someone with anxiety, high blood pressure, and difficulty sleeping at nighttime, it's best to limit your daily caffeine consumption to two hundred milligrams or less (about one and a half cups of coffee). Pregnant women are also advised to limit or even avoid coffee consumption.

2. **Berries.** Berries of all types—strawberries, blueberries, raspberries, and so on—are rich in nutrients, particularly antioxidants (especially the polyphenols that give them their rich color) and fiber, and they tend to be some of the fruits with the lowest glycemic loads around. Berries have an extensive body of research to

BETTER BEVERAGES

Among our colleagues, the general wisdom is that adults get metabolically unhealthy because they eat too much, and kids get metabolically unhealthy because they drink too much—meaning, they over-consume sweetened beverages such as soda, fruit juice, sports drinks, and sweetened iced teas.

The best beverages for kids (and adults who like sweet beverages) are water and unflavored milk. Seltzer is OK if your kid has a craving for something with bubbles—it comes in many flavors without added sugars. You can even add a little lemonade or fruit juice to a glass of seltzer (two parts seltzer, one part juice). Unsweetened iced or hot tea are also good options.

Avoid swapping in diet soda for regular soda, as diet sodas have been shown to be disruptive to the microbiome in a way that reduces glucose tolerance, increases insulin resistance, and leads to weight gain and fatty liver.[5] They actually cause your gut bacteria to produce ethanol—or alcohol— meaning it affects your liver in the same way as alcohol without the buzz.[6] And both regular soda and diet soda have been shown to have an association with fatty liver disease, suggesting that it's not just the sugar in regular soda that's problematic for the liver, but the combination of fructose (in regular soda), aspartame (in diet soda), and other ingredients such as coloring agents that trigger insulin resistance and liver inflammation.[7]

Again, just as no foods are "bad" and totally off-limits, soda and diet soda aren't verboten, but you want to treat them like a dessert or a burger and fries—something to have only on occasion, and not more than about once a week.

If you have an older child (at least age ten), you can try giving them one cup of coffee in the morning, as coffee can be like medicine for the liver. Try not to add sugar, but you can add some milk or half-and-half to make it more palatable.

demonstrate their benefit on heart health. While there are fewer studies examining the impact of berries on liver health in particular, fruit fiber in general is good for the liver.

How to eat them: Berries are great on their own (a generous handful is a good serving size) or served with unsweetened cream or whipped cream, on top of plain low-fat yogurt (whole yogurt if it's for a kid), or sprinkled on top of salads or oatmeal. If berries aren't in season where you live, they can be expensive—but frozen berries are a great, lower-cost option that's available year-round. Kristin's kids love eating frozen berries just as they are, or you can throw them straight into oatmeal or yogurt—they will dissolve a little bit and perhaps turn your whole bowl blue or red. That's part of the fun. Pro tip: buy fresh berries in season and freeze them for later use.

3. **Kiwi.** Kiwi is an excellent source of pyrroloquinoline quinone, or PQQ, an antioxidant also found in breast milk, soy, parsley, and celery. In an animal study, PQQ was shown to protect offspring of obese mothers from developing NAFLD, even when the offspring were fed a typical Western diet high in fat and carbohydrates. It's also high in vitamin C, which is important for your immune system.[8]

   How to eat it: Eating kiwi with the skin on is best, if you can tolerate the slightly furry texture (if you can't, try putting an unpeeled kiwi into your next smoothie). The skin contains much of the fruit's fiber, meaning that consuming the skin helps bring down the net carbs of a medium-sized kiwi from ten grams to about eight grams. Just make sure you wash kiwi before eating it (refer to page 94 for instructions on how to use baking soda to reduce pesticide content).

   Once they're ripe enough to yield to gentle pressure when you squeeze them, kiwis are great sliced and eaten as is. Or, slice the top off (where it was once attached to the stem) and scoop out the insides with a spoon. You can also freeze slices (laid out on a piece of parchment paper or waxed paper) for a cooling snack during the summer.

4. **Edamame.** Soybeans (also known as edamame) are a mainstay of many Asian cultures, including in the blue zone of Okinawa—a fact that's not surprising when you learn just how many health

benefits soy has. Soy is an excellent source of plant-based protein, as well as fiber, omega-3 essential fatty acids, iron, zinc,
and B vitamins. The compounds that give soy its real power,
though, are a category of antioxidants known as isoflavones,
which are known to play a role in preventing bone loss and certain cancers.

A 2020 Chinese study found that regular soy consumption
was protective against the development of NAFLD and that protection started with as little as one serving per week (and rose
with each additional weekly serving).[9] An animal study found
that obese mice fed soy protein reduced their triglycerides and
the fat in their livers by 20 percent—researchers believed this
happened because the soy protein activated a pathway that
helps with the metabolism of fat.[10] Soy also contains PQQ,
the antioxidant in kiwi, making it a multipurpose addition to
your diet.

> *How to eat it:* Edamame makes a great snack—you can buy
> it frozen in the shell then defrost it in the microwave and
> season with a little salt and pepper before using your front
> teeth to pop the beans out of the pod and into your mouth.
> Peeled edamame can be used in place of chickpeas to make
> hummus, mixed in with quinoa, or eaten on their own
> (they're great mixed with a little mint, feta cheese, and
> extra virgin olive oil!). Other ways to eat soy include as tofu,
> tempeh, and miso. We recommend buying organic soy.

5. **Dark Chocolate.** Yes, you're reading that right: chocolate can be a
health food. After all, it's made from the cocoa bean, which is a
plant, and a healthy, deeply hued plant at that. (It's only when it's
combined with a lot of milk and/or sugar that it falls more in the
treat category.) Cocoa is high in fiber, iron, and the category of
antioxidants known as polyphenols. And it also appears to have
particular benefit for the liver: a 2021 study done on obese mice
with fatty livers on a high-fat diet found that the mice who were
given cocoa had lower inflammation, less liver fat, and lower

levels of DNA damage to liver cells.[11] While we don't necessarily advocate for you going out and eating ten tablespoons of cocoa powder per day (the human-sized equivalent of what the cocoa-eating mice in the study ate), these findings do speak to the liver-protective properties of cocoa powder and dark chocolate.

> *How to eat it:* You can stir two tablespoons of unsweetened cocoa powder into a cup of your favorite milk that you've warmed on the stove or in the microwave. Sweeten with a few drops of liquid stevia and you've got a delicious pick-me-up that doubles as a snack (and that kids will also love). If you want to eat dark chocolate, make sure that it is at least 70 percent cocoa and has five grams or less of sugar per serving. Ideally, you'd choose a brand sweetened with stevia, monk-fruit, or erythritol (sweeteners that don't impact blood sugar). Lily's Chocolate is such a brand that's widely available, and thanks to an increased consumer interest in the keto diet, there are more options appearing on shelves all the time. Remember that you still need to watch your dark chocolate servings—a typical serving should be one-quarter or one-third of a bar, not the whole thing. To get even more bang for your nutritional buck, choose bars with nuts in them as well to add in even more fiber as well as healthy fats.

6. **Legumes.** Legumes are anything that grows in a pod, including lentils, chickpeas, soybeans, black beans, black-eyed peas, white beans, and kidney beans. They are great for gut health because they are high in fiber, which promotes digestion. Fiber also feeds your friendly gut bacteria, which play a role in many components of health, especially immunity and brain health, including mental health. Legumes are also rich sources of folate, and folate is a key part of your body's detoxification process.

   People who eat more legumes have been found to have a lower risk of developing fatty liver.[12] Legumes also contain spermidine, a type of compound called a polyamine also found in mushrooms, aged cheese, and soy, which has been found in animal studies to significantly prevent fibrosis and liver cancer, and even to promote longevity.[13]

> *How to eat them:* Beans and legumes are great for adding heft to a soup, salad, or plant-based meal. If you buy them dried, it's best to soak them overnight and pressure-cook them (if you have an Instant Pot) to make them more digestible; if you buy them canned, you want a BPA-free can. The brand Eden Organics presoaks its beans and then pressure-cooks them right in the cans. Rolling some adzuki beans up in a lettuce leaf with avocado slices, a little cilantro, and a squeeze of fresh lime is a terrific snack or meal. Buying precooked lentils (usually kept in the refrigerator case in the produce section) means you're only opening a packet away from a filling and tasty snack—a little drizzle of extra virgin olive oil, red wine vinegar, salt, and pepper turns the lentils into a simple yet scrumptious salad.

7. **Garlic.** Lovingly known as the stinking rose, garlic is part of the allium family and a rock star on the health front: it has been found to reduce the duration and severity of colds, lower high blood pressure, reduce total and LDL cholesterol levels, protect brain health, and promote blood flow. In terms of liver health, specifically, research has shown that garlic powder can lower weight and body fat even if you make no other changes to your diet or exercise routine![14] Considering that NAFLD can often begin to reverse after losing only 5 percent of body weight, this is exciting news indeed.

> *How to eat it:* It's better to get nutrients through whole foods when possible, so while you could start taking a garlic powder supplement, you could also just start prioritizing garlic in your daily diet. Use garlic powder on salads, quinoa, roasted chickpeas, or nuts. Finely chop or mince garlic and add it to salad dressings or homemade salsa

(Kristin's favorite way to use tomatoes in the height of summer when they are abundant). Add it to the oil you sauté your vegetables in, or stir it into soups. Truly, there are few savory foods that don't taste better with a little garlic, extra virgin olive oil, salt, and pepper. If peeling and chopping the cloves seems like one step too far, you can buy pre-cut garlic in jars (usually in the refrigerated case of the produce section, or perhaps near the oils and vinegars), or even frozen pressed garlic—just pop a cube or two into your pan.

8. **Green Tea.** Made from the same plant as black tea, green tea is processed quickly, before its leaves are allowed to darken and oxidize (think of a cut apple turning brown), as black tea's leaves are. When it comes to the liver, research shows that mice fed a high-fat diet who are given an extract of green tea develop one-half the amount of liver fat as mice who are fed the same diet but do not receive the green tea extract. (When the green-tea mice exercised as well, they developed only one-quarter the liver fat of the control group.) Researchers theorize that the polyphenols in green tea block the breakdown and absorption of carbohydrates, protein, and fat.[15]

Regular consumption of green tea has also been found in controlled studies to be accompanied by a decrease in abdominal fat, total body weight, BMI, and waist circumference, and an improvement in metabolic syndrome.[16] Honestly, with all these benefits—both directly to your liver and indirectly to many of the metabolic risk factors that go hand in hand with fatty liver disease—why *wouldn't* you devote some energy toward developing a green tea habit?

How to consume it: Aim for a cup of strongly brewed green tea most days (steep the tea in water just shy of boiling for at least two and up to ten minutes). Green tea does contain caffeine, but only about half as much as a cup of coffee, so if you aren't super caffeine-sensitive, you can enjoy a cup in the afternoon when you need a pick-me-up. If you don't like the taste, there are some great green tea blends that offer different flavor profiles—one with toasted rice or barley added to it has a nice nutty flavor, while mint green tea has a fresh sweetness. You can also take green tea extract either in pill form or as a liquid that you can stir into a glass of water. You can also cook with it—matcha is a powder made of very finely ground green tea leaves that offers a concentrated dose of the antioxidants found in green tea that you can add to yogurt or smoothies, or use in recipes for quinoa, granola, or chia seed puddings. (There is also impressive research that evaluated a Mediterranean diet plus the addition of green tea and found that it reduced visceral fat by 14 percent, as opposed to only 7 percent in a typical Mediterranean diet that did not include regular green tea consumption.[17])

9. **Extra Virgin Olive Oil.** This staple of the Mediterranean diet is jam-packed with beneficial phytonutrients and healthy fats, which is likely why so many studies have found extra virgin olive oil to be protective of heart health and to boost immune function. It's such a potent health protector that a 2022 study found that the more olive oil you add to your diet, the less your risk of death from several diseases, particularly when it's used to replace butter, margarine, mayonnaise, and dairy fat. Authors found that half a tablespoon or more per day led to a decreased mortality risk.[18]

Metabolically speaking, a diet rich in olive oil has been shown to reduce the amount of fat stored in the liver and improve insulin resistance.[19] Olive oil is a great source of monounsaturated fat that contains small amounts of polyunsaturated fats as well. Both types of fat help improve your blood lipid profiles, reduce blood pressure, and increase insulin sensitivity, which is a key part of preventing fatty liver disease.[20] They have also been shown to increase HDL cholesterol levels (the good kind of cholesterol) that offer preventative benefits for a range of long-term diseases.[21]

Olive oil is also a rich source of polyphenols, which help your body get rid of diseased cells and decrease the growth of cells and blood vessels associated with tumors. It's for these reasons that olive oil consumption has been linked to a reduction in the risk of cardiovascular disease and dying from all causes.[22] Animal studies have found it to be protective against oxidative damage to the liver after exposure to chemical pesticides.[23]

> *How to eat it:* Look for the words "extra virgin olive oil" on the label, which means the oil is made from the first pressing of the olives, as extra virgin olive oil has been shown to have significantly higher levels of antioxidants than what's labeled simply "olive oil." It's easy to add olive oil to just about everything. You can simply drizzle it and some vinegar over your greens in your salad. You can use it over vegetables, to fry eggs, or as a replacement for butter on whole grains (such as in baked goods).

10. **Cruciferous Veggies.** Like most vegetables, cruciferous ones—including arugula, bok choy, broccoli, Brussels sprouts, cabbage, cauliflower, collards, daikon radish, kale, kohlrabi, radishes, turnip, and watercress—are rich in fiber and various phytonutrients that help your metabolic health. What sets them apart from other veggies, both in taste and in health benefits, is one particular group of compounds known as glucosinolates, which are sulfur-containing phytochemicals. When you cook, chew, and digest cruciferous veggies, your body breaks those glucosinolates into biologically active compounds including sulforaphane, which is hailed for its anti-cancer properties, and indole-3-carbinol, which has been shown to have unique liver-protective properties. Lower indole-3-carbinol is associated with severe obesity and higher levels of fat in the liver. When researchers administered indole-3-carbinol to liver cells in a group of study participants, levels of both fat and inflammation were reduced.[24]

How to eat them: Broccoli and cauliflower are delicious raw and good vehicles for hummus, olive oil, or dips; they're also both great drizzled with a little extra virgin olive oil and roasted until they brown in spots. (Try our Baba Ganoush recipe and Krissy's Keto Broccoli and Cheese Casserole in the Recipes section.) Cabbage is the primary ingredient of coleslaw—skip the sugar and opt for a dressing anchored by extra virgin olive oil instead of mayonnaise and this common side dish becomes a tonic for your liver. Brussels sprouts are also amazing roasted—or you can thinly slice them when raw and add them to salads. Add chopped cruciferous vegetables to every salad and soup you make. Try kale and arugula in place of or in addition to lettuce in your salads. They are both great sautéed in olive oil with a little chopped garlic, too. The thick white stems of bok choy are delicious sliced and eaten raw or added to stir fries or soups. There's really no limit to how to incorporate cruciferous veggies—aim to buy at least one every time you go to the grocery store (or two if you do weekly shops), and experiment!

11. **Chicken and Turkey Breast and Fatty Wild Fish.** In general, protein is your liver's friend. Eating protein helps you feel full and naturally helps you crowd out some of the carbs from your plate. And protein has special powers for the liver. In yet another piece of evidence that it's not the amount of calories that counts but the type, research has found that reduced-calorie diets rich in protein are significantly better at reducing liver fat stores than reduced-calorie diets that are low in protein. German researchers divided obese patients into two groups—while both groups were given a reduced-calorie diet for three weeks, one group's diet contained high amounts of protein, while the other group's had little protein. After three weeks, both groups had lost an average of approximately eleven pounds. While the low-protein group saw no change in their liver fat, the high-protein group had *40 percent less liver fat* than when the diet began. The

researchers analyzed the genetic code of the liver cells and found that many genes responsible for synthesizing, storing, and absorbing fat were less active in the high-protein group.[25]

Our favorite sources of animal protein are chicken and turkey breast and fatty wild fish, such as salmon, halibut, and rainbow trout. Wild-caught fatty fish include salmon, sardines, cod, and lake trout, all of which are rich sources of omega-3 fatty acids. Omega-3 is a polyunsaturated fat and probably the most import-ant fat for liver health because it alters the expression of genes involved in the synthesis and storage of fat in the liver.[26] You can eat these kinds of fish in moderate amounts (two to three times a week) on any of our plans.

> *How to eat it:* These forms of animal protein can be parts of a wide range of meals—but keep in mind that you still want low-glycemic vegetables and fruits to be the stars of the show, with protein and carbs as supporting players. Eat your grilled chicken breast on top of a big salad or have your piece of salmon with a pile of your favorite sautéed vegetables.

12. **Nuts and Seeds.** Nuts are one of nature's perfect foods; they are rich in protein, fiber, and healthy fats, and—mostly—low in net carbs. Specifically, nuts are high in both monounsaturated and polyunsaturated fatty acids, in vitamins such as niacin, folic acid, and vitamins B6 and E, as well as in minerals such as potas-sium, calcium, and magnesium. Studies show that nut consump-tion can provide cardio-protective effects—such as lowering LDL cholesterol. These benefits are due to their unique composition: nuts are high in plant phytosterols, which compete with choles-terol and therefore aid in cholesterol management. The preva-lence of antioxidants, including phenolic compounds, in nuts likely explains why they have a strong record of being helpful in losing weight and in reducing markers of inflammation. These health protections extend to the liver, too. A 2019 study pub-lished in the journal of the International Association for the

Study of the Liver found the more often people ate nuts, the lower their risk of developing fatty liver—and this is after adjusting for age, weight, blood lipids, glucose levels, and markers of inflammation. Benefits could be seen even going from never eating nuts to eating them once a week.[27]

However, there are some nuts that are better than others. Walnuts, for example, are the whole food with the highest content of the omega-3 fatty acid alpha-linolenic acid (ALA). On the other end of the spectrum, peanuts—which are technically the seed of a legume—have the highest amount of net carbs of any nut.

Our top five liver-friendly nuts are:

1. Walnuts
2. Almonds
3. Pistachios
4. Brazil nuts
5. Pine nuts

Of the seeds we love because they're high in fiber and nutrient-dense, too, our favorites are:

1. Pumpkin seeds
2. Sunflower seeds
3. Chia seeds
4. Flaxseeds
5. Sesame seeds

How to eat them: Nuts and seeds make a great snack—but they are calorie-dense, so think one or at most two handfuls, not several. In addition, you can:

- Chop and sprinkle them over other foods, such as salads, stir-fries, quinoa, yogurt, or steel-cut oatmeal.
- Use them in a pesto that you serve on top of bean-based pasta.
- Use nut oils in sauces and salad dressings.

- Grind nuts into flour that you can then bake with (or buy nut flours such as almond or hazelnut), or grind seeds into a powder that you can add to oatmeal, yogurt, or baked goods to add extra nutrition.
- Puree them into smooth and creamy nut or seed butters using a food processor (or buy nut or seed butters, ideally low- or no-sugar ones like Joe's) and add them to smoothies, yogurt, or oatmeal.

Cautions about nuts and seeds: There are a few groups of people who should take care when eating nuts and seeds:

- Of course, anyone with a nut allergy, whether to tree nuts (such as almonds, pecans, walnuts, and cashews) or legumes (peanuts) should avoid those foods.
- People with a history of diverticulitis will want to take care with nuts and especially seeds. While the association between eating nuts and diverticulitis has been challenged in the literature, as nuts can be chewed well, seeds are still a concern, as they are smaller and can more easily get trapped in the diverticula.
- Sometimes older people have problems with chewing nuts and seeds. If you have issues with dentition, stick to nut or seed butters and nut flours.

Upgrading Your Snacks

Chips, Popcorn, and Pretzels

With chips, look for bean-based options (ones made with lentils or chickpeas, for example), root vegetable chips (such as beets, sweet potato, or cassava), popcorn (it is a whole grain, with enough fiber to make it low on the glycemic index), or protein-enhanced chips, as they are more nutrient-dense than standard potato or tortilla chips. Also look for chips with the shortest list of ingredients, as they are less likely to contain flavor enhancers that make them hyperpalatable. If you're shopping for pretzels, opt for whole-grain versions.

Protein Bars

Ideally, any protein bar you eat or give your child will have five grams or fewer of added sugars and five grams or more of either fiber or protein (bonus points for both!). Nut-based bars often check these boxes. For kids, what you don't want to see are any added herbs (such as chlorophyll or turmeric) or large amounts of vitamins (such as vitamin C or E) as kids require smaller doses than adults, and the makers may not have formulated these bars for children. As always, the shorter the ingredient list, the better.

Yogurts

Most flavored yogurts are loaded with sugar. Whenever possible, buy yogurt—whether in cups, tubes (especially for kids), or drinkable form—that has five grams or fewer of added sugar per serving. The added sugar distinction is important because the milk that yogurt is made from contains the natural sugar lactose. Avoid yogurts with artificial ingredients. (That rule about a short ingredient list applies here, too.)

The Scoop on Dairy

Moderate amounts of dairy are part of the traditional Mediterranean diet, and they are part of our plans, too. We both hear from patients who have heard they should avoid dairy because it is inflammatory, but dairy itself is neutral—whether it causes an inflammatory response depends on your physiology. Many people do have an intolerance to a sugar and a protein found in dairy products—lactose and casein, respectively.

Lactose intolerance, in particular, is very common and can get more pronounced with age. While lactose intolerance isn't harmful, it can negatively impact your quality of life by causing gas, bloating, and diarrhea. If this is something you've noticed after eating dairy, you may want to try lactose-free dairy products, fermented forms of dairy such as yogurt and kefir (as the friendly bacteria consume a lot of the lactose, lowering the amount), or dairy products made with sheep's or goat's milk (as those types of milk tend to cause fewer reactions).

Dairy is a good source of protein, and in fermented forms it has friendly probiotics that support gut health and immunity. One component of dairy that doesn't deliver a lot of benefit is the fat. Dairy fat is mostly saturated, and we advise everyone to consume less saturated fat for the sake of both their liver and their heart. While you don't need to seek out low-fat cheese, or switch from using half-and-half in your coffee, you do want to keep your consumption of high-fat dairy to moderate amounts. This goes for ice cream, too, which you should be having as a rare treat anyway, thanks to its sugar content. If you have yogurt, cottage cheese, or milk several days a week, opt for low-fat versions. (If you only have them once a week or less, it's fine to keep them full-fat if that's a taste or texture you prefer.)

As for that low-fat yogurt and even cottage cheese, we recommend that you buy it plain so that you avoid a lot of added sugar, and use berries, cinnamon, and maybe a little stevia and/or vanilla extract to add sweetness and flavor. You'll train your taste buds to appreciate a different form of sweetness, and you'll also get the polyphenols from fruit.

Reset Your Appetite

If you've been eating a pretty typical carb-heavy (high-glycemic) diet, you have probably become acclimated to hyperpalatable foods. While the liver-friendly and low-glycemic-load foods that we have introduced you to in this chapter and in our eating plans are delicious—and so are our recipes!—you will probably have to go through a period of adjustment where you recalibrate your palate a little bit. After all, the process of limiting carbs in the body leads to a metabolic shift of fuel as well.

But what could be a harder adjustment to make is to get used to eating fewer calories.

To be clear, we are *not* suggesting you do any calorie counting or caloric restriction—studies have shown over and over that taking this approach doesn't work to help lose weight, keep weight off, or improve metabolic health. In fact, we've seen that when our patients focus only on calories, they tend to focus more on quantity over quality. And yet, going lower carb definitely doesn't mean "eat whatever you want, and however much you want, so long as it's low carb." We are not issuing an open invitation for you to make bacon one of your major food groups or to eat bagsful of snacks marketed as keto friendly.

To find and maintain a healthy metabolic profile, you need to learn how to avoid over-fueling yourself. Think of it this way: eating more calories than you truly need to maintain your weight and fuel your level of activity is like going to fill your car up with gas and continuing to pump after the tank is full. That extra gas doesn't help your car go farther; it just spills out onto the ground and creates a fire hazard. It's the same with overeating—the extra calories aren't necessary and aren't helping you fuel your body. They're likely just getting stored as fat.

If you've been eating hyperpalatable and/or high-glycemic-load foods, you've likely been eating a high amount of calories, for two reasons. First, those foods tend to be more caloric than low-glycemic-load foods—for example, a half cup of high-glycemic white rice has 107 calories while the same-sized serving of cauliflower rice has 14 calories. A serving of hyperpalatable potato chips has 154 calories while a small baked sweet potato has 52. Second, those foods are designed to be so tasty and so convenient that you don't even notice when you've eaten a triple-sized serving. To adjust to a more liver-friendly way of eating, you'll have to recalibrate your appetite. But don't panic—we've got a few powerful tools to help you do just that.

Painless Portion Control—and More Pleasure

How do you adjust your eating without counting calories or getting hung up on serving sizes?

The first step is to change what you eat. If you're eating high-fiber, nutrient-dense foods, you'll get fuller more quickly than when you were eating primarily high-glycemic-load, hyperpalatable foods.

You can also change *how* you eat. Many of us are guilty of mindless eating, when you can hardly remember what you ate because you were also scrolling through your social media feeds, checking your email, or watching a show. When you aren't consciously paying attention to your body and your food when you're eating, you tend to eat more

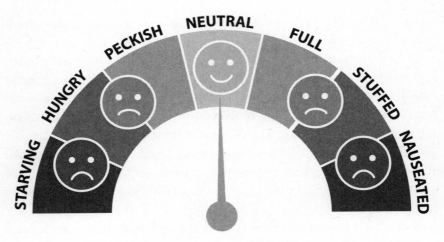

Figure 5.1. Hunger Scale

because you don't notice that you're getting full. Mindless eating also deprives you of a lot of pleasure, because it's likely that you may not even notice the taste of your food. A super useful tool that can help you be aware of your portions and enjoy your food more is mindful eating.

Rather than seeking to restrict calories or to follow a certain diet, mindful eating teaches you to tune in to the experience of eating—the tastes, sights, and sounds—as a way to deepen your awareness of how it feels to nourish yourself. Mindful eating helps you enjoy and appreciate your food. It can also help you recognize when you're truly hungry and realize when you've had enough.

More than just a nice idea, mindful eating has research to support its health benefits. A review of fourteen different studies found that mindful eating was successful in reducing binge eating and emotional eating.[28] And a 2018 study found that when participants in an online weight-loss program received coaching on incorporating mindfulness practices, they lost more weight as their mindfulness scores rose.[29] And participants in an eight-week mindful eating intervention showed a significant reduction in food cravings and negative body image.[30]

Refer to the simple visual to the left to help you assess how hungry you truly are (or aren't).

Think About Your Throwaway Foods

We all have "throwaway foods" that we typically eat—food we consume when we're not really hungry. It could be the extra handful of nuts you grab to take with you in the car after you've already had a handful. Or the candy that gets passed out at the school meeting that you're really not hungry for but you eat because it's there. Avoid the distracted eating that's not about needing to fuel yourself. You'll naturally cut out some calories that you won't even miss.

Getting to Know Your Hunger Signals

While it is true that you want to satisfy your hunger before it gets to the ravenous or starving state so that you avoid creating the conditions that lead to binge eating, we also know that not every sensation that registers as hunger is a true need for food.

When you first notice what you perceive as hunger, take a moment to ask yourself what preceded it. Are you physically feeling hunger? Or did you have a tough call with your boss? Or are you about to start on a project that you'd maybe like to distract yourself from? If there's something that's triggering your emotions more than your actual hunger, try writing down your thoughts for a couple of minutes to help your feelings—and therefore, your cravings—settle down.

Then ask, how long has it been since your last meal? If it's been less than three hours, give yourself twenty minutes to see if it subsides, because a lot of times it will. You can have a cup of coffee, or herbal tea if you want to avoid caffeine because it's later in the day, perhaps with a little half-and-half or your favorite plant-based milk, to help you make it to your next mealtime. Even drinking a glass of water can help you ride out a craving.

And if you wait and are still hungry, have something with a low glycemic load, such as a handful of nuts or a few baby carrots with

MINDFUL EATING HABITS

- *Check in with your hunger.* It's really common for people to not pay attention to their hunger until it is peaking. By the time you're ravenous, it's practically impossible to not overeat. That's because when your blood sugar level gets super low, your body will trigger hunger as a survival mechanism. When this happens, you're beyond thinking about what to eat or being able to notice if you're full; you're just sticking whatever you can get your hands on in your mouth. On a physiological level, your body is trying to avoid death by getting you to eat whatever it takes to get your blood sugar back up—quick. If you have NAFLD and type 2 diabetes, you have a much higher risk of hypoglycemia (the official term for very low blood sugar), which means your tendency to binge eat may be higher. Mindful eating teaches you to get familiar with the different stages of hunger (see Figure 5.1 for a helpful visual) and to check in with yourself throughout the day to see where you are on the hunger scale. Eating when you're actually hungry—not in a neutral state but also not so famished that your stomach is growling—will help you not overeat.

- *No more multitasking while eating.* Put your phone away, close your computer, and turn off the TV. Not only do these things distract your attention away from your food, but a lot of times they create stress. If you're sitting down to eat while the nightly news is on, you're going to be focused on all the horrible things going on in the world, and when you're stressed, your body diverts resources away from digestion and toward getting ready to fight or flee. When you sit down to eat, make sure you have nothing to do but enjoy your food and the company of anyone you might be eating with. If you have to eat in a short window while on the job, try to stay off your phone and/or computer and let yourself enjoy the process of eating. Maybe you can remember to take a breath between bites to help you stay present. That being said, not every meal needs to be mindful. If it's a hectic workday and you need to eat while using a screen, it's OK. You can try again tomorrow.

- *Elevate mealtimes.* We're all so overscheduled that food is often what we try to squeeze into the cracks, but we need to go back to food being the main focus and everything else fitting into the cracks. Sitting down at a table that has papers, keys, and mail cleared off it, maybe even with a placemat and a place setting, helps you focus on your meal. Even if you're having a very casual meal or snack (no cooking involved), resist the urge to eat it while standing at the counter or even the fridge. Take it to an actual table where you sit down to eat. You'll still have to eat in the car or at your job sometimes, but do what you can to make mealtime a sacred space in your day. If that is still hard, try to carve out one day a week to put this into practice.

- *Plate your meals.* Instead of serving dinner family style, have everyone make a plate in the kitchen for themselves and then carry it to a table. If you don't have extra food within arm's reach, you will be less likely to eat a second helping simply because it's there.

- *Use smaller plates.* The bigger your plates, utensils, and serving spoons, the more food you're likely to pile on your plate without even realizing that you're doing it. Aim to make the amount of food on your plate be about as much food as you could hold in your two cupped hands.

- *Appreciate your food.* Before you dig in, take a few moments to appreciate the fact that you have food to eat and all the people who were involved in bringing that food to your plate.

- *Tune in to your senses.* Digestion starts with your eyes and even your nose. Spend a little time looking at your food and savoring its aroma—it will help you slow down and will help get your digestive enzymes flowing. As you're chewing, see how many flavors you can identify.

- *Take your time.* Aim to chew every bite until it's fully liquefied and to put your fork down between bites. This allows more time for your brain to register that your stomach is getting full and naturally helps you keep your portions and total calories down without ever feeling deprived.

- *Keep going.* Any new skill takes practice. Science suggests it can take between ten and fifteen times of trying something new before you really get it, so give yourself a week or two to experiment with mindful eating before you decide how well it's working for you.

- *Be OK with imperfection.* Realize you won't be perfect 100 percent of the time. If you enjoyed the experience, honor it and don't beat yourself up. If it didn't make you feel good, recognize why it happened so that you can better avoid it happening again.

hummus. Because if you quench that small feeling of hunger with something that has a high glycemic load, you will only feel hungrier after your blood sugar crashes.

It's also helpful to assess what else might be triggering your hunger, such as whether you had enough protein, fiber, and healthy fat in your previous meal or how well you slept the night before. Knowing these things will help you make changes that will help you avoid future cravings. Some of our patients have found success in keeping a journal of these occurrences.

Now that you know the pillars of all the plans and foods you'll be avoiding (or replacing with lower-carb versions), we want to explain the differences among the plans so you can pick the right one for you at this time.

Preparation Check-In

Throughout the rest of the book, we'll encourage you to do some reflecting at the end of each chapter, because the more awareness you have about the choices you're making, progress you're achieving, and results you're experiencing, the more likely you'll be to keep going. Add your answers to your Regenerative Health notebook, or wherever you are tracking your progress.

Reflections
*   The mindful eating techniques I've tried are:*
*   My favorite mindful eating technique is:*
*   The throwaway foods I've identified, or even been able to stop eating, are:*

When I reorganized my kitchen to put healthy foods front and center, I learned:

The liver-friendly foods I've stocked up on are:

When it comes to minimizing processed foods that I have on hand or buy at the store, I've learned:

chapter 6

Pick Your Plan

Now that you know the foundational steps to regenerating your health, it's time to dive deeper into the plans to help you figure out if you're ready to move forward with a new eating plan or if it's better for you to stick with Your Checklist for Change, which we covered in Chapter 4, for now. Both are good choices. In this chapter, we'll talk you through the things you need to consider in order to choose the best course of action for you.

While we dive more into the specifics of each plan in the next few chapters, it's helpful to get a preview of what's ahead. Here are the primary features of our plans all in one place. All four of these plans are based on the Mediterranean diet; the main variable between each of the plans is what percentage of the calories come from carbs. Basically, the lower your metabolic health and the more severe your fatty liver disease is, the more you stand to benefit from reducing your carb intake.

Renew Your Liver Food Plans at a Glance

	Modified Mediterranean Plan	Moderate-Carb Plan	Low-Carb Plan	Family Plan
In a Nutshell	Primarily designed for prevention of fatty liver disease and maintenance of benefits you create after following one of the other plans for a couple of months.	Primarily designed for reversing NAFLD and NASH.	Takes aim at reversing fibrosis and cirrhosis and improving liver cancer.	Designed for those of you with kids who need to avoid or reverse the "good" stages of fatty liver disease, and guidance on how to encourage kids to eat healthier without focusing on losing weight.

	Modified Mediterranean Plan	Moderate-Carb Plan	Low-Carb Plan	Family Plan
Primary Goals	Prevention of NAFLD, reversal of NAFLD or NASH, mitigation of NASH-fibrosis or cirrhosis	Reversal of NAFLD or NASH, mitigation of NASH-fibrosis and cirrhosis, prevention of NAFLD	Reversal of NAFLD, NASH, and NASH-fibrosis; potential reversal and mitigation of cirrhosis; management or even reversal of type 2 diabetes; prevention of NAFLD; improving metabolic health	Prevention of NAFLD, reversal of NAFLD, mitigation of NASH-fibrosis and cirrhosis; not meant to restrict but to provide choices the whole family may enjoy
Best Metabolic Type Match	Preventer	Fine-tuner and Recalibrator	Regenerator	Can be a mix of profiles—it's designed to help the whole household take better care of their health
Benefits	Most doable and sustainable of all the plans, better management of type 2 diabetes, reduction of risk of cardiovascular disease	Better management of type 2 diabetes; more focus on losing excess weight and/or reducing blood sugar levels; still very doable and sustainable; can prevent type 2 diabetes, cardiovascular disease, and certain cancers	Quickest results of all the plans, short-term weight loss, reduced hunger, improvement in insulin sensitivity	May help to manage mood disorders such as depression and anxiety, models a healthy lifestyle for kids and establishes good habits, shifts attention and discussion away from a child's weight and toward better health
Carb Targets	40–50 percent of daily calories from carbs	26–40 percent of daily calories from carbs	10–26 percent of daily calories from carbs	No targets—just eat better!

	Modified Mediterranean Plan	Moderate-Carb Plan	Low-Carb Plan	Family Plan
Grams of Carbs	130–175 grams per day (the size of a tennis ball per meal, or roughly half your plate)	100–130 grams per day (the size of a lacrosse ball per meal, or just less than half of your plate)	10–100 grams per day (the size of a golf ball per meal, or one-quarter of your plate)	N/A

A NOTE ABOUT THE DEFINITIONS OF THE DIFFERENT CARB PLANS

In truth, there are no standardized definitions of what "moderate carb," "low carb," and "very low carb" mean. If you read the scientific literature that compares the effects of these diets, you'll see that they each define them slightly differently. To come up with our meal plans and their suggested carb targets, we consulted numerous studies, various health organizations (such as the National Lipid Association), and leading researchers.

To recap, the carb targets we settled on are:

- Modified Mediterranean—40 to 50 percent of daily calories from carbs
- Moderate-Carb—26 to 40 percent of daily calories from carbs
- Low-Carb—10 to 26 percent of daily calories from carbs

The Food Pillars

In addition to the Twelve Liver-Friendly Foods you read about in Chapter 5, there is more to know about the foods that will become pillars of your diet after adopting one of the four plans. You can eat these foods with all of our Renew Your Liver plans, although if you choose the Low-Carb plan, you may need to moderate the quantity of intact grains that you eat so that you keep your carb intake on the lower side. (Note that if you're used to the carb restrictions of a ketogenic diet, you'll be pleasantly surprised that you have a lot more leeway on our Low-Carb plan.) They are:

- Lots of deeply hued fruits and vegetables
- Beans and legumes

- Extra virgin olive oil
- Nuts and seeds
- Wild-caught fatty fish
- Intact grains
- Green tea and coffee

All of our plans also encourage intermittent fasting—giving your-self at least twelve hours between your last meal of one day and the first meal of the next. Let's look at each of these components and how they specifically fit into the plans.

Deeply Hued Fruits and Vegetables

Basically, you want colorful fruits and vegetables to take up a much higher percentage of your daily diet than you would find in a typical American diet. Colorful produce is nutrient-dense, high in fiber, and rich in anti-inflammatory phytochemicals. Unless you're following the Family plan, which places no restrictions on carbs, you do want to pay attention to the net carbs in the fruits and vegetables you choose, but on the Modified Mediterranean plan, you don't need to be too careful. On the Moderate-Carb and Low-Carb plans you'll need to be more mindful of choosing fruits and vegetables with lower levels of net carbs in order to stay within the carb parameters of those plans.

Beans and Legumes

Beans and legumes—such as chickpeas, black-eyed peas, edamame, black beans, cannellini beans, pinto beans, and lentils—are great sources of plant-based protein and essential nutrients such as folate and fiber. They are mainstays of the diets in the blue zones where people have a higher tendency to live past one hundred. They *do* come with some carbs, but again, unless you're on the Low-Carb plan, you don't need to worry too much about their carb content since their fiber content is so high (and thus, this lowers the total net carbs, as shown on page 81). If you are on the Low-Carb plan, you'll want to keep your bean and legume consumption to a generous handful a couple of times a week at most.

Olive Oil

As we said earlier, you want to look for extra virgin olive oil. Use it to cook with and also to drizzle on salads and vegetables in every plan.

Nuts and Seeds

As you read, nuts and seeds are great sources of protein, fiber, and yes, some carbs, but they also have polyunsaturated fatty acids just as extra virgin olive oil does.[1] Overall, nuts and seeds provide high nutrient density and help you feel full on every plan.

Wild-Caught Fatty Fish

You can eat these kinds of fish, which are rich in healthy fats, in moderate amounts (two or three times a week) on every plan.

Intact Grains

The traditional Mediterranean diet emphasizes whole grains; we like to take this idea one step further by focusing on grains that are intact, which means that they are as close as possible to the form they were grown in. That may mean trying grains that are new to you, such as quinoa, millet, amaranth, teff, sorghum, or buckwheat. It may also mean changing the grains that you're already familiar with—such as going from instant oatmeal to steel-cut oats, or from white rice to brown or wild rice. Aim to make half the grains intact that you eat regularly, and you will reap the benefits of more fiber, protein, B vitamins, and nutrient density while also lowering the glycemic load of your grains.

While we are following the main tenets of the Mediterranean diet in this book, we have layered in a few basic modifications that make the diet even more liver friendly. One of them is to eat fewer grains overall and, for the grains you do eat, to reduce your total carb consumption and improve your nutrient density by upgrading your carbs. By which we mean: swap out non-nutrient-dense carbs made from grains for carbs that are more nutritious—for example, a nut-based cracker instead of one made with refined white flour, or sprouted 100 percent whole wheat bread instead of typical white bread.

The one exception is our Low-Carb plan, where we advise minimizing even intact grains so as to keep overall carb content low. Even then, you can still have a little quinoa, or even steel-cut oats, so long as your other food choices that day are lower in carbs, but having some intact grains at every meal will likely bump you up into Moderate-Carb territory.

Any option throughout the book that is appropriate for the Low-Carb plan is also included on all the other plans.

Simple Swaps to Upgrade Your Carbs

Traditional Carb	Upgraded Carb
Regular pasta	All plans except Low-Carb: Bean-based pasta
Standard crackers	All plans:* Nut- or seed-based crackers *Check the net carbs if you are on the Low-Carb plan and determine your serving size accordingly
Instant oatmeal	All plans except Low-Carb:* Steel-cut oatmeal *If you want something similar on the Low-Carb plan, try chia pudding—we have several options in the Recipes section
White bagel	All plans: Low-carb or keto bagel Modified Mediterranean or Family plans: Whole wheat bagel or sprouted-grain bagel
White bread	All plans: Low-carb or keto bread Modified Mediterranean or Family plans: Whole wheat bread or sprouted-grain bread
White rice	All plans: Quinoa, cauliflower or broccoli rice, or wild rice Modified Mediterranean or Family plans: Brown rice
White flour tortilla	Modified Mediterranean plan: Sprouted wheat tortilla Modified Mediterranean, Moderate-Carb, and Family plans: Almond flour tortilla All plans: Keto, egg-white, or other low-carb wraps (see table on page 187)
Hamburger bun	All plans: Low-carb, keto, cauliflower, or broccoli bun (or no bun at all) Modified Mediterranean and Family plans: Sprouted whole wheat bun
Regular pizza crust	All plans: Cauliflower or almond flour pizza crust (or no crust at all! Also, see the recipe for No-Carb Pizza in the Recipes section) Modified Mediterranean or Family plans: Thin crust or whole wheat crust
Potato chips	All plans: Kale or seaweed chips Modified Mediterranean, Moderate-Carb, and Family plans: Beet chips, sweet potato chips

Coffee and Green Tea

While coffee and green tea aren't explicitly part of the typical Mediterranean diet, they are both liver-friendly beverages that are acceptable and encouraged on all four plans. Since green tea has about one-third the amount of caffeine that coffee has, you can drink it well into the afternoon. It's also great served iced with a squeeze of lemon (and maybe a little liquid stevia or powdered monkfruit if you find it to be bitter). If you want kids to try some coffee, add a little half-and-half and stevia, if necessary, to make it more palatable, but don't give it to them past noon. Since green tea has about half the caffeine of coffee, they can have it up until about 2:00 p.m., and it shouldn't interfere with their sleep.

Intermittent Fasting

To offer even more benefit to your blood sugar and insulin levels, in addition to eating fewer carbs and upgrading the carbs that you do eat, we recommend that you build into your daily routine a doable fast, or limiting your eating to a certain window of time, as we outlined in Chapter 2. **Note that this is applicable to all plans except the Family plan, as intermittent fasting is not suitable for children.**

Choosing the Best Bread

Traditional (that is, wheat-based) bread and buns (and wheat-based tortillas) *can* be a healthy part of a liver-friendly diet, but they're not on all of our Renew Your Liver plans.

The Modified Mediterranean and Family plans include bread, but not your typical white bread and buns. (For the Moderate-Carb and Low-Carb plans, luckily there are many lower-carb wrap and tortilla options—we'll give you guidance on how to choose them on page 187.) If you are on either the Modified Mediterranean or Family plan, the things you want to look for in a loaf of bread are the following:

- *The word "whole."* A kernel of wheat has three components: the bran, the germ, and the endosperm. To make white flour, the bran and the germ are stripped away—as are the protein and vitamins

The Pillars and Plans at a Glance

	Modified Mediterranean Plan	Moderate-Carb Plan	Low-Carb Plan	Family Plan
Deeply hued fruits and vegetables	You want colorful fruits and vegetables to take up a much higher percentage of your daily diet than you would find in a typical American diet; otherwise, no restrictions	You want colorful fruits and vegetables to take up a much higher percentage of your daily diet than you would find in a typical American diet; you'll need to be more mindful of choosing fruits and vegetables with lower levels of net carbs in order to stay within the carb parameters (refer to page 318 for a list)	You want colorful fruits and vegetables to take up a much higher percentage of your daily diet than you would find in a typical American diet; you'll need to be more mindful of choosing fruits and vegetables with lower levels of net carbs in order to stay within the carb parameters (refer to page 318 for a list)	You want colorful fruits and vegetables to take up a much higher percentage of your daily diet than you would find in a typical American diet; otherwise, no restrictions
Beans and legumes	You don't need to worry too much about their carb content; since their fiber content is so high, the total net carbs are moderate	You don't need to worry too much about their carb content; since their fiber content is so high, the total net carbs are moderate	You'll want to keep your bean and legume consumption to a generous handful a couple of times a week at most	You don't need to worry too much about their carb content; since their fiber content is so high, the total net carbs are moderate
Extra virgin olive oil	Up to 3 tablespoons per day; use it to cook with and also to drizzle on salads and vegetables	Up to 3 tablespoons per day; use it to cook with and also to drizzle on salads and vegetables	Up to 3 tablespoons per day; use it to cook with and also to drizzle on salads and vegetables	Up to 3 tablespoons per day; use it to cook with and also to drizzle on salads and vegetables
Nuts and seeds	A couple handfuls of nuts and seeds per day	A couple handfuls of nuts and seeds per day	A couple handfuls of nuts and seeds per day; be more mindful of choosing nuts with lower levels of net carbs in order to stay within the carb parameters (refer to page 319 for a list)	A couple handfuls of nuts and seeds per day

	Modified Mediterranean Plan	Moderate-Carb Plan	Low-Carb Plan	Family Plan
Wild-caught fatty fish	Eat in moderate amounts two or three times a week	Eat in moderate amounts two or three times a week	Eat in moderate amounts two or three times a week	Eat in moderate amounts two or three times a week
Intact grains	Aim to make half the grains you eat regularly intact, eat fewer grains overall, swap out non-nutrient-dense carbs made from grains for carbs that are more nutritious	Aim to make half the grains you eat regularly intact, eat fewer grains overall, swap out non-nutrient-dense carbs made from grains for carbs that are more nutritious	Minimize intact grains so as to keep overall carb content low; focus on quinoa, or even steel-cut oats, so long as your other food choices that day are lower in carbs	Aim to make half the grains you eat regularly intact, eat fewer grains overall, swap out non-nutrient-dense carbs made from grains for carbs that are more nutritious
Green tea and coffee	No limitations, being mindful of your sensitivity to caffeine and whether you have high blood pressure, acid reflux, or anxiety (as coffee can exacerbate these conditions)	No limitations, being mindful of your sensitivity to caffeine and whether you have high blood pressure, acid reflux, or anxiety (as coffee can exacerbate these conditions)	No limitations, being mindful of your sensitivity to caffeine and whether you have high blood pressure, acid reflux, or anxiety (as coffee can exacerbate these conditions)	A cup a day of either one is acceptable for kids (skip the sugar); avoid giving kids coffee after noon and green tea after 2:00 p.m.
Intermittent fasting	Work your way up to going ten to twelve hours without nourishment	Work your way up to going ten to twelve hours without nourishment	Work your way up to going ten to twelve hours without nourishment	N/A (intermittent fasting isn't appropriate for kids)
Pastas, breads, and sugars	Whole-grain and bean-based pastas; whole-grain breads, buns, and tortillas; and even some natural sugars (like honey and maple syrup) are acceptable in moderate to small amounts; see plan chapter for details	Bean-based pastas; low-carb or sprouted-grain breads, buns, and tortillas; and even some natural sugars (like honey and maple syrup) are acceptable in moderate to small amounts; see plan chapter for details	Avoid typical pastas, breads, and sugars as much as possible because of their carb content; there are many lower-carb pasta, bread, tortilla, and bun options available, explore substitutes on page 187	Whole-grain or bean-based pastas, whole-grain breads, and even some natural sugars (like honey and maple syrup) are acceptable in moderate to small amounts; see plan chapter for details

they contain—and all that's left is the endosperm, which is primarily carbohydrate. Because all bread is made with wheat, seeing "wheat bread" on the label doesn't necessarily mean that the germ and the bran of the wheat kernel were included in the processing. "Whole wheat," on the other hand, implies that all three parts of the kernel were included.

- *A percentage, such as "100 percent whole wheat."* This is even better than the word "whole" alone, as it connotes that the manufacturer went to the trouble to use all three parts of the kernel and they want you to know it. A high percentage of whole wheat will naturally also mean that the bread has a good amount of fiber and is more of an intact grain than just regular wheat flour.
- *A short ingredient list.* The shorter the ingredient list, the fewer fillers and preservatives there will be. Also, some breads will list whole wheat flour as the first ingredient but simply wheat flour as the second or third—the fewer the ingredients on a bread that calls itself whole wheat, the more likely that the majority of the flour used was ground from whole kernels of wheat.
- *Sugar does not appear in the first three ingredients.* It's hard to activate yeast—which is essential for most forms of bread—without sugar, so it's hard to find bread without some amount of added sugar. But you want it to be far down the ingredient list.
- *The word "sprouted."* Sprouting a grain makes its nutrients more bioavailable and increases the protein and fiber content of the bread made with that grain. Ezekiel is a well-known brand that sprouts its grains before making them into bread—it's typically in the freezer section. (They make tortillas, too.)

With these guidelines, you can find a loaf of bread that is nutrient-dense and a healthy part of your Modified Mediterranean plan.

Alternative Pastas

Pasta has become a mainstay of the typical Western diet. And since Italy is on the Mediterranean Sea, pasta is also closely associated with the Mediterranean diet. In addition, there is pasta-like couscous in the Middle East, and noodles appear in cuisines from around the world—rice noodles in Southeast Asia, ramen in Japan, wontons in China, and various dishes riffing on spaghetti throughout the world (Jollof spaghetti in Senegal, makrouna in Tunisia, Filipino spaghetti in the Philippines, tallarines in Peru, espagueti in Cuba). Whether it's made with white wheat flour or white rice flour—the two most popular forms—pasta is also, sadly, high in carbs and, because it's low in fiber, high in net carbs.

Thankfully, you don't have to give up pasta altogether in order to love your liver. There is a wide array of pastas made with alternate main ingredients, and in addition to being lower in net carbs, they also deliver a spectrum of additional nutrients. Granted, different pastas will have different flavors, and you may not like all of them. But there are enough different options that, if you keep an open mind and taste test a few different versions, you will find at least one that you like. You may also find that you like different alternative pastas for different dishes.

All of the following types of alternative pastas have the benefit of creating better blood glucose control—a huge benefit that is great for your liver and your overall health.

Ways to Use Pasta Alternatives

You can replace any pasta with a pasta alternative in just about any dish. Some examples include:

- Cold pasta salads
- Stir-fries (Kristin loves brown rice noodles with date-sweetened chili sauce, mango, jalapeño, sesame seeds, and mixed Asian veggies)
- As an addition to green salads to add protein, fiber, and texture
- As an addition to soups and stews to make them more of a meal

A Quick Guide to Healthy Sugars or Sugar Alternatives

Refined sugar in all its forms—granulated, brown, or powdered—is something you want to minimize (saving it only for the rare splurge

Types of Alternative Pastas

Main Ingredient	Benefits	Notes	Meal Plans
Almond flour	Good source of fiber, magnesium, manganese, vitamin E.	Has a very palatable taste and smooth texture. Unlike most pastas, which are dried, almond flour pasta is sold fresh (look for it in the freezer case, from the brand Cappello's); as such, it cooks in boiling water in only a minute or two.	All except Low-Carb
Black bean	Black bean pasta is very high in protein and fiber. Black beans are also one of the richest sources of antioxidants, so you're covering a lot of nutritional bases in one serving of these dark brown noodles.	There's no denying that this pasta alternative does have a bean-y taste, but it lends itself well to bold flavors—sun-dried tomatoes, cilantro, and garlic sautéed in extra virgin olive oil is a good pairing, as is your favorite curry paste dissolved in a little coconut milk.	All except Low-Carb
Brown rice	Brown rice noodles have a similar taste to white rice noodles, but with 4 grams of fiber per serving (compared to white rice noodles' 1 gram); that means fewer net carbs than traditional rice noodles.	Using brown rice noodles is a great way to add more nutrition (in the form of fiber) to your favorite Asian stir-fries and noodle soups.	Modified Mediterranean plan, Family plan
Buckwheat	Good source of protein and fiber as well as minerals, including potassium, phosphorus, magnesium, calcium, and iron.	Also called "soba noodles," buckwheat and buckwheat flour are naturally gluten-free, but if gluten is something you're sensitive to, read the label carefully as most soba noodles are a blend of buckwheat and wheat. Buckwheat has a nice, nutty flavor that may remind you of pancakes (as buckwheat flour is often used in recipes for that breakfast staple).	All except Low-Carb

Main Ingredient	Benefits	Notes	Meal Plans
Chickpea	High in protein and soluble fiber, also a good source of iron and polyphenols.	Chickpea pasta comes in a wide range of different shapes and sizes. You can even find boxed mac and cheese made with chickpea pasta.	All except Low-Carb
Edamame	Rich in soy isoflavones, potassium, and protein; in general, soybeans are a good source of complete protein for vegans and vegetarians.	Neutral taste that pairs well with a variety of sauces. Because it is so high in protein and fiber, it's very filling.	All except Low-Carb
Heart of palm	Very low calorie (about 20 calories in one serving).	If you've ever had heart of palm in a salad, you know it has a flavor similar to artichoke hearts and a firm yet easy-to-chew texture. This alternative pasta is simply slices of actual hearts of palm (the core of palm plants), so there is no cooking required. Heart of palm typically comes in the form of spaghetti or lasagna noodles.	All
Kelp noodles	Low carb and low calorie as well as a good source of iodine (important for thyroid health) and calcium.	For something made from seaweed, kelp noodles have a surprisingly mellow flavor—what may come as a surprise is their crunchy texture. Requires no cooking.	All
Lentils (green or red)	High in protein, soluble fiber, iron, a variety of B vitamins, and zinc.	Has an agreeable taste that isn't too far off from regular pasta, making it a family-friendly option.	All except Low-Carb
Quinoa	High in protein, decent amount of fiber; quinoa is an excellent source of complete protein for vegans and vegetarians.	The New York Daily News called quinoa pasta "the best pasta alternative, full stop." Just read the label, as some quinoa pasta actually contains a lot of corn flour, which reduces the health benefits and ups the carbs considerably.	All except Low-Carb

Main Ingredient	Benefits	Notes	Meal Plans
Shirataki	Low carb and very low calorie (a 4-ounce serving has about 10 calories).	Also called miracle noodles or konjac noodles, these are made from glucomannan, a type of fiber found in the root of the konjac plant. Shirataki noodles come packaged in water (they are often kept in a refrigerated case near tofu in the grocery store)—you want to rinse them well before you heat them in a nonstick skillet over medium heat.	All
Vegetable "noodles"	All vegetable noodles are rich in antioxidants, fiber, and polyphenols. They have a high water content (meaning they are hydrating) and are low calorie, and they work well either cold or hot. Carrot, butternut squash, and sweet potato noodles are also high in beta carotene, an important player in eye health.	Not actually pasta, but vegetables cut into small noodle shapes, including beets, butternut squash, carrot, spaghetti squash, sweet potato, and zucchini.	All, although noodles made from beets, butternut squash, carrot, and sweet potato do contain carbs, so if you're on the Low-Carb plan, you'll want to keep your serving sizes small.

once or twice a month, ideally) because it is highly inflammatory and has a dramatic negative effect on your glucose and insulin levels. Luckily, we have a lot of healthier natural sugars and sugar alternatives to choose from.

Stevia

Derived from the leaves of the stevia plant, stevia can come in liquid or powdered form. It won't impact your blood sugar, which is a big upside. The downside is that a lot of people feel it has a bitter aftertaste. For this reason, we advise you not to try baking with it or even adding it to oatmeal.

Best for: Adding to beverages such as coffee or iced tea or to plain yogurt to sweeten it

Plans: All

Local Maple Syrup

Let's be clear: while maple syrup is natural, it's still sugar. Because of maple syrup's rich taste, a little goes a long way. And maple sugar will definitely impact the environment more than traditional sugar derived from sugar cane will, which you might want to consider.

Best for: Sweetening oatmeal and buckwheat pancakes, some baking

Plans: Modified Mediterranean and Family

Manuka Honey

This form of honey comes from Australia and New Zealand and is made by bees that feed on the pollen of the manuka bush. Like maple syrup, honey is a natural sugar that will raise your glucose and insulin levels. But honey has medicinal properties, and manuka honey in particular has been shown to be a powerful antibiotic that promotes the healing of wounds and sore throats.

Best for: Baking, sweetening oatmeal or plain yogurt

Plans: Modified Mediterranean and Family

Monkfruit

Made from the flesh of a fruit that is native to China and also known as Luo Han Guo (after the Luo Han monks who tended the trees that grow the fruit), monkfruit comes in granulated or powdered form. With a similar sweetness to stevia, monkfruit has less of an aftertaste than stevia does, which makes it better for baking. It is found in many keto-friendly products, from cookies to chocolate syrup. Kristin loves the maple-flavored syrup made by Lankato, which is sweetened with a blend of monkfruit and erythritol.

Best for: Baking, maple syrup alternative

Plans: All

Erythritol

This is a sugar alcohol that comes in granular, brown, or powdered form and is a solid alternative for regular white, brown, and powdered sugar in baking. It does not impact your blood sugar. Erythritol could produce some bloating or changes to elimination, so it's best to start with small, infrequent amounts and let your digestive system adjust to it.

Best for: Baking

Plans: All

Allulose

Allulose is a naturally occurring monosaccharide that has a sweet taste but is considered noncaloric because it does not impact blood sugar levels. First identified as a component of wheat in the 1940s, allulose is finally becoming more popular as researchers have only recently discovered how to mass produce it. Like erythritol, allulose could produce some bloating or changes to elimination.

Best for: Baking and adding to beverages

Plans: All

Alternative Sweeteners to Avoid

Here are some nonsugar sweeteners we *don't* recommend:

- *Agave syrup.* While natural, it has a very high glycemic load.
- *Brown rice syrup, coconut sugar, turbinado sugar.* Again, they are natural, but they impact your blood sugar and insulin the exact same way as traditional white sugar—there are just too many decent alternatives to justify using these.

- *Sucralose and aspartame.* While artificial sweeteners such as these have been linked to adverse health effects, many of these studies were conducted using amounts not typical in human consumption. If you enjoy a packet of Splenda with your coffee every day, it won't kill you. However, we recommend using some of the other options we just covered for baking and cooking.

Putting It All into Practice

Here are some other hallmarks of all of our plans:

- **A focus on how to eat (meal suggestions), not what to eat (recipes).** You don't have to be a chef to take better care of your liver. You can definitely be more of a short-order cook who can whip up something nutritious and tasty with a small amount of time and effort. As a result, we made our recipes easier, using products you can get everywhere (no need to stick to only the fancy organic supermarket!). We also included plenty of meal suggestions for each plan out of what we call no-recipe cooking—which is more putting something together and less following step-by-step instructions. We do still have plenty of recipes to make it crystal clear how to cook some of our favorite liver-friendly foods, but you don't need to follow them unless you want to.
- **Everything in moderation.** Real-life eating isn't about restricting; it's about appreciating how your body feels and acts when you eat a certain way and even allowing yourself indulgences here or there without going overboard. We don't believe in restriction— but we do believe in boundaries. Everyone has a non-negotiable food or two—something you love that you can't get behind completely cutting out of your diet. For example, Ibrahim loves ice cream, while Kristin loves bacon. We still eat these foods, but we only have them once a week and focus on really enjoying them as treats.

  Figure out what your non-negotiable is, factor it in at some point in your week, and know that over time you may get to a week where you don't even want it anymore.

- **Benefits to your liver.** You can't make a bad choice here—all of the plans in this book are good for liver health! While we can and do recommend specific plans for different metabolic profiles and stages of disease, it doesn't matter how carefully we have designed those plans to help your liver get healthier if they aren't something you can stick to. The single best eating plan for you is the one you can sustain.

To that end, you want to consider a few things before picking a plan, or frankly, before deciding if you're ready to adopt a new eating plan at all. It might be better for you to stick with making smaller changes for now and then move into a more formal plan once you've had some initial success.

Here are the things to take into consideration when picking a plan:

- Your metabolic profile
- Your stage of liver disease
- An intuitive sense of what will work best for you
- Your capacity for change
- Your motivation and goals
- And maybe even your genes!

Let's look at these one by one.

Your Metabolic Profile

We covered how to determine your metabolic health profile in Chapter 2. Now we're sharing our guidance on which plan is most customized to each of the profiles, as you can see in Figure 6.1.

Your Stage of Liver Disease

You can and should also factor in your stage of fatty liver disease when assessing your next move. In general, the further your liver disease has progressed, the lower your carb intake should be, as giving your liver a break from processing glucose and your insulin resistance a

How to Choose an Eating Plan for Your Metabolic Profile

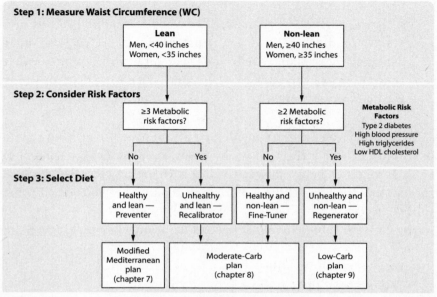

Figure 6.1. Renew Your Liver Plans: How to Choose an Eating Plan for Your Metabolic Profile

chance to heal will help your liver more quickly regain the tissue and capacity to devote to regenerating. Again, though, the best plan is the one you can stick to.

Figure 6.2 shows a visual breakdown of how—all other things being equal—the eating plans correspond to the stages of fatty liver disease.

You'll notice that the Family plan is not included in this graphic—remember that the Family plan is a less conservative approach for people at any stage of fatty liver disease. We've really designed it for individuals under the age of eighteen, or households with children, who want to focus on establishing healthy eating habits instead of on losing weight.

Developing an Intuitive Sense of What Plan Will Serve You Best

Now that you've used the previous two graphics to see what plan or plans your metabolic profile and stage of liver disease suggests

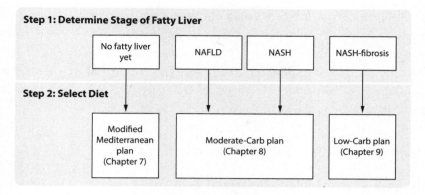

Figure 6.2. How to Choose an Eating Plan Based on the Stage of Fatty Liver Disease

might be best, it's time to bring a deeper understanding of you—your life, your taste buds, your emotional health, your hunger—into account.

While it's true that if you want different results, you've got to take different actions, making change doesn't stop there—you also need to make peace with the thoughts and conditions that led to your current results in the first place. When the behavior you want to change is eating, it's important to understand how everything you've learned and internalized about dieting and health in the past has contributed to where you are today.

As Ibrahim's mentor at the Cleveland Clinic always told him, "The barriers to liver health are not in the belly; they're in the mind." An example is one of Kristin's patients who had worked with her for a few months. He knew exactly what to eat and was good at figuring out the logistics that can be a barrier for some people—things like shopping, cooking, and making a plan for when he got extra busy—but still, he struggled to change his behavior. It was only once he started working with a holistic therapist that he connected the dots between his early life experiences and his current relationship to food. He recalled that his parents used to leave him in a high chair with an ample amount of food so that he would be occupied while they were doing other things. It helped him understand why he was a chronic overeater, and that awareness helped him change those ingrained habits.

If you were food insecure as a child, or grew up in poverty, or were made to feel bad about yourself because you were told you were overweight, or even if you experienced other trauma that's not related specifically to food, it can be hard to rewire the coping mechanisms you developed to help you get through those times. Kristin has seen patients with trauma in their past make big strides after seeking out the support of a mental health professional. If you have an idea that you might benefit from some mental health support, for whatever reason, know that taking care of your psychological health will also benefit your physical health, as it will help you make new choices and adopt new habits that are more nourishing.

To help our patients untangle the way their thoughts, beliefs, and past experiences might be influencing their current food choices and overall health, we introduce them to the principles of intuitive eating. These principles inform an approach to eating and health developed by Evelyn Tribole and Elyse Resch, two registered dietitians and coauthors of the book *Intuitive Eating*, which was first published in 1995 and has had multiple editions published since then. Tribole and Resch founded intuitive eating on the principle that diets don't work and that diet culture is harmful. Intuitive eating helps you reconnect to a respect, appreciation, and understanding of your own body and hunger so that you can find your way to a sustainable approach to eating and a joyful level of health. There are ten principles of intuitive eating that are all helpful, but there are three that we find most applicable to liver health:

- *Accept your emotions with compassion.* Everyone experiences unpleasant emotions, such as anger, boredom, loneliness, and fear, and it's very natural to want to distract yourself from them. Emotional eating can numb your feelings or take your attention away from them, but it cannot solve the things that are causing them. Over the long term, emotional eating will only make those feelings more intense and the situations that trigger them more entrenched. When you find ways to experience and move through your unpleasant emotions—whether that's talking with a therapist or other mental health professional, journaling, movement, or channeling them into something creative—you won't have to rely on food to keep them at bay, and you open up the possibility of developing a new, healthier relationship to food.

- *Acknowledge that size is not health.* We have covered the importance that overall metabolic health plays in liver health. This then gives you permission to stop focusing so much on finding that perfect beach body (whatever that means). If you feel you need to make reductions in belly fat to enhance liver health, we encourage that. But reducing belly fat does not necessarily mean you need to look like a model or that you should be able to get back into your skinny jeans from high school. Embracing health first can help you change the way you see your body and can assist with overall respect for it.

- *Give yourself a break and recognize that you are human.* A patient once told Kristin, "I don't want to ever fall off the wagon." Her reply to this patient, and to you, is that we *all* fall off the wagon every once in a while. You are human, and because you are human, you are imperfect. Instead of planning for perfectionism, plan instead on what you do when life gets in the way. It's not about being perfect, or following any eating plan to a T, but about continually discovering what makes you feel best, making progress toward your health goals, and loving yourself along the way. Lose the shame and guilt, and get right back on the wagon at your next meal. Doing so will help to shape your long-term sustainability in changing—and maintaining—your health goals.

By tending to your emotions, letting go of the idea of having a picture-perfect body, and cutting yourself some slack when you don't follow your plan to the letter, you give yourself a lot more freedom to find a way of eating that feels good *to you* and therefore is sustainable and maintainable.

When you consider these intuitive eating principles, is embarking on a structured eating plan healthy for you at this moment? There is no right or wrong answer here, only the one that is true for you.

An Honest Assessment of Your Capacity for Change

Everyone can change, but how long it takes will depend on your capacity for taking on new things. If you are already overwhelmed by the demands of your life, it will be next to impossible to also revamp your diet and lifestyle. That's not to say you should put this book down and do nothing until life calms down—because you could be waiting too long. It only means that you should probably stick to incorporating one or two small changes.

To determine if you're ready to move forward with a new eating plan, think about what you have going on in your life right now. Are you in the midst of a move, taking care of a loved one who is ill, in the weeds of parenting, or experiencing a really busy time at work? Is your sleep suffering, or are you in pain or having low energy because of your health? If you answered yes to any of these questions, definitely start small. Review Your Checklist for Change (pages 89-94), choose one or two of the items with an asterisk as they are the most important, and stick with those smaller changes for now.

Also think about your social environment: Is your partner not supportive of eating healthier? Are most of your friends or family members big drinkers? Is eating high-glycemic foods a big part of your family culture? If so, starting low and slow makes sense. Focus on what you can control, let go of what you can't, and get creative about the best way for you to move forward given where you currently are. Get some successes under your belt and you'll be more rooted in your devotion to making more changes. Think about what you can commit to, and be realistic. Don't aim for perfect; aim for progress.

If you're sleeping pretty well, have a supportive community, and have a strong why, it will be a lot easier—you can go ahead and choose the eating plan that makes the most sense for you and your health.

Two Crucial Ingredients for Success: Your Why and Your Goals

It's wonderful to research and read books that can help you face a health problem. But, of course, you have to do more than read. You have to actually start doing things in your life differently. And to find, and keep, the motivation to take those different actions, you need two things—you need to know why you want to do them in the first place, and you need goals to help you know what to do and to monitor your progress.

Let's start with your why. Having one strong why (or two, or three) will help you make the changes you're embarking on now more sustainable so that they become an everyday part of your life.

Kristin tells her patients that they need three reasons why they want to get healthier and only one of them can be related to vanity. It's fine to want to look great at your college reunion or other big event, but that event will come and go, and you don't want the results you've gotten to come and go, too.

Some of her patients who have seen the best results have also had the strongest whys. Two of her patients had central obesity (with their excess fat accumulated in their abdomen), type 2 diabetes, and NAFLD. One of them had seen her mother suffer with dementia and didn't want to follow her on that path. Another was an older gentleman whose daughter was having her first child. He wanted to be able to get on the ground to play with his grandchild and be around to see the child graduate from high school, grow up, and get married. Family really can be a very strong why. Maybe one of your parents suffered with cirrhosis or liver cancer, and you want to avoid the same fate. Maybe you have kids and want to be around well into their adulthood.

Kristin had a patient in her sixties who had NAFLD, type 2 diabetes, and high blood pressure. This woman's husband had just been diagnosed with cancer, and her why was that she wanted to stay healthy enough to be the one to take care of him. She followed a moderate-carb diet; her liver health, blood sugar, and blood pressure all improved; and she was able to reduce many of her medications.

There are other reasons for a strong why. Remember Jon, whose story we shared in Chapter 2? His incentive was that he wanted to open himself up more to socializing and dating, which he has started doing.

Your why may be that your doctor told you that you need to lose weight or else you will soon be facing serious health consequences. This can be a strong motivator, but it is also based in fear. And while fear may get you into action, it's not going to get you across the finish line. Let your why be something that inspires you and calls you forward, not something that makes you want to run away.

You absolutely have a why. If you don't already know what yours is, it's not that it doesn't exist; it's that you haven't yet looked deeply enough to determine what it is. If you don't care about yourself, do you care about the people who love you? Do you care about breaking some hearts if something happens to you?

Once you've identified the thing(s) that's going to keep you motivated and engaged, you want to back that up by setting some doable goals that will help you move toward your why. When it comes to setting goals, weight loss doesn't need to be one of them. A goal could be to eat three servings of colorful vegetables a day, which will make you healthier but not necessarily thinner (although it might, especially if those vegetable help retrain your palate away from hyperpalatable, high-carb foods and crowd out some of those less healthy options on your plate and in your belly). Remember, our aim in writing this book is to help you improve your metabolic health, not necessarily to lose weight. Our method is to teach you how to eat, not just what to eat.

If you do want to set a goal around weight loss, that is OK. Just keep it very moderate and very doable—for example, to lose 5 percent of your body weight over the next two months. Ibrahim finds that his patients tend to do better when their goals are simpler. One patient of his with NASH ended up losing fifty pounds, but gradually—her official goal was to lose one to two pounds a week.

One variable you can experiment with when it comes to goal setting is the timeframe. Some people may do better with a longer-term goal—such as losing 2.5 percent of their body weight in a month—because it gives them some flexibility if they have a challenging week to get back on track without missing their goal. You might need something with a shorter timeframe so that you stay present with your aims. If so, you might set a weekly goal to exercise three times, or even a daily goal, such as eating a certain number of servings of vegetables.

If you can, get your family members or housemates on board with your goal, too—it provides accountability and camaraderie. And if it spurs a little health competition, well, that can be helpful, too.

Whatever your goals are, Kristin advises you, as she does her patients, to write them down somewhere you will see them every day. You often hear the advice to write it on a Post-it note that you stick on your computer, but Post-it notes can fall off and get crumpled. She likes to write her goals and/or her why with a dry erase marker on her bathroom mirror—it will stay there until she makes a point of wiping it off.

No matter what your goal is, check in with yourself at least every other week to see how you are progressing—assess if you are indeed moving closer to your why and how you are meeting your goals. And if you realize you really haven't made any progress, you'll be able to regroup and get going again before too much time has passed.

Bonus Option: Learn More About How Your Body Interacts with Specific Nutrients

As we covered in Chapter 4, your genetics can be helpful in revealing your predispositions to certain diseases and conditions, although they are also modifiable via your diet, lifestyle, and environment thanks to the influence of epigenetics (which determines which genes are turned on and which are turned off). However, there is a field of genetic testing, known as nutrigenomics, that provides insights into how your particular genetics influence how your body reacts to specific foods and nutrients. This information can help you tailor your eating plan to your unique physical makeup.

Using a saliva sample—similar to the genetic testing offered by companies such as 23andMe and Ancestry.com—a nutrigenomics test will generally assess about seventy of your genes to look for specific variants on these genes that have been identified as having an influence on how your body interacts with food, as well as the best dietary and exercise approaches to achieve better health.

For example, a nutrigenomics report can help identify food intolerances, such as lactose or gluten; or it may look at how your body breaks down certain compounds (such as caffeine). The test can also better identify which nutrients you need to prioritize, either through food or supplementation. Your nutrigenomics report can also provide insight on what macronutrient ratio—what percentages of fat, protein, and carbs—work best for you, and whether you have a proclivity toward type 2 diabetes.

In addition to giving you helpful insights on how to structure your diet, a nutrigenomics report can be very validating. Perhaps you've read the research on the ketogenic diet, but when you've tried it, it hasn't really helped you lose weight or has made you feel sick. Your nutrigenomics report might show that you have the genotype that does better with less saturated fat. Or perhaps you've heard that drinking coffee is good for your liver, but it makes you jittery; you may discover that you have the genetic variant that makes you more sensitive to caffeine, and so you'll know that you should stick to decaffeinated or half-caffeinated if you want to keep drinking it.

In relation to liver health in particular, vitamin E has been shown in studies to help treat fatty liver when taken in large doses. But large doses of vitamin E over a long period of time have also been shown to raise the risk of cancer. A nutrigenomics report can show if you have the genetic variant associated with vitamin E and cancer or not, helping you and your health care provider decide if vitamin E supplementation is a wise course of action for you.

Of course, we do need to note that there is also the very real possibility that you'll get the report and find you don't have any of the variants that relate to diet and weight loss. While nutrigenomics *can* provide insights that help you tweak your diet to your unique physiology, it's not a guarantee that it will. But research is still in process; researchers are continually identifying new genetic variants that govern how your body interacts with nutrition. When Kristin first trained in nutrigenomics, the tests assessed seven genes. Now, a few years later, they look at over seventy of them. Nutrigenomics is the wave of the future as it helps people get personalized medicine.

If you're interested in getting a nutrigenomics test and report, you can do an online search for "nutrigenomics test" (you can also flip to the Resources section at the end of this book for a couple of specific recommendations). You'll get a lot of different results from different companies that offer different types of reports and consultations. Some will take a previous genetic testing report and give you more information about the genetic variants you may have that relate to nutrition; others offer the testing and a basic report, while still others will offer a consultation with a dietitian or nutritionist.

It's important to remember that even though the information on a nutrigenomics report can be insightful, thanks to epigenetics, it isn't set in stone. Your environment and lifestyle and eating choices can change how genes are expressed. Still, Kristin has seen patients become motivated to implement a beneficial change after seeing what is on their nutrigenomics report—such as avoiding gluten, or bumping up their exercise—and it has helped them feel better and move closer to their health goals. Sometimes knowledge really is power.

What Is the Best Choice for You?

Taking all these things that we've just covered into account, what do you sense is the best choice for you? To choose an eating plan now or to stick with Your Checklist for Change? There is no one-size-fits-all approach to health. Listen to your body, as it is trying to tell you something! This is where you get to choose what your research, your diagnosis, and your intuition tell you will fit you best.

Of course, you can and should read through each of the plans so that you can gauge what you can stick to. Let's take a deep dive into the plans so that you can do just that.

Reflections

Take a moment to reflect on these questions/prompts and write your thoughts in your notebook or journal.

Which intuitive eating principles are good for me?
What are my reasons for wanting to take better care of my liver?
What are my goals?
What is the plan that seems to make the most sense for me at this point?

part three

The Renew Your Liver Plans

chapter 7

The Modified Mediterranean Plan

Metabolic Type(s) It's Good For: Preventers (healthy and lean)

Stages:
- Prevention
- NAFLD
- NASH

Goals:
- Prevention of NAFLD
- Reversal of NAFLD or NASH
- Mitigation of NASH-fibrosis and cirrhosis

As we've mentioned, all of the eating plans that we share in this book are based on the Mediterranean diet. Why? The Mediterranean diet is just a slam dunk for your liver—it's been shown to reverse fatty liver disease in many studies.[1] The authors of a 2021 review of fourteen studies that examined the effect of the Mediterranean diet on non-alcoholic fatty liver disease concluded, "After reviewing the litera-ture, the Mediterranean diet can be considered a major step forward in NAFLD management. It promotes health by replacing saturated fats and carbohydrates and plays a direct role in eliminating NAFLD pathology."[2] It reduces inflammation, insulin resistance, triglycerides, and accumulation of liver fat.[3]

But the Mediterranean diet benefits more than the liver, because again, when you help one organ, you help all organs. This classic diet also has a body of science behind it in terms of reducing the risk of type 2 diabetes, Alzheimer's and dementia, and certain cancers. It is also demonstrated to be protective against cardiovascular disease—and remember that the most common cause of death in people with fatty liver is heart attack and stroke.

There have been so many studies on the health benefits of the Mediterranean diet, Kristin jokes with her patients that in ten years, we may be looking back at it and other popular diets and questioning why we adopted the others so widely. She believes that the Mediterranean diet, which has existed and fostered health for centuries, will stand the test of time. It is the gold standard of diets and the perfect choice if you're looking to impact and support your entire body.

The main way that our plans deviate from the Mediterranean diet is by lowering the overall carb content (to varying levels, depending on which plan you select) and upgrading the grains that you do eat so that they are more nutrient-dense. Let's talk about why we're advocating for a lower consumption of carbs first.

In the last handful of years, there have been many studies showing that moderate carb consumption lowers blood sugar and leads to better lipid management—based on the carbohydrate insulin model we covered in Chapter 4. You get the best of both worlds when you combine the Mediterranean diet with a more moderate intake of carbs (something we think of as reducing your carb intake but focusing more on upgrading the carbs that you eat—a concept we introduced earlier but will explain further in this chapter).

There have also been new products introduced in the last few years that offer typically carb-heavy favorites—such as rice and pasta—made out of more healthful ingredients—such as cauliflower and beans. These products make it a lot easier to eat more nutrient-dense, fiber-rich, and lower-carb options. As one specific example of how the Renew Your Liver plans are different, where the straight-up Mediterranean diet would suggest that you switch from white flour pasta to whole-grain pasta, we acknowledge that while that's still a good switch, if you really want to take it one step further, we recommend you switch to bean-based pasta because it's got more fiber, more protein, and fewer net carbs. Our Modified Mediterranean plan is an enjoyable, intuitive eating pattern that you can stick to over the long term. It is designed with the prevention of fatty liver in mind, but it can also be used to reverse NAFLD and NASH and to mitigate

NASH-fibrosis. If you have one of the "bad" or "ugly" stages of NAFLD, you may see faster results from the Moderate-Carb or Low-Carb plans. However, the Modified Mediterranean plan can be like an on-ramp to a different way of eating—you can start here, get comfortable, see some initial results, and then take it to the next level with one of the other plans if you like. Or it can be what you downshift into after spending a couple of months on a more carb-restrictive plan, such as the Low-Carb or Moderate-Carb plans.

If you are already carb-conscious, you may think that this plan is pretty permissive with the amount of carbs it allows. But the evidence shows that you *can* have a decent amount of carbs each day and still improve your blood sugar and insulin levels and reduce the risk or symptoms of type 2 diabetes. The standard American diet is very carb heavy, and the carbs we eat more often aren't of great quality—with a bagel for breakfast, sandwich and fries for lunch, and pasta for dinner—while this plan is more in line with healthier dietary patterns.

For some folks, jumping into a low-carb plan, or even a moderate-carb plan, can be too aggressive, especially if you've been eating a lot of carbs at most meals. Starting with the Modified Mediterranean plan will help you feel better and maybe even lose a little weight if you're carrying some extra pounds, both of which are very motivating. Best of all, you'll realize that it's not that hard or won't feel like too much of a sacrifice—you can still go out to dinner or to a barbecue and not feel like the odd person out.

The Modified Mediterranean Plan: Goals, Precautions, Benefits, and Carb Totals

Metabolic type: Preventer (healthy and lean)
Primary goals: Prevention and maintenance
Secondary goals: Reversal of NAFLD or NASH or mitigation of NASH-fibrosis or cirrhosis, in addition to better management of type 2 diabetes and reduction of risk for cardiovascular disease
Precautions: None

Benefits: Prevents fatty liver disease, type 2 diabetes, cardiovascular disease, and certain cancers; most doable and sustainable of all the plans

Carb level: About 45-50 percent of total; 130-175 grams per day, which can be almost half of your plate at each meal

Foods of the Modified Mediterranean Plan

The traditional Mediterranean diet features the following foods, which you have read about.

Plenty of (Every Day)
- Colorful fruits and vegetables, especially leafy greens and berries
- Beans and legumes
- Nuts and seeds
- Whole, preferably intact, grains
- Extra virgin olive oil
- Coffee (up to three cups per day, unsweetened)
- Green tea (up to four cups per day, although if you're also having three cups of coffee, stick to decaf green tea to keep your overall caffeine consumption moderate)

Moderate Amounts
- Fatty wild fish such as salmon, cod, or lake trout (two or three times a week)
- Lean poultry such as white meat chicken and turkey, and eggs (twice a week)
- Whole, intact grains such as quinoa and brown rice (half to three-quarters of a tennis ball at each meal)
- Dairy, up to two servings a day, preferably low fat to keep the saturated fat content down and fermented (such as yogurt or kefir) to support gut health
- Dark chocolate, one-quarter of an average-sized bar (at least 70 percent cocoa content with stevia or other natural sweetener instead of sugar) (three to five times a week)

- Red wine (no more than two five-ounce glasses per day for men and one five-ounce glass per day for women; however, cutting alcohol will benefit your liver health even further)

Small Amounts

- Lean red meat, as close to wild as you can get, such as bison, and if you're going to eat beef, grass-fed (no more than four ounces once a week)
- Sweets (the traditional Mediterranean diet says small servings and no more than three times per week)

A HEALTHY CARB YOU CAN EAT OFTEN: OATMEAL 101

As a whole grain, oatmeal is a great part of the Mediterranean diet that makes a filling and healthy breakfast. But there are a few different types of oatmeal, and some of them are better for your liver than others. There are steel-cut oats, rolled oats, quick-cook oats, and instant oats. Because they are more intact, more nutrient-dense, and higher in fiber, we recommend that you stick to steel-cut—although if you just can't get behind the texture of steel-cut, rolled oats are OK, too.

Steel-cut oats (also called Irish oatmeal) are simply oat groats that have been roasted and then cut into smaller pieces. They are the most intact version of oats that you can buy. They have the lowest amount of net carbs.

Benefits: Intact grain, fewest net carbs

Drawbacks: Take longer to cook than other forms and have a chewier texture than you may associate with oatmeal

Rolled oats (also called old-fashioned oats) are what most people typically think of when they think oatmeal—they're also what are used in most oatmeal cookies and granola bars. Rolled oats are oat groats that have been roasted, then steamed and run through a flattening machine to make them thinner than steel-cut oats.

Benefits: A good source of fiber and protein; quicker cooking, good for baking and making overnight oats (see page 254), familiar texture

Drawbacks: Slightly higher net carbs and glycemic load, more processed

For great oatmeal ideas, look in the Recipes section for **Breakfast of Champions: Five Ways to Prepare Oatmeal.**

**IF YOU PREFER CEREAL
TO OATMEAL . . .**

Sometimes, you just want some crunch with your breakfast, and you don't want to have to cook at all. In that case, stick to cereals with five grams or less of added sugars and five grams of protein and/or fiber. Often, cereals labeled "keto," such as those made by Catalina Crunch, meet these criteria. Have them with either low-fat milk (unless you're serving to a kid, then make it whole milk) or your favorite unsweetened nut or seed milk.

Meal Suggestions

We've included a list of meals and snacks—some that you pull together on your own, others that follow the recipes we've provided—for each of the plans in the back of the book, starting on page 229. For the Modified Mediterranean plan, you can also eat anything on the Moderate-Carb and Low-Carb plans, as they won't throw you off your carb targets.

What to Expect

If you've been eating a super-high-carb, processed diet you may notice that your energy levels are low for the first ten days or so. That's because your body will be making a metabolic shift from relying on an ever-present and large supply of glucose and stored glycogen and learning to regulate its blood sugar and insulin levels differently.

Even though you may be feeling fatigued, getting some movement will help burn your stored glycogen and help your body adjust to its new normal more quickly. While taking a daily walk will, paradoxically, help you have more energy, now is probably not the time to do intense workouts, which can leave you feeling more tired afterward.

A TYPICAL DAY ON THE MODIFIED MEDITERRANEAN PLAN

All the meal plans and recipes in the world won't help if you can't figure out how to fit your new style of eating into your life. Here is a "day in the life" picture of the Modified Mediterranean plan to help you envision what incorporating it into your life will look like—this is Ibrahim's typical daily schedule.

5:45 a.m.: Wakes up and drinks a glass of warm water.

6:15 a.m.: Thirty-minute workout: rotate between riding a stationary bike or running on the treadmill and lifting weights; on strength-training days he also incorporates interval training.

7:30 a.m.: Breakfast—two boiled eggs followed by a cup of fresh-brewed black coffee.

8:00 a.m.: Begins workday.

9:30 a.m.: Has a second cup of black coffee.

12:00 p.m.: Lunch—Greek salad with grilled chicken.

1:30 p.m.: Has a third cup of coffee.

3:30 p.m.: Snack—usually an orange or an apple.

6:00 p.m.: Dinner—tabbouleh with two slices of pizza (ideally cauliflower crust pizza but sometimes regular dough) and a glass of red wine. (Occasionally he adds a piece of dark chocolate for dessert.)

7:30 p.m.: Snack—small handful of cashews.

10:00 p.m.: Bedtime.

Reflect on Your Progress

Studies show that an important component of adopting a healthier diet is to check in on how well you're adhering to your nutritional guidelines and how what you are eating is making you feel. Many studies actually give their participants a scorecard to assess adherence. While we aren't going to go that far, we are taking inspiration from this evidence-based practice so that you can see how you're doing and whether you're on track.

Each week you are on the Modified Mediterranean plan, find ten minutes to ask yourself the following questions, jotting your answers down in your Regenerative Health journal or notebook or wherever you are keeping tabs on your progress. Building this habit of self-reflection and assessment will help you stick to your goals for the long term.

1. *Have I tried a new nutrient-dense food in the past week?*
2. *What's one substitution that I made this week (for example, quinoa for white rice or bean-based pasta for regular pasta)?*
3. *How many servings of deeply hued vegetables and fruits did I eat on a typical day in the past week?*
4. *How many days did I have fast food or takeout food in the past week?*
5. *How many days did I eat typical sweets in the past week?*
6. *How many days did I eat fried foods in the past week?*
7. *How many days did I consume at least two tablespoons of olive oil?*
8. *How many days did I eat seafood or fish in the past week?*
9. *How well did I do in the last week on eating whole or intact grains versus refined grains?*
10. *How much coffee and/or green tea did I have in the last week?*
11. *How many sweetened beverages (soda, juice, lemonade) did I have in the last week?*
12. *Did I take a few minutes this past week to assess how I feel mentally, emotionally, and physically after eating this way?*
13. *How many days did I work out in the past week?*
14. *Overall, on a scale of one to ten, with one being the worst and ten being the best, how well did I do on sticking to my plan this week?*

chapter 8

The Moderate-Carb Plan

Metabolic Types It's Good For: The Fine-tuner (healthy and non-lean); the Recalibrator (unhealthy and lean)

Stages:
- NAFLD
- Early-stage NASH
- NASH-fibrosis
- Cirrhosis

Goals:
- Reversal of NAFLD or NASH
- Mitigation of NASH-fibrosis and cirrhosis
- Better management of type 2 diabetes
- Prevention of NALFD with a greater focus on losing excess weight and/or reducing blood sugar levels

Many people are surprised that taking a moderate-carb approach can have big therapeutic effects on metabolic health—most people tend to think you've got to take drastic measures to see results. Another common belief is that adopting a healthier eating pattern is complicated. These are the two things Kristin's patient Brenda believed.

When Kristin and Brenda started working together, Brenda was sixty-four and fit the profile of larger-bodied yet still metabolically healthy person to a T. Yet her waist size had crept up and her total cholesterol, triglycerides, and LDL cholesterol were at the high end of the normal range. Brenda tried to eat healthfully during the day but would go on jags of eating at night. And she often found herself eating when she wasn't hungry—maybe because she felt she hadn't gotten enough protein at her earlier meal and sometimes just because food was there. She described herself as having an addiction to sugar that was as strong as the addiction she once had to cigarettes.

Brenda had gained her weight after her father had died twenty-five years earlier, when eating helped her cope with her grief, and ever since then, she'd been trying to get to a healthier place. While she was relieved to discover that her lipid profiles were still considered healthy, she could tell that her health was precarious. By now, she was experiencing knee troubles that had her on the path to a double knee replacement. And if her metabolic numbers trended upward at all, she would become vulnerable to cardiovascular disease, diabetes, and fatty liver disease. She had tried "everything under the sun," as she put it, to get healthier, including some pharmaceuticals designed to help with weight loss.

Because Brenda had a history of restricting herself from certain foods only to binge-eat them later, Kristin suggested a moderate-carb approach for Brenda so that she could still enjoy plenty of carbs and not feel deprived. Kristin also encouraged her to adopt the habit of eating only when you're hungry—which means stopping when you're no longer hungry (instead of when you're full). And the final eating strategy Brenda adopted was intermittent fasting. She began delaying her breakfast until 11:00 a.m. and then finishing dinner by 8:00 p.m. She became a fan of avocado toast (one small avocado mixed with a little lime juice and chopped red onions and cherry tomatoes on whole wheat bread) with two eggs for breakfast. This meal kept her full until midafternoon, when she'd have a small bowl of plain yogurt with frozen wild blueberries and a little bit of granola for lunch. Then she'd have soup and grilled shrimp for dinner and a piece of chocolate or a Quest bar if she wanted something sweet.

As she acclimated to her dietary changes, over time Brenda also started walking more and going to Pilates twice a week and a restorative yoga class once a week.

"Just focusing on carbs—and not calorie counting—and eating only when I was hungry made it so simple," Brenda says now. She's also experiencing significantly less pain in her knees and has reduced her sleep meds several times ("I keep having to get out the pill cutter," she reports). And her skin is clearer. The changes Brenda has made are showing up in her lab results, too. After six months, her total cholesterol and triglycerides are both down fifty points, while her LDL is down by nearly thirty points.

Brenda still has her favorite foods—she and her husband live in Florida, and they love fried grouper fingers, but they have them only once a week. And maybe best of all, she reports, "I'm not as stressed about food. If I'm doing the right thing most of the time, a slip-up isn't going to undo all of that. I know I can get back on track because I've done it before."

Easy to do, simple, forgiving, stress-reducing, and yet still powerfully impactful—these are all the reasons why we love the moderate-carb approach. Let's take a closer look and see if this plan makes sense for you.

The Basics of Our Moderate-Carb Plan

As you might expect, our Moderate-Carb plan has fewer carbs than our Modified Mediterranean plan and more than our Low-Carb plan. We designed it with two metabolic profiles in mind—the Fine-Tuner (healthy and non-lean, which was Brenda's profile), and the Recalibrator (unhealthy and lean). This plan offers a middle-of-the-road approach that is both a preventative and effective treatment for the early stages of fatty liver (NAFLD and NASH).

In addition to your stage of fatty liver disease and your metabolic profile, other factors that might point you toward the Moderate-Carb plan include the following:

- You would like to jump-start your health benefits (including improved insulin sensitivity, improved metabolic health, and losing weight, if that's a goal of yours) without having to go low carb.
- You've tried low carb and it doesn't work for you for any reason—difficulty, don't like the way it makes you feel (physically, emotionally, or energetically), not delivering the results you expect.

- You value nutrient-dense, high-fiber carbs (such as fruit, sweet potatoes, and intact grains) and don't want to severely restrict your intake of these foods simply because of their carb content.
- You already follow a mostly Mediterranean diet plan (maybe you even say, "I eat pretty healthy") and would like to take your efforts a step further and see what turning down the dial on your carb intake can do for you.
- Or really, you're just curious.

We've said it before, and we'll say it again: you can't go wrong with any of our plans. Any of them will help you love your liver. So if the middle-of-the-road approach of the Moderate-Carb plan appeals to you, that's the only reason you need to give it a try.

If doing the Modified Mediterranean plan is like taking the steps to get into the pool, and the Low-Carb plan is jumping off the diving board, the Moderate-Carb plan is hopping into the shallow end.

The Benefits of Moderate-Carb Intake

Low-carb and keto diets tend to get a lot more attention from the media and in conversations with friends than moderate-carb diets. Moderate-Carb is like the middle child of our plans—the most likely to be overlooked. But it has a strong record of research to suggest that it has better long-term health benefits than either average- (meaning, high-) carb intake or low-carb diets.

In 2018, researchers from the Harvard T. H. Chan School of Public Health tracked fifteen thousand Americans who lived in four diverse communities for twenty-five years. They found that the people who ate a moderate amount of carbs (defined in this instance as 50–55 percent of their daily calories) were less likely to die of any cause than those who ate either high-carb (70 percent or more of their caloric intake) or low-carb diets (40 percent or fewer of their calories came from carbs).[1] The researchers compared their results to several other studies of populations from around the world and found that they were aligned. And other studies have found similar benefit to a moderate-carb, or balanced-carb, approach,[2] including an Australian study[3] and a Korean one.[4]

The Harvard T. H. Chan School of Public Health study suggests that there is what's known as a U-shaped curve to the benefit of carbohydrates (Figure 8.1). Risk of mortality is high on both the low and high ends of the daily carb intake spectrum—meaning, keeping carb intake moderate appears to be the sweet spot in terms of living long and healthy. You can also think of a moderate approach like Goldilocks—not too much, not too little, but *just right.* Many things related to health have a similar, U-shaped curve of benefit, including alcohol consumption and even exercise. There truly is so much wisdom in the adage "Everything in moderation."

Why would following a low-carb diet, which has been held up as such a popular and healthy choice these last several years, put someone at a higher risk of dying? The researchers theorize that it's because the people who kept their carbs that low also ate a lot of animal protein, which has been associated with an increased risk of cardiovascular disease and cancer. And remember, the single biggest killer of people with non-alcoholic fatty liver disease isn't liver failure or liver cancer; it's heart disease. So over-relying on meat and dairy is even riskier for those with a fatty liver. The researchers also noticed that the people who ate low carb but ate vegetables, plant oils, nuts, and legumes didn't experience the same spike in mortality as those

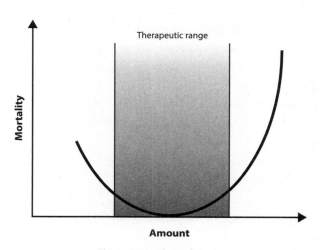

Figure 8.1. U-Shaped Curve

who replaced most of their carbs with meat and dairy. No matter what, whether you eat low carb or moderate carb, it's important to make most of your protein plant based.

Unlike a ketogenic diet, the Moderate-Carb plan—or, as we also like to think of it, a balanced-carb approach—*is* something you can stick to for a long time. After all, this Harvard study followed people for twenty-five years. Of course, you don't have to commit to it for twenty-five years! You only need to get started and take it day by day, continuing to come back to your reasons for wanting to improve your health. But it is more than just a meal plan for right now. It can be a way of life, *for* life.

A moderate-carb, plant-based approach also aligns with what's known as the Longevity diet, as studied and popularized by Dr. Valter Longo, professor of gerontology, cell biologist, and director of the Longevity Institute at the University of Southern California. Longo and his team evaluated the dietary strategies that increase life span with very few side effects in single-cell organisms and mice; population-based data; and several large, clinical diet trials. Their review of such a wide range of research led them to conclude that the diet that consistently provided the best outcomes for longevity has the following features:

- Moderate carb
- Low to moderate protein (with slightly higher protein levels for older folks, who are otherwise prone to losing muscle)
- Protein that comes primarily from fish and plants—one meta-analysis found that people who ate the most animal protein, even though they also ate low carb, had a 23 percent higher risk of dying from any cause, a 14 percent higher risk of dying from heart disease, and a 28 percent higher risk of dying from cancer.[5]

Other research-backed insights on cutting carbs to a moderate level include the following:

- **Stricter isn't necessarily better in the long run.** After two years of following overweight participants on either a low-carb or balanced-carb diet, there was little to no difference between the two approaches in terms of lost weight or cardiovascular risk factors. Even whether they had type 2 diabetes or not didn't significantly change their outcomes.[6]

· **What you replace those carbs with matters.** It's important to remember that you don't want to start eating all the steaks and bacon you want because you're "going low carb" (or even moderate carb). As we've mentioned—but it's so important that it bears repeating—you want to swap out the carbs you're currently getting from refined, un-intact grains and flours, fries, and chips and replace them with nutrient-dense foods, such as legumes, nuts, seeds, vegetables, fruit, fish, and limited amounts of animal protein (chicken, dairy, etc.).

· **Moderation cuts through the noise.** While different macronutrients have fallen in and out of favor—for example, our obsession with low fat in the 1990s morphed into a fascination with high fat (with the rise of keto) in the 2010s. A meta-analysis of studies that examined the effects of diets with varying macronutrient breakdowns led researchers to conclude, "Taking all the studies into account, the message of moderation is perhaps the most convincing one of all—diets that focus too heavily on a single macronutrient, whether extreme protein, carbohydrate, or fat intake, may adversely impact health."[7] When in doubt, stick to the middle of the road. (If you're wondering what this means for our Low-Carb approach, we'll unpack that in the next chapter.)

The Makeup of a Moderate-Carb Approach

In general, people are surprised to hear how many carbs there are in a moderate-carb diet. It's not that this plan is all that restrictive in the amount of carb-rich foods you can eat; it's more that our typical diet is so high in carbs to start with!

Particularly if you've been eating a pretty high-carb diet, the Moderate-Carb plan will likely help you see some weight loss in the first few weeks. If that's a goal of yours, this weight loss can be very motivating, as will realizing that you can live a normal life without a lot of sacrificing or advanced planning to stick to your plan. You could start here, get comfortable, then take it to the next level with the Low-Carb plan to really make some quick progress or if you start to plateau. But again, you really can't go wrong with any of our plans. There is nothing wimpy about choosing the Moderate-Carb plan! You will still be changing your palate, retraining your cravings and hunger level, and upping your nutrient density while also taking better care of your liver and your overall health.

The Moderate-Carb Plan:
Goals, Precautions, Benefits, and Carb Totals

Goals
- Reversal of NAFLD or NASH
- Mitigation of NASH-fibrosis and cirrhosis
- Better management of type 2 diabetes
- Prevention of NALFD with a greater focus on losing excess weight and/or reducing blood sugar levels

Precautions
- If you have chronic kidney disease, stage 3 or higher, or if you are taking insulin for diabetes, touch base with your physician before you reduce your carb intake. Why? Your kidneys clear insulin from the bloodstream. If you have kidney disease, your kidneys are less efficient at reducing insulin levels, meaning you have more insulin on hand. And if you reduce your carb intake, your blood sugar will naturally lessen. With the abundance of insulin on hand, your body could clear too much glucose and your blood sugar could go too low. If you take insulin for type 2 diabetes, the same thing could happen—you could experience hypoglycemia (the technical term for blood sugar that is too low).
- If you are pregnant or breastfeeding, your nutritional needs are different. Also, pregnancy can trigger gestational diabetes, so you want to have a talk with your physician before you start changing your intake of carbs in a significant way.
- If you're under eighteen, refer to the Family plan.

Benefits
- Can reverse early stages of fatty liver disease and prevent type 2 diabetes, cardiovascular disease, and certain cancers.
- Highly doable and sustainable—you can easily go out to eat or to a barbecue and stay within your carb targets (unless it's a rare occurrence and you decide to go for it—we do believe in the value of a weekly cheat meal!).

Carb Level
- Carbs should provide between 26 and 44 percent of daily calorie intake—about 100 to 130 grams per day.
- At each meal, the carbs should be roughly equal to the volume of half a tennis ball, just shy of half the food on your plate.
- It's important to note that your carbs should be spread out throughout the day—saving up all your carbs for dinner and dessert can impede your efforts to reduce insulin and encourage your liver to burn the fat it has stored.

Pillars of the Moderate-Carb Plan

The Moderate-Carb plan shares the same pillars of the Modified Mediterranean plan, which we outlined in Chapter 7. The major difference from the Modified Mediterranean plan in terms of what you put on your plate is that you're going to eat smaller servings of grains. Don't worry—you won't go hungry. Prioritizing high-fiber foods—including nuts, seeds, colorful vegetables, and richly hued fruits—to fill that empty space will help keep you happily full.

Moderate-Carb Meal and Snack Options

Refer to our list of suggested meals and snacks, starting on page 231. You can choose from anything listed under the Moderate-Carb headings, as well as from the Low-Carb plan, as those foods won't throw you off your carb targets.

A TYPICAL DAY ON A
MODERATE-CARBOHYDRATE PLAN

Kristin eats according to a Moderate-Carbohydrate plan. Here's her typical daily schedule.

5:45 a.m.: Wake up and drink an eight-ounce glass of water.

6:00 a.m.: Cup of fresh-brewed coffee with one drop liquid stevia.

6:30 a.m.: Second cup of coffee with hazelnut NutPod creamer (no sweetener in this cup).

7:00 a.m.: Take kids to school.

8:00 a.m.: Begin workday (occasionally around this time, she will have a flavored seltzer).

11:00 a.m.: Breakfast/lunch: Four slices of turkey bacon with melted cheddar cheese on a low-carb tortilla.

12:30 p.m.: Forty-five-minute workout (she alternates among stationary bike rides, outside walks, and light weightlifting).

1:45 p.m.: One more cup of coffee with a sugar-free creamer, typically with a hazelnut or cinnamon flavor.

2:00 p.m.: Handful of Savory Rosemary Cashews (they are easy to grab on the way to get her kids from school and they keep Kristin full until she gets home from kids' sports, appointments, and other after-school activities).

6:00 p.m.: Dinner: Sautéed mixed vegetables (onions, mushrooms, Brussels sprouts, and broccolini) with pre-cooked lentils and Tahini Sauce.

6:50 p.m.: Zero-sugar whipped cream in a miniature ice cream cone.

7:45 p.m.: Put the kids to bed and brew a cup of caffeine-free cinnamon tea for her husband and herself.

10:00 p.m.: Bedtime.

Throughout the day, Kristin will typically drink two to three large (forty-six-ounce) bottles of water.

Reflect on Your Progress

Each week you are on the Moderate-Carb plan, find ten minutes to ask yourself the following questions. You can write your answers in your Regenerative Health journal or notebook, or keep track of them in a spreadsheet or in the Notes app on your phone if you're more digitally inclined. Whichever method you choose, building this habit of self-reflection and assessment will help you stick to your goals for the long term.

1. *Have I tried a new nutrient-dense food in the past week?*
2. *What's one substitution that I made this week (for example, quinoa for white rice or bean-based pasta for regular pasta)?*
3. *How many servings of deeply hued vegetables and fruits did I eat on a typical day in the past week?*
4. *How many days did I have fast or takeout food in the past week?*
5. *How many days did I eat typical sweets in the past week?*
6. *How many days did I eat fried foods in the past week?*
7. *How many days did I consume at least two tablespoons of olive oil?*
8. *How many days did I eat seafood or fish in the past week?*
9. *How well did I do in the last week on eating whole or intact grains versus refined grains?*
10. *How much coffee and/or green tea did I have in the last week?*
11. *How many sweetened beverages (soda, juice, lemonade) did I have in the last week?*
12. *Did I take a few minutes this past week to assess how I feel mentally, emotionally, and physically after eating this way?*
13. *How many days did I work out in the past week?*

chapter 9

The Low-Carb Plan

Metabolic Types It's Good For: Regenerators (unhealthy and non-lean)

Stages:
- NAFLD
- NASH
- NASH-fibrosis
- Cirrhosis

Goals:
- Reversal of NASH-fibrosis
- Potential reversal and mitigation of cirrhosis
- Management or even reversal of type 2 diabetes
- Reversal of NAFLD or NASH with a greater focus on seeing results quickly
- Prevention of NAFLD
- Improving metabolic health

When Frank first came to see Ibrahim, he was grieving the death of his mother from complications related to metabolic syndrome, diabetes, and cardiovascular disease, and he was scared.

At fifty-seven, Frank felt his life had seemed great up until now. He was a successful businessman with a lot of friends in the food and beverage industry. He was a big bourbon and beer drinker who loved nothing more than hanging out in his friends' restaurants and bars, having a few drinks and eating lots of burgers and fries. One of the last things Frank's mother said to him was a request—she wanted Frank to take better care of himself so that he didn't die of the same complications she did. So although he was in a painful period of his life, he was motivated to make changes.

Keeping his promise to his mother, Frank scheduled an appointment with his primary care physician, who diagnosed Frank with NASH (although technically Frank had BASH, which stands for "both alcoholic and non-alcoholic steatohepatitis," and which is increasingly common). In other words, Frank had fatty liver disease secondary to both excessive alcohol and excessive carb intake. He was also diagnosed as having prediabetes and high cholesterol. Frank's doctor put him on cholesterol-lowering medication and was strongly suggesting medication to help prevent full-on type 2 diabetes, but together they decided to hold off to see how much of an impact Frank could make with lifestyle changes first. That's when Frank made an appointment with Ibrahim for guidance on reversing his fatty liver disease.

Although Frank was going through a hard time, in a way, his mother's dying wish was a gift because it had extra power behind it. As a result, Frank was committed to stop drinking altogether and to revamp his eating habits. Because Frank was very motivated, Ibrahim suggested a low-carb diet so that he could make a lot of progress relatively quickly.

And that is exactly what happened. Over the next year, Frank lost fifty pounds. At his follow-up visit, his blood tests came back entirely normal. His blood sugar levels and insulin levels had stabilized, and he was no longer prediabetic. Although his cholesterol was still a little on the high side, he was able to reduce his cholesterol meds by half.

Just as importantly, Frank reported that he felt more energetic than he ever had. He said that he'd been able to pour the energy into his family and his work. He'd gotten a new job and had already been promoted since his first visit with Ibrahim.

Ibrahim asked him how he'd done it, and Frank replied that he and his wife, who did most of the cooking, had adopted a low-carb diet until he'd lost the weight that he wanted to lose, which took him about five months. Then they loosened up a bit to a more moderate-carb plan. Although he's still not drinking alcohol, he is having his beloved French fries once a week.

Frank was in the perfect position to realize that he needed to do things differently in order to take better care of himself, and he was motivated to make those changes, so going low carb was a great choice for him. And it can be a great choice for you if you, too, are motivated. Let's take a look at what a low-carb plan is and who it's good for.

The Benefits of Keeping Carb Intake Low

When you cut your carb intake to about a quarter of your daily caloric intake, studies show that you lower your blood glucose levels, which in turn lowers your insulin levels. If a typical high-carb diet puts you on a blood sugar roller coaster—where glucose levels spike after every carb-heavy meal or snack and then plummet as the pancreas releases insulin, causing you to crave more carbs—following a low-carb eating plan is more like a drive through rolling hills. After a few days of acclimating to a lower carb intake, your cravings will start to diminish as you won't have such big blood sugar dips that can cue hunger and a desire for carb-heavy food.

In addition, going low carb can help you make progress more quickly than either a Moderate-Carb or Modified Mediterranean approach. That momentum can be very motivating to help you stick with a healthier eating pattern.

Other research-backed benefits of cutting carbs include the following:

- **Greater improvements in lipid profiles** such as reduced triglycerides, LDL (the "bad" cholesterol), and inflammatory markers when compared to moderate- and high-carb diets.[1]
- **A bigger reduction in diabetic medication** than diets with higher levels of carbs.[2]
- **A more significant reduction in long-term blood glucose levels and greater weight loss** than diets that get about 50 percent of daily calories from carbs.[3]
- **Increased metabolism,** which means you'll be able to burn fat better. This is especially good news in terms of your liver health,

because it means you'll be better equipped to reduce the fat that's been stored in your liver.[4]

- **Improved mental and cognitive health.** There is an undeniable link between physical and mental health—after all, it is hard to feel up emotionally if you don't feel well physically. More specifically, there is also a link between type 2 diabetes, cardiovascular disease, and fatty liver disease and mental health, as well as a connection between poor metabolic health and dementia or Alzheimer's (which is often referred to as "type 3 diabetes"). Giving your body a break from too many carbs and too much glucose and insulin can lead to improved cognitive health, including a decline in dementia and an increase in overall mental health.

Although, again, anyone will see benefits from following any of our plans, in general, we recommend a low-carb eating plan for people whose fatty liver disease has progressed to either fibrosis or cirrhosis as it provides the biggest benefit in the shortest time.

Here are some very good reasons to choose this Low-Carb plan:

- You're highly motivated, as Frank was, to make changes.
- You're a dive-off-the-diving-board type of person who likes and responds well to more dramatic changes in your habits (more so than if you were to take a gradual wade into the pool using the steps in the shallow end, which equates with adopting the Modified Mediterranean plan, or hopping into the low end, which correlates to the Moderate-Carb plan).
- You've been following a Moderate-Carb or Modified Mediterranean plan for a while, and your results have plateaued.
- Or, again, you're just curious.

Keep in mind that it is also entirely possible—and still beneficial—to start with the Low-Carb plan, reap a few benefits, establish a new way of eating, and then shift into the Moderate-Carb or Modified Mediterranean plan, as Frank did. Or you could follow the Low-Carb plan the majority of the time, and loosen the reins a bit one or two days a week to more of a Moderate-Carb or Modified Mediterranean approach.

This is how both Ibrahim and Kristin tend to eat; low carb during the week and moderate carb on the weekends.

The Low-Carb Plan:
Goals, Precautions, Benefits, and Carb Totals

Goals
- Reversal of NASH-fibrosis
- Potential reversal and mitigation of cirrhosis
- Management or even reversal of type 2 diabetes
- Reversal of NAFLD or NASH with a greater focus on seeing results quickly
- Prevention of NAFLD; improvement of metabolic health

Precautions
- If you have type 1 diabetes, or chronic kidney disease at stage 2 or higher, or if you are taking insulin for type 2 diabetes, touch base with your physician before you reduce your carb intake. (Refer to page 174 for more info on why chronic kidney disease is a consideration.)
- If you are pregnant or breastfeeding, your nutritional needs are different. Also, pregnancy can trigger gestational diabetes, so you'll want to have a talk with your physician before you start changing your intake of carbs in a significant way.
- If you're under eighteen, refer to the Family plan.

Benefits
- Greater short-term weight loss, reduced hunger, and improvement in insulin sensitivity.[5]
- Quickest results of all the plans.

Carb Level
- Between 10 and 26 percent of daily calorie intake—so anything between about 10 to 100 grams per day (less than 10 percent carbs is technically a very-low-carb, or ketogenic, diet; that is lower than we are recommending).

- At each meal, your carbs should equal roughly the same volume as one-quarter of a tennis ball, or one-quarter of your plate.

Low Carb Does Not Equal Keto

It's important to note that a low-carb meal plan is not the same thing as the ketogenic, or keto, diet. A ketogenic diet is a *very*-low-carb diet, with only 10 percent or less of daily calories coming from carbohydrates.

In addition to being very low carb, the ketogenic way of eating is typically also high fat—because it is designed to nudge your body into burning fat for fuel instead of glucose, and eating high levels of fat helps your body make that metabolic switch. Our Renew Your Liver Low-Carb plan does *not* place an emphasis on significantly boosting your fat intake. Rather, we suggest you replace the carbs that you're omitting from your diet with foods that are nutrient-dense, plant based, and primarily a blend of proteins, fats, and fiber, such as nuts, seeds, and deeply hued vegetables and fruits (the latter in moderation).

To be clear, there is nothing inherently wrong with a very-low-carb diet like keto—it is very helpful for losing weight and restoring insulin sensitivity in a relatively short timeframe. If you're highly motivated and want to focus on really getting your liver enzymes down and your metabolic health up for the next three to six months, a keto diet can absolutely be helpful. However, if you are pregnant, breastfeeding, a type 1 diabetic, or a heart failure or kidney patient, check with your physician before embarking on a ketogenic diet.

You can do the keto diet with the foods included on this low-carb eating plan, but by making sure that the carbs take up no more than about one-eighth of your plate: an amount the size of a golf ball. After a few months, you can then increase your carb intake to either a low-carb or moderate-carb approach and still maintain the majority of your benefits.

The goal of a ketogenic diet is to get your body into ketosis, or the metabolic state of burning fat for fuel instead of glucose. You may not have realized that you could burn different types of fuel—like a hybrid vehicle!—but the human body is truly amazing. Its goal is to keep you in a state of normalcy (or homeostasis). Really, it doesn't care what you feed it, or even if you don't feed it (for a short time), as it will switch to burning your fat stores in order to keep going. That being said, your body's preferred fuel is glucose because that is easily converted into glycogen (the stored form of glucose) and therefore easy to keep around. It's also easy to burn, like kindling, whereas fat requires more energy to burn, like a log.

In addition, your brain loves glucose. So when you restrict the amount of food that the body can metabolize into glucose and glycogen—basically, that means carbohydrates—the first thing your body will do is seek out any remaining droplet of glycogen left *and* try to get more by triggering the liver to form new glucose from protein. This process is called gluconeogenesis—a fancy way of saying the new formation of glucose. It will take your body several days to give up the dream of running on glucose and start burning fat. This can be a difficult time for a lot of people because the brain can't burn fat—it has to wait for your body to transform fat into ketones, which are a fatty acid by-product of the metabolization of fat.

Even once you get into ketosis, for some of our patients, we've noticed it can be a challenge to stick to the diet plan beyond just a few months. Here are a few of the downsides to the keto diet that we see:

- **It's strict.** Keto is as close to no-carb as you can get. It requires planning and attention to maintain, and it is possible that it could lead to some disordered eating. Beyond that, there is an eating disorder that has recently become so popular that it has been given a name—orthorexia, which is an unhealthy obsession with eating healthfully. People with orthorexia can cut out so many types of foods that they become malnourished. This is, of course, an extreme example, but eating disorders of all types are becoming more common and are something to be aware of.
- **It's not sustainable for everyone.** Even with all the keto-friendly products on the market, it can be challenging to avoid carbs to this level and still be able to live your life, eating out at

restaurants or other people's homes, attending celebrations—and even preparing your everyday meals.

- **It can make you feel physically worse before you feel better, and that can be a turnoff for some people.** There is a phenomenon known as the "keto flu": while your body goes through the transition from burning glucose to burning fat, you may feel tired and woozy.
- **It may lead to the consumption of too much animal protein.** Cutting out all carbs means you have a lot of calories to replace. And people often think that "keto" is the same thing as "eating bacon all day."

For all these reasons, while we are supportive of your trying a keto diet if it's calling to you (and, again, you aren't pregnant, breastfeeding, diabetic, or someone with chronic kidney disease or cardiovascular disease), we stop short of recommending the ketogenic diet as a preventive measure or dietary treatment for fatty liver disease. If you want to see results quickly and have them last a long time, we suggest starting with a low-carb (but not very-low-carb) diet.

Avoiding All Pastas, Breads, and Sugars

On the Low-Carb plan, you will want to avoid pastas, breads, and sugars entirely or as much as possible because of their carb content. There are some crackers and wraps for sandwiches you can eat, as you'll learn.

Raising Your Protein Quotient

Because a high intake of saturated fat from animal proteins is linked to a higher risk of cardiovascular disease, following a low-carb diet isn't a permission slip to load up on steak, hamburgers, and sausage. And while lean poultry and wild-caught fish are good sources of protein, thanks to the impact of animal farming on the environment and climate change, plus the health benefits of plant-based sources of protein, most of us could benefit from getting more of our protein from plants.

Plant-based cheeses, butters, and even meat substitutes such as Beyond Meat and Impossible Burgers are typically high in saturated fat (there are six grams of saturated fat in a Beyond Meat burger). And even though beans and legumes are great sources of protein that don't contain saturated fat and have a host of other health benefits, including being high in fiber, they also contain a fair amount of carbs. Chick-peas, for example, have about twenty-five grams of net carbs in a one-cup serving. So you'll want to limit your bean consumption to about one cup per day if you want to stay within the parameters of a low-carb diet.

Luckily, there are many plant-based sources of protein that are also low carb.

Low-Carb, Plant-Based Protein Sources

Food	Serving Size	Protein	Net Carb
Almonds	1/4 cup	7 grams	1.5 grams
Almond butter	2 tablespoons	7 grams	4 grams
Chia seeds	1 tablespoon	2 grams	1 gram
Edamame	1/3 cup	4.6 grams	1.5 grams
Flaxseeds	2 tablespoons	3.6 grams	0.3 grams
Hemp seeds	2 tablespoons	6.3 grams	0.2 grams
Pecans	1/4 cup	4 grams	1.3 grams
Pumpkin seeds	1/4 cup	10 grams	2.6 grams
Tempeh	1/4 cup	19.9 grams	7 grams
Tofu	3.5 ounces (about 1/4 block)	9 grams	1.5 grams
Walnuts	1/4 cup	5 grams	2.3 grams

The Secret to Low-Carb Sweet Treats

Clearly, following a low-carb plan with a goal of improving your metabolic and liver health means omitting as many added sugars as you possibly can, as sugar is both high carb and contributes to so many of the risk factors for fatty liver disease (including insulin resistance and type 2 diabetes). But that doesn't mean you can never have a traditionally sweet treat ever again. There are many sugar alternatives derived from plants that lend a sweet taste to food without the big spike in blood sugar and insulin that comes from eating traditional sugars. Refer to the Quick Guide to Healthy Sugars or Sugar Alternatives in Chapter 6 for a list of the ones we recommend—and the ones we don't.

In time, your palate can adjust to less sweet foods, and you'll appreciate the sweetness of fruits even more. Still, with fruits, you want to favor the ones that have the lowest net carbs, such as blackberries, raspberries, strawberries, watermelon, peaches, and cantaloupe.

Low-Carb Wraps

A good low-carb wrap can help you make tasty, portable foods—like a sandwich—without all the carbs found in most breads. Thanks to the popularity of the ketogenic diet, there are now loads of wraps made from a wide variety of ingredients, including seaweed, almond flour, coconut flour, and eggs. It may take some trial and error to find the low-carb wrap that you like best, as they all have different textures and flavors, but once you have your favorites, you'll be ready to make all manner of easy meals.

Below is a general guide to your options, based on the main ingredient. There are many, many more types of low-carb wraps. For any that you find in your local store, a quick read of the nutrition information will help you decide if it's worth trying. They should have about twenty net carbs or less, and the shorter and simpler the ingredient list, the better.

A Guide to Low-Carb Wraps

Wrap Type	Nutrition Info	Notes
Egg-white wraps	<1 carb per serving; high in protein and low in calories	There are several different brands, available at Walmart and Trader Joe's
Jicama wraps	1 net carb per serving (two wraps)	Available at Trader Joe's; vegan

Wrap Type	Nutrition Info	Notes
Nori wraps	1 net carb per serving	These are the seaweed wraps used in sushi rolls—they taste best after you heat them by briefly placing them in a hot pan or by holding them directly over a lit burner on your stove; vegan
Coconut wraps	4 net carbs per serving; good source of fiber	These are made with coconut flour and are as pliable as a standard flour tortilla; brands include Julian Bakery's Paleo Thins and Nuco; vegan
Cactus and corn tortillas	4 net carbs per serving	Similar to traditional corn tortillas, made lower carb with the addition of cactus (nopales); vegan
Spinach or kale wraps	9 net carbs per serving	Made by Raw Wraps, these foldable wraps are strengthened by psyllium seeds and the flavor's rounded out with apples and onions
Cauliflower tortillas and sandwich thins	10 net carbs per serving for tortillas; 2 net carbs per serving for sandwich thins	Made by Mission and Outer Aisle
Almond flour tortillas	8–17 net carbs per serving	Made by Mission and Siete; use them as tortillas or cut them into wedges, spray them with a little olive or avocado oil, and toast them (they make great chips!); vegan
Cassava flour tortillas	20 net carbs per serving	Made by Siete and La Tortilla Factory; cassava flour is high in resistant starch, which benefits gut health; vegan
Chickpea flour tortillas	22 net carbs and 5 grams of protein per serving	Made by Siete; these wraps are a little higher in net carbs but provide a decent amount of protein; vegan

Low-Carb Crackers

Crackers are a versatile food that can be a base for snacks and light meals. Most traditional crackers are high in carbs and not well-suited to a low-carb eating plan, but luckily, there are many new types of crackers that have fewer carbs. Below are a few of our favorites. Pair them with one of the many dips in our Recipes section, such as Warm Ricotta Dip, Buffalo Chicken Dip, or Baba Ganoush.

Low-Carb Cracker Options

Cracker Type	Nutrition Info	Notes
Parmesan crisps	<1 net carb per serving	Made by many different brands, including Whisps and Parm Crisps, these crunchy, salty, and savory crackers are generally nothing more than Parmesan cheese. They don't really stand up to a dip, but they are a tasty snack on their own
Flaxseed crackers	1 net carb per serving; high in fiber and rich in the omega-3 fatty acid ALA	Sold under the brand name Flackers, these hearty crackers stand up to the thickest dips and spreads; vegan
Almond flour crackers	Anywhere from 1 to 23 net carbs per serving; high in protein	Brands include Simple Mills (which also includes tapioca starch and cassava flour, bumping up the net carbs to 16 per serving), Blue Diamond (which also includes rice flour, making for a crispy cracker but also more net carbs—23 per serving), Highkey (which only has three ingredients and 1 net carb), and Fat Snax (2 net carbs per serving)
Egg white crisps	4 net carbs and 8 grams protein per serving	Sold by Quevos, these high-protein crackers include a little cassava flour, flaxseeds, and psyllium husks for structure (and fiber)
Whole-grain rye crisp breads	4–5 net carbs per serving	Made by Wasa, Ryvita, and Finn Crisp, these big, hearty crackers make a great platform for cottage cheese, hummus, tomato and mozzarella slices with a smear of your favorite pesto, and more; rye flour is lower in gluten than wheat (helpful for those seeking to eat less gluten but not appropriate if you have celiac disease), and rich in minerals including selenium and manganese; vegan
Brown rice cakes/crackers	12–23 net carbs per serving; whole grain	Rice crackers and rice cakes have been around a long time, but unless they're made with brown rice, they're not whole grain and they're pretty high in carbs. Lundberg makes a "Thin Stackers" brown rice cake that keeps net carbs to 23 per serving (which is four cakes); Quaker's rice cakes are made with whole-grain brown rice and have 7 net carbs per cake (unless you get a sweet flavor, like apple cinnamon, which contains sugar and 11 net carbs per cake); and Edward & Sons makes a traditional brown rice cracker that is 12 net carbs per serving

Cracker Type	Nutrition Info	Notes
Whole-grain, gluten-free crackers	17–18 net carbs per serving	Mary's Gone Crackers put great-tasting, whole-grain, gluten-free crackers on the map, made from a blend of brown rice, quinoa, flaxseeds, and sesame seeds; Quest also makes a low-carb, high-protein cheese cracker

Chia Pudding: The Low-Carb Version of Oatmeal and Dessert

If you've read the chapter about our Modified Mediterranean meal plan, you'll know that we are big fans of oatmeal—a whole grain (and, in the case of steel-cut oats, an intact grain) that is easy to prepare and serves as a vehicle for all kinds of healthy add-ons, including nuts, seeds, and berries. That said, oatmeal with toppings is a little heavy on the carbs for a low-carb meal plan.

Enter chia seed pudding. This sweet yet healthy dish makes a great start to your day or end to a meal (although it is filling, so if you want to have it for dessert, you might want to pair it with a lighter dinner). Chia seed pudding is endlessly customizable and also lends itself well to incorporating a lot of healthful additions, whether that's cocoa powder, strawberries, chopped walnuts, or a combination of toppings.

Chia seeds contain antioxidants, potassium, fiber, calcium, omega-3, iron, protein, and magnesium. The best health benefits come from grinding the seeds down and soaking them in liquid—they will absorb the liquid and transform it into a thick consistency. We've included several recipes for chia pudding, starting on page 309. Find your favorite or customize your own, and you will always know how to make something that fills your belly, satisfies your sweet tooth, and sticks to your food plan.

Meal and Snack Suggestions for the Low-Carb Plan

We've included a list of meal ideas and snack suggestions starting on page 235 of this book. While you're on the Low-Carb plan, it's best to stick with the things on the Low-Carb lists—foods from the suggestions for the other plans are likely to push you out of the low-carb range.

Checking in on Movement

Sometimes when Kristin's patients start on a low-carb plan, they report feeling low energy. That makes sense, especially when they've been eating a large amount of carbs every day. They simply don't have as much glucose on hand to burn for energy, and it can take the body a little while to adjust.

While you're acclimating to your new eating plan, you may want to focus on scheduling your movement sessions for the time of day when you tend to be more energetic. For many people, this is in the morning. The good news is that exercise tends to give you more energy immediately after you do it, and it also helps you sleep more soundly at night, which then gives you more energy the next day. So keep moving, even if you need to keep the intensity low while you adjust.

Reflect on Your Progress

As we mentioned earlier, studies show that an important component of adopting a healthier diet is to check in on how well you're adhering to your nutritional guidelines and how what you are eating is making you feel. We are taking inspiration from this evidence-based practice so that you can see how you're doing and whether you're on track.

Each week you are on the Low-Carb plan, find ten minutes to ask yourself the following questions. You can write your answers in this book or in a notebook—or maybe you are a spreadsheet fan and want to track your data digitally. Whichever method you choose, building this habit of self-reflection and -assessment will help you stick to your goals for the long term.

1. *Have I tried a new nutrient-dense food in the past week?*
2. *What's one substitution that I made this week (quinoa for white rice or bean-based pasta for regular pasta)?*

3. *How many servings of deeply hued vegetables and fruits did I eat on a typical day in the past week?*
4. *How many days did I have fast or takeout food in the past week?*
5. *How many days did I eat typical sweets in the past week?*
6. *How many days did I eat fried foods in the past week?*
7. *How many days did I consume at least two tablespoons of olive oil?*
8. *How many days did I eat seafood or fish in the past week?*
9. *How well did I do in the last week on eating whole or intact grains versus refined grains?*
10. *How much coffee and/or green tea did I have in the last week?*
11. *How many sweetened beverages (soda, juice, lemonade) did I have in the last week?*
12. *Did I take a few minutes this past week to assess how I feel mentally, emotionally, and physically after eating this way?*
13. *How many days did I work out in the past week?*
14. *Have I met my goals for a Low-Carb plan? Is it time to switch to the Moderate-Carb or Modified Mediterranean plan?*

chapter 10

The Family Plan

Metabolic Types It's Good For: All types
Stages:
- Prevention
- NAFLD
- NASH
- NASH-fibrosis

Goals:
- Prevent fatty liver disease
- Treat fatty liver that has been diagnosed
- Manage mood disorders such as depression and anxiety
- Model a healthy lifestyle for your children and establish good habits that can last a lifetime
- Shift attention and discussion away from a child's weight and toward better health

Many people are inspired to take better care of their liver because a family member has been diagnosed with fatty liver disease, and they want to avoid facing the same fate. Their concern makes sense, because fatty liver does have a genetic component—particularly if you are a mother and you had fatty liver or gestational diabetes during pregnancy, which puts your kids at higher risk of getting diabetes or fatty liver. But genetics is only one piece of the equation. Environment also plays a huge role in liver health and overall health.

One of the most important ways we learn about how to take care of ourselves is through our family—the types of foods we think are normal, the way we prepare them and the way we eat them, how we manage stress, and the kinds and amount of movement we get.

These ideas and habits are passed down as surely as our DNA is. Environment plays such a strong role that research shows that when dog owners have metabolic diseases, such as type 2 diabetes, their dogs are also likely to have them.[1]

Maybe it's you who has recently been told that your liver enzymes are high or that you have fatty liver disease. Maybe it's one of your parents. Or perhaps it's your child who has been told they have fatty liver disease. Whoever or whatever is inspiring you to take better care of your metabolic and liver health, it's a real opportunity for the entire family to adopt healthier habits.

You can't do much about the genetic hand that was dealt to you or that you've passed on to your children, but this Family plan helps you control what you can—your behaviors and your environment.

We wrote the Family plan with kids in mind, but it's not a kids' plan per se. It's a plan for helping you to step up as a leader in your family and be an example for your children, all while helping them learn new ways to eat and habits that will get them moving. The earlier you start your kids on healthy habits, the easier it will be to maintain them. But it's never too late to get started.

Food-wise, the focus of the Family plan is on upping nutrient density and reducing added sugars. Adding in more fruits, vegetables, nuts, seeds, beans and legumes, lean poultry, dairy, and wild fatty fish will naturally crowd out some room on their plate and in their belly for the more processed, sugary stuff.

The Family Plan:
Goals, Precautions, Benefits, and Carb Totals

Goals
- Prevent fatty liver disease if it hasn't yet been diagnosed
- Treat fatty liver that has been diagnosed
- Manage mood disorders such as depression and anxiety
- Model a healthy lifestyle for your children and establish good habits that can last a lifetime
- Shift attention and discussion away from a child's weight and toward better health

Precautions

- If you or anyone in the family is pregnant, diabetic, or has a chronic medical condition, you should check in with your doctor before starting the plan.
- This plan does *not* take into account food allergies that your child may have, such as a nut allergy or a non-celiac gluten sensitivity, so you will need to adjust the food recommendations contained in this chapter to your child's specific needs (and consult with their doctor before you start).
- While the Family plan's focus is not on restricting certain foods— it's more of a guideline on how to upgrade the foods you eat to be more supportive of metabolic health in general and liver health in particular—you do have to take care when talking about changing eating habits with kids. You don't want to label foods "good" or "bad," or monitor portion control, because you don't want to inadvertently encourage any thoughts or behaviors that could potentially blossom into disordered eating. If your child is displaying signs that could be associated with disordered eating (cutting out certain types of foods, skipping meals, or talking about their body in a way that doesn't jibe with reality, things like "I'm so fat"), put the Family plan on hold and speak with your child's physician.
- We do not recommend that kids under the age of eighteen engage in intermittent fasting. It's too restrictive for them. Also, the caloric needs and metabolism of kids are different than adults, and they typically benefit from having three meals and a snack every day.

Carb Level

When kids are involved, we really shy away from focusing on any kind of measuring of food intake, whether on the percentage of carbs—or fat or protein, for that matter—or on total calories. The focus of this plan is on being healthier, which entails:

- Increasing nutrient density
- Reducing added sugars (not including natural sugars in fruits and vegetables)

- Reducing refined grains and processed foods
- Honoring your body's signals of hunger and fullness
- Getting more movement

Who the Family Plan Is Good For

Here are some reasons for choosing the Family plan:

- You and/or another adult in your family has been diagnosed with fatty liver or metabolic syndrome and you want everyone in your household to start eating and living healthier.
- You, as a mother, were diagnosed with fatty liver or gestational diabetes when you were pregnant (studies show that children whose mothers had either of these diseases during pregnancy are more likely to develop diabetes or fatty liver than kids whose mothers did not).
- Fatty liver, type 2 diabetes, or metabolic syndrome runs in your family, and you want to avoid this same fate for yourself and/or your kids.
- You simply want to keep your family healthy.
- You and/or your children are living with depression and anxiety—there is a well-established connection between food and mood, and following this commonsense eating and lifestyle plan is also a plan for managing these very common psychiatric conditions.
- You are looking for a way to support your larger-bodied child or spouse (or both) in getting healthier without focusing on weight, and you want to do it as a family so that no one has to follow a "special diet."

This last point leads us to a very important caveat to the Family plan . . .

Focus on Health, Not on Weight

When you are gearing up to make changes to your family's eating patterns and movement habits, you want to be very careful when choosing how you talk about it with your kids. You want them to know that you're suggesting it because you want everyone in the family to be healthier, *not* because you think they or anyone else needs to lose weight. Using sensitivity around discussing weight and avoiding labeling certain foods "good" or "bad" is vital to helping your child make better decisions without mistakenly encouraging disordered thinking around food and their bodies.

A good way to approach it is to explain that the family is changing their habits so that everyone will feel better, have more energy, take better care of the liver, and reduce the risk of developing fatty liver disease (or can manage it or even reverse it if it's already present).

Talking to Kids About Health

While kids may be attached to their current way of eating, it is possible to avoid making your efforts to get healthier a negative experience for your kids. You don't want to have to tell them "no" all the time, nor do you want to try to force them to eat something or tell them that they're eating too much. Use the guidelines below to make your adoption of the Family plan a positive experience for them.

Tips for Talking to Kids About Health and Nutrition

Instead of Saying . . .	Try Saying . . .
You need to lose weight.	We are focusing on being healthier as a family so we can have more energy and feel better.
You're eating too much / you've had enough / no, you can't have more.	Are you still hungry? Let's take a little break, and then we can all have more if any of us is still hungry.
You have to eat this.	You don't have to like this new food; you just have to try it.
Don't eat that! (or) That food isn't on our diet.	That's a once-in-a-while food / eat a piece of fruit or some vegetables with it / take a walk (or go play basketball, or ride your bike) first, and if you still want it, you can have it.
No, you can't have dessert.	Let's divide this piece of dessert among everyone at the table. Then everyone can have a taste.
Slow down—it's not a race!	Dinner is a time for us to spend time together as well as to eat. Let's stay at the dinner table until everyone is finished.

Modeling the Way

Terah, a registered nurse, was inspired to take better care of her health when she was still only a teenager. At sixteen, Terah lost her dad—who was only forty-five—to complications from smoking and type 1 diabetes, which he didn't manage all that well. "Seeing how poorly he took care of himself when he really should have done a better job taught me the power of prevention," she says. Now she's the cochair of the wellness committee for the company where she works. She's also the unofficial wellness director for her husband and two kids, who fit the description of selective eaters.

Terah cites her two biggest tools in terms of getting your family to adopt healthier habits: modeling and prepping.

As someone who experiences anxiety—one panic attack felt so much like a heart attack that she called 911—Terah has noticed that her mental health improves when she's eating well and working out regularly. So she set up a simple home gym in the basement and started doing workouts with weights five days a week. It didn't take long for her kids to ask her to wait to work out until they're home from their after-school activities so they can exercise with her. Thanks to the contagiousness of seeing the people you love take better care of themselves, her husband is using the home gym regularly, too.

On the food front, Terah swears by the power of meal prepping: "When I spend an hour or two on Sundays prepping our food, there's less chaos during the week." Keeping their meals simple during the week means that Terah can precook hard-boiled eggs and chicken breasts for ready-to-go proteins, steel-cut oats for breakfasts, brown rice or quinoa for intact grains, and maybe one slow cooker meal (such as chickpea tikka masala or vegetarian chili for a meatless meal). She also chops vegetables for salads and portions fruit into little bags that her kids can grab when they want a snack. Having the building blocks of their meals pre-cooked means Terah has more time in her workdays for things like exercise, getting to bed at a decent hour, or just having time to herself to decompress after work.

In terms of getting her kids to stick to a mostly whole-food diet, Terah makes it a point to have them try dishes, even if they don't want to make a meal out of them—they are free to eat something else that she's pre-prepared. She also swears by having a rotisserie chicken around. But she uses a light touch: "I don't tell them that there's any food that's not healthy. I tell them it's OK to eat everything in moderation," she says, which is the exact approach we recommend so as not to make eating a battle, or to label any foods as "good" or "bad."

Terah's husband, who loves his chips and ice cream, took a little longer to come around. "He finally got to the point where he was like, 'I think I need new pants. Can I do what you're doing?'" Since that day, he has started eating more nutrient-dense foods and moving more. After two months, his waist size has come down to the point that it's no longer a risk factor for metabolic disease.

There are times when Terah has gotten away from eating well and exercising regularly—she admits that eating at night after the kids have gone to bed is something she struggles with, and sometimes she'll decide to take the summer off from her usual eating habits. But Terah has learned that setting up some kind of structure that holds her accountable to other people always helps. Whether it's consulting with a nutritionist, getting a step challenge going with her family members, or getting her coworkers to all commit to having two servings of a vegetable a day and offering little rewards—like a gift card—to everyone who meets their goal, she says, "Incentives, competition, and seeing other people stepping up their game is really motivating." And underneath it all, her dad's example is the biggest motivation there is. "He taught me that prevention is key—you don't need to treat something if you can prevent it." Now his example is also influencing his grandkids' habits and understanding of health.

We love Terah's story because it's a great example of how the behaviors of the adults in the household absolutely influence the behaviors of the children in the home. Science backs this up: one study that followed North Carolina families over a period of four years found that when parents modeled healthy eating behaviors, children ate more healthy foods and decreased consumption of junk foods. Of course, there's more to parenting than simply modeling—you've got to enforce some guidelines, too. This same study found that when parents enacted policies of getting regular physical activity, the kids moved more; and when they had limited access to junk foods, the kids ate less of the unhealthy stuff.[2]

Just increasing your health knowledge can help your children be healthy, too. A Swedish study found that when parents of six-year-olds were given health information then interviewed about their motivation for helping their children get healthier (the kids were also taught about healthy habits by their teachers as part of the intervention), all kids consumed fewer unhealthy foods and beverages, and those who met the clinical definition of obese also lost weight.[3]

Important Pieces of the Family Plan

While we're providing thirty days of suggested meals for the Family plan in the back of the book, we also wanted to outline the pillars of a healthier approach to eating and moving.

Not Outlawing Any Foods

No matter what they're eating, you want your kids to enjoy their food. That means turning off the TV and no screens at the table whenever possible. It also means not cutting any favorite foods completely out of their diet—whether that's a candy bar or a bacon cheeseburger—so that they don't end up craving it and binge-eating it once their willpower runs out (or they're at a friend's house or a birthday party).

Encouraging Them to Get in Touch with Their Feelings of Hunger and Fullness

There are many reasons we eat that aren't related to hunger—boredom, upset, habit, and so on. Teaching your kids to pay attention to their body's expressions of hunger can get them more attuned to when they truly need food. (The hunger scale shown in Figure 5.1 can help—encourage them to pick which level they're at before they have a snack.)

Respecting Their Bodies

This, again, is about being clear that the goal of eating better is *not* about losing weight but about taking care of your body so that it can take care of you for a long, long, long time.

Better Beverages

As you learned earlier, kids too often drink sweetened beverages. Water, seltzer, and even perhaps a little unsweetened coffee, green tea, or herbal tea (because they are so liver supportive) for kids over ten are better choices.

Share these principles with your kids, and let them see you putting them into action, too. You can model this behavior for them by saying, "I'm not going to have a snack right now because I'm just not hungry." Or, "I'm making us a healthy dinner so that we can take good care of our livers." Or, "Let's go for a bike ride and then get ice cream tonight."

FOUR STRATEGIES TO SHIFT OUT OF HABITUALLY EATING UNTIL YOU'RE STUFFED

In order to avoid saying, "You've had enough!" to your kids, try these four tactics:

- Offer more nutrient-dense foods first—such as apple slices with a nut or seed butter, or popcorn that you've seasoned with a little extra virgin olive oil and grated Parmesan cheese. The fiber, healthy fats, and protein in these foods will help kids feel their fullness. The packaged junk foods so many kids love are designed to taste so good that they drown out the cues their bodies send that it's time to stop eating.

- For those times when your kids have chips, either buy them in single-serving bags or teach them to pour the chips into a bowl instead of eating straight out of the bag.

- Have your family make their plates in the kitchen instead of setting out bowls of food, family style, on the table so second helpings will be mindful.

- Encourage kids to wait twenty minutes before having second helpings of anything; this will help give their brains a chance to hear the signals of fullness their stomach might be sending (this is great advice for adults as well).

Close the Kitchen

We don't want kids to implement intermittent fasting because it can feel restrictive, and it often doesn't jibe with school schedules (children should have something to eat before school so that they are fueled for learning and socializing). However, it's good for a child's liver to get a little bit of a break sometimes so that it doesn't become overwhelmed.

The approach we recommend with kids is to set a boundary of not eating after dinner is finished until the next morning—especially if your child has been diagnosed with any stage of fatty liver disease. This simple practice will give their liver some time off and will help dissuade the formation of a habit of late-night eating.

A tactic Kristin uses in her own household, and shares with patients, is to tell the kids "the kitchen is closed" once you have cleared the dinner plates. That means no more cooking—if they're truly hungry before bed, go for something with fiber in it, like an apple with peanut butter or a piece of whole-grain toast with almond butter instead of something high glycemic, like ice cream. It's a good practice for the whole family.

Get Enough of These Specific Liver-Friendly Nutrients

While the Family plan aims to be nutrient-dense, there are two specific nutrients that you want to ensure you and your family are eating plenty of. They are:

- **Omega-3 fatty acids.** These essential fatty acids—meaning, your body requires them but can't make them on its own—help your liver in three ways: they aid in the reversal of later stages of fatty liver disease; they assist in reducing inflammation in the liver; and they lower levels of triglycerides, high levels of which are a risk factor for fatty liver.
  Good sources of omega-3s include wild fatty fish—such as salmon—walnuts, chia seeds, hemp seed, and flaxseeds.
- **Vitamin E** is anti-inflammatory and an antioxidant, and it helps improve insulin resistance. Studies also show that it helps reduce the amount of fat in the liver. The only hitch is that these studies

used large doses of vitamin E, and over the long term, high-dose vitamin E supplementation has been associated with a higher risk of all-cause mortality and prostate cancer in adults.[4] (Research suggests that a variant of the gene catechol-O-methyltransferase, or COMT, may influence how beneficial vitamin E supplementation is as well as whether it will increase or reduce cancer risk—this is the type of information you can get from a nutrigenomics report, as discussed at the end of Chapter 6.)[5]

Good sources of vitamin E include almonds (including almond butter), sunflower seeds (including sunflower butter), avocado, and peanut butter.

With kids, we recommend getting nutrients from food instead of supplements. That said, your child may not touch fatty fish, nuts, or seeds, in which case you might want to think about supplements. But the decision to supplement should come as a result of a conversation with your child's doctor as they have insight into the full spectrum of your child's health, including the results of their blood work, and can also recommend proper dosages for your child.

Family Meals

If you don't already have a habit of eating together as a family, let your dedication to eating healthier be your inspiration for starting one. Even if your schedules are busy enough that you can only eat together once a week, it still counts.

Eating together as a family is important for many reasons:

- It's a prime way that you model healthy eating habits to your kids and teaches them social skills.
- It fosters communication among family members—you learn more about what's going on with everyone, and if there's anything that's bothering someone, being able to talk about it helps everyone feel better emotionally.
- Research found a laundry list of benefits to family meals—kids whose families eat together regularly have been found to have higher self-esteem, academic success, and mental resilience, and

less depression, substance abuse, disordered eating, violent behavior, and suicidal thinking.[6] This doesn't mean that if you can't make family meals happen every night due to an inflexible job/work schedule or other non-negotiables, you are a bad parent! Do the best you can and follow our other suggestions to help your kids on their healthy path.

It's important to note that a study in 2020 involving more than 250 adults found that family meals were more likely to happen when family members weren't discouraging about making healthy eating choices and when communications in general were high. It also found that family meals were more likely when children were younger—so while family meals are helpful no matter how old your children are, this research suggests that starting when kids are little will make establishing the habit a little easier.[7] (But if your kids are older, remember that parental guidelines are helpful and make it a non-negotiable at least once a week!)

Move More

Just as you don't want to use the phrase "lose weight," you also want to avoid the word "workout"—you don't want kids to feel like they need to burn calories. This is just about them being up, moving around, blowing off steam, and having fun. Movement can also be a great way to spend time together as a family. Keep homing in on what they—and you—enjoy doing, and encourage them to get movement so it won't feel like a fight. Again, you're not exercising to lose weight; your goal is to help build lifelong skills, habits—and, yes, memories—for your kids so that they will always view physical activity not as a chore but as something they love.

- The pediatric team in Ibrahim's office counsels their patients to do at least twenty minutes of brisk walking every day. That's a pretty low bar and doable for most. Those twenty minutes can be broken up into two ten-minute periods—such as to and from the bus stop.

- Whenever Kristin's kids are fighting, she transitions them toward a family walk. She says that some weeks it feels like they are taking a family walk every night!
- Kids are very similar to adults in that they will be engaged by things they actually enjoy. You may wish your child were a rising tennis star, but they love playing kickball. Get a kickball and some bases and play with them at the park or in the backyard.
- If they want to go somewhere—to get ice cream, to the playground, to the toy store, even the gas station to buy junk food—say it's fine, as long as we walk or ride bikes there.
- Plan family trips that have activity built in, such as hiking in a national park, walking most of the day at an amusement park, or visiting a city where you walk everywhere.
- As Terah suggested, start a friendly family competition with your kids. Get everyone a pedometer (or Fitbit, or Apple watch, depending on your budget), and whoever has the most steps in a day, week, or month gets a prize.
- If your child loves video games, find games that build in a lot of movement, whether it's Just Dance, virtual reality boxing, or Wii tennis.
- If at all possible, let your kids walk to and from school instead of giving them rides or taking the bus. Building movement into their daily routine is the best way to ensure that it happens automatically.
- A family dog is a great (and non-negotiable) reason to go out on walks every day; you can also take them to the woods or the dog park on weekends. Let the kids bring a friend along on these outings to make them even more enjoyable.
- If your kid is a sports kid, team sports are a great option. There are also disciplines like martial arts and yoga that they may enjoy. A lot of kids whose parents Kristin works with aren't into sports but really embrace track and field, swimming, or dance. If they don't like the first experience they have with organized physical activity, keep trying—there is likely something that will stick.

What to Look for When Buying Kid-Friendly Foods

With school lunches and after-school snacks, it's convenient to have packaged foods on hand. If your child has a favorite snack, they don't have to give it up completely—just give them healthier options most of the time and they can have the candy, doughnut, sugary cereal, or whatever their favorite packaged snack food is on Saturday.

In general, you want to avoid foods geared toward kids that claim to be low calorie (there's probably something artificial in there to make up for the lost flavor of reducing the number of calories). And pay more attention to the nutrition label and ingredient list on the back of the package than the marketing claims on the front, as those claims can be confusing and are more aimed at getting you to buy than in truly supporting health. For example, Kristin recently took her son with her to Target, where he saw a package of juice boxes that advertised, "Now with 25 percent less sugar than soda." He got so excited and said, "Can we get it? Can we get it?" But the juice still had way too much sugar! (About thirty grams per serving.) For this reason, although it's helpful to give kids a voice in what they get to eat, it can be better to go to the grocery store on your own. Food manufacturers spend a lot of money to get their products placed at a kid's eye level, and your kids won't have the knowledge that you do about what's truly healthy and what only sounds like a healthier choice.

If you do want to or end up taking your kids to the store with you, take them to the produce department and tell them to pick out foods in five different colors, and explain that in the inner aisles of the store you're going to stick to what's on your grocery list.

Getting Kids to Try New Foods

It's entirely possible that you have all the best intentions of changing the way your family eats, and your kid will want none of it. Selective eaters are a real thing, and it can be challenging to get some kids to expand their repertoire.

In general, the more you can engage your kids in the process, the more ownership they'll feel, and the more likely they'll be to try new foods. Here are a few ideas to get them to open up to broadening their food choices:

- Show them three recipes and ask them to choose their favorite to try.
- Get them to help you cook (in an age-appropriate way, of course).
- Watch some cooking competition shows together and talk about the recipes and ingredients.
- Offer to make a video of your child cooking something, whether from a recipe or by giving them a few ingredients and challenging them to make something.
- Reward them for trying new foods. Kristin found a helpful toy that is a little like an advent calendar crossed with a carnival game: it's a wheel divided into little compartments. Every time her kids try a new food, she has her boys spin the wheel to determine which compartment they get to open to reveal a little treat, like a few chocolate chips or a piece of paper that says they get to pick the next show that they watch together. She says, "I know they will grow out of it, probably sooner than I'd like, but for now it motivates them to try things that might otherwise get them to turn up their noses. And you don't need an actual toy to make this work—you could write up a few rewards on pieces of paper to keep in a jar and then let your child choose one each time they try something different."
- When you serve something new, don't make them eat all of it; just ask that they try it. You may need to serve something new three or more times before they actually eat more than a bite, so don't give up too soon.
- If a wholesale switch to some of these healthier options doesn't fly with your kids, try mixing their usual food with the new, healthier option. For example:

  - Serve a mix of half white rice and half brown, or try a mix of half cauliflower rice and half white rice.
  - Blend a bean-based or whole-grain pasta with regular pasta.

- Pair something super healthy—like zucchini noodles with Red Sauce—with something delicious and more familiar, like whole-grain garlic bread.

We're not asking you to be sneaky or try to hide the healthier foods—unless you know that's the only way your child will eat them. It's better to get their buy-in.

Nutrient-Dense Desserts

While there's no food that is absolutely off the table (metaphorically and literally) forevermore, there are certain foods you want to have only occasionally. In Ibrahim's practice, the pediatric team advises parents that kids only have a classic dessert, like cookies or ice cream, once or twice a week.

When the family is going to have a traditional dessert, try to have everyone get some extra movement either during that day or the next morning. On other days, try these nutrient-dense desserts when you want something sweet after dinner:

- Berries and whipped cream
- One-ingredient sorbet (blend two cups partially thawed frozen blueberries or two frozen bananas until smooth)
- Melted dark chocolate and strawberries
- A piece of fruit, such as an apple, pear, clementine, or kiwi
- Fruit kabobs
- Watermelon chunks (you might try tossing them with lime juice and chopped mint)
- A square or two of dark chocolate

Try our recipes for sweet treats:

- Peanut Butter Chocolate "Chaffles" (page 252)
- Peanut Butter Mousse (page 308)
- Apple Crisp (page 304)
- Protein-Powered Cookie Cream (page 305)
- Low-Carb Peanut Butter Cups (page 306)

- Miraculous Chocolate Chip Cookies (page 307)
- Any of our chia puddings (see pages 309-311)

Meal and Snack Suggestions

We've included a list of meal ideas and snack suggestions for the Family plan starting on page 241. You can also choose options from the Modified Mediterranean and Moderate-Carb plans, but take care when selecting from the list of Low-Carb plan meals and snacks. Kids don't need to be eating cauliflower buns, for example, and they need plenty of carbs. Stick to the options from the Low-Carb list that are whole foods, or recipes made from whole foods, and choose mainly from Modified Mediterranean and Moderate-Carb.

Reflect on Your Progress

Thinking about how you're doing in your efforts to create healthier habits will help you stay on track, pinpoint where you may need to place more focus, and celebrate your successes.

Each week you are following the Family plan, answer the following questions. You can even start a weekly family ritual for talking together about your efforts. You can write your answers to these questions in this book, or in a notebook—or maybe you are a spreadsheet fan and want to track your data digitally. Whichever method you choose, building this habit of self-reflection and -assessment will help you stick to your goals for the long term.

1. *What's one new nutrient-dense food everyone in the family has tried in the past week? Did you like it? Are you open to trying it again even if it wasn't your favorite the first time out?*
2. *How many servings of deeply hued vegetables and fruits did everyone eat on a typical day in the past week?*
3. *How many days did everyone have fast or takeout food in the past week?*
4. *How many days did everyone eat typical sweets in the past week?*
5. *How many days did everyone eat fried foods in the past week?*

6. *How many times did you eat salmon, oysters, or other fatty fish, or walnuts, chia seeds, hemp seeds, or flaxseeds in the past week?*
7. *What whole or intact grains did everyone eat this week?*
8. *How many sweetened beverages (soda, juice, lemonade) did everyone have in the last week?*
9. *Did we take a few minutes this past week to assess how everyone is feeling—mentally, emotionally, and physically?*
10. *How many days did everyone move for at least twenty minutes this past week?*
11. *How many days did you eat a meal together as a family this week?*

chapter 11

Love Your Liver for Life: Moving Between Plans

A S STATED BEFORE, we've designed the plans in this book to be flexible. You may start with the Low-Carb plan and then down-shift into the Modified Mediterranean plan, which may be more doable over the long term. Or you may start with the Modified Mediterranean plan, get the hang of eating differently, and then decide to move into a Moderate-Carb or Low-Carb plan to take your efforts further. Or you may start on the Family plan but then switch to Low-Carb when the kids are at their dad's, visiting relatives, or off to camp or college. Whatever your reasoning, you don't have to stick with one plan for-ever and ever, amen.

That being said, it's really helpful to be clear on a few things before you make a change from one plan to another (feel free to reflect on these and take notes in your journal):

- **Why you're switching things up.** Do you need to relax your focus on eating? Or do you need to get more mindful about it? Did your circumstances change? Did your goals change? Are you bored with the meal and snack options? Did you or your doctor notice that your liver enzymes have increased compared to prior years, which might warrant a different dietary approach?
- **What worked well in your previous plan that you want to con-tinue.** It's always important to celebrate your successes—it helps reinforce the behaviors and habits that contributed to them. Also, when something works for you, you want to stick with it. As the saying goes—if it ain't broke, don't fix it. Maybe there were reci-pes you loved or a concept that really spoke to you. Keep the good parts with you in your new approach.

- **What didn't work so well.** This is where your brain will likely want to focus—the pieces of your previous plan that you didn't stick to or the parts that were hard. These could also be the aspects of the plan that lessened your joy—maybe you missed the pasta dish at your favorite takeout place, for example. We all have the things that we didn't do so well and the things that we miss. By acknowledging them, you can figure out what you need to change in your new approach. If you're on a plan that will help your liver, but it's not helping your mental health, it's not the right plan.

Addressing these points will help you personalize the plan for you, your goals, and your specific situation.

Making a Successful Shift into Maintenance Mode

The truth is, getting healthy is much different than staying healthy. In fact, maintaining the benefits of any new diet and lifestyle program is unlikely: studies show that only about 10 percent of people are able to maintain weight loss for longer than a couple of years. It's yet another reason to shift your focus from losing weight to developing healthy habits.

And should you ever feel like you fell off the wagon and erased all your benefits, keep in mind that the health improvements you achieved when you were following a Renew Your Liver plan were still beneficial; you gave your liver a break. Even if you fall back into old habits, you don't totally erase those benefits or negate the fact that you gave your liver a chance to regenerate. If you relapse—or rather, when you relapse—just start again.

Of course, that doesn't mean you shouldn't do what you can to stay on track with your healthy habits. Below is a list of tactics that we've seen help patients in our own practices, which studies have determined are typically used by people who maintain positive changes in their metabolic health.[1] We have divided them into practices (the practical strategies that keep you on track) and mindsets (the thoughts and beliefs that can make sticking to those habits easier or harder).

Practices

- **Track your food intake.** Keeping a food diary is a common strategy of people who maintain their health benefits after making a change to their diet and lifestyle.
- **Get moving.** An exercise routine is key for helping you maintain your new level of metabolic health. Keep moving in a way you enjoy and it will become a valued part of your life—and not just one more obligation to complete. Go on solo walks or swim laps if you need solitude, or team up with friends to play pickleball or go dancing to give yourself a social outlet. It's not about burning calories; it's about having fun and protecting your health.
- **Keep shopping and storing foods strategically.** It's so much easier to eat what you see when you open your fridge, so keep buying fruits and vegetables and storing them front and center. That also means continuing to *not* buy the highly processed, hyperpalatable foods that are too easy to eat too much of, and if you do bring them into the house, keep them relatively inaccessible and out of sight. There's an old joke about the "seafood diet," which means "if I see it, I eat it." It's silly, but it's also true, as we eat with our eyes first. Put that truth to good use by keeping beautiful healthy foods on hand and in view.
- **Measure your waist.** If not literally, then try on a piece of clothing that buttons at your waist at least weekly, which makes it easier to determine when you need to be more mindful of how what you are doing is affecting your waistline. Awareness is a powerful tool that helps you know what you need at this moment.
- **Tell someone you're struggling.** If you're finding it challenging to stick to your plan, tell someone who wants the best for you and believes in you. Just saying out loud how you're feeling and the specific things that you feel are difficult to do or achieve can help to ease your mind and let you see things more clearly.

Mindset

- **Love and accept yourself now.** Don't wait until you reach a goal to feel good about yourself. Start with a sense of self-worth and compassion. As Ibrahim likes to say, "What's on your mind is as important as what's on your plate." Beating yourself up is not helpful; it's demotivating. Eating healthier and moving more is something you do for yourself because you're valuable and you're worth taking care of. Make transformation a positive process, not a punitive one.

· **Trust that it will get easier over time.** Many of the people who have been able to maintain their improvements in health report that, with time and practice, ignoring cravings and sticking with their positive habits became less effortful. That doesn't mean they will require *no* effort—just that they will become part of your routine.

· **Remember—everything in moderation.** Maybe you've been too restrictive with your eating and now you're rebelling against that restriction. Giving yourself some grace can help you to not be too hard on yourself. Perfection is not realistic and can be self-defeating. Those who successfully maintain their new habits know there will be lapses. But they also know they can recover from lapses and how to get back on track.

· **Remind yourself of your progress.** It's easy for the human brain to focus on what it perceives to be failures. It's part of our negativity bias, which means we tend to pay more attention to what goes wrong than what goes right. To counteract the negativity bias, make it a practice to remind yourself of the ground you've gained. You might look at numbers-based successes, such as improved lab results, inches lost, or average number of steps you take. Or you might think of more subjective successes, such as recalling how you used to feel before you started taking better care of your health compared with how you feel now, or what you are able to do now that you weren't able to do then. Research suggests that once you are well into a journey toward change, thinking about how far you've come and why you don't want to revert back to the way things were can be more motivational than visualizing success. The latter is typically more motivating at the start of the process of change.[2]

Things to Keep an Eye on for Maintenance

As you continue on in maintenance mode, you want to stay mindful of how you are doing in terms of your health. Most of us rely on two things: the scale and our annual physical. For too long, we've tried to determine the success of our efforts to get healthier in pounds lost, but now you have learned that weight loss doesn't necessarily mean improved liver health. And while checkups are important opportunities to pinpoint issues, you don't have to wait for your once-a-year appointment to come around. Here are other things to keep your eye on to determine if your current eating plan and movement habits are keeping you in a healthy zone or if perhaps you need to recommit yourself to making positive changes:

- **Blood test results.** You can check trends in your blood work at your annual checkup or perhaps your six-month check-in (which your doctor is likely to recommend if you have already been diagnosed with fatty liver). The test results you want to monitor are liver enzymes, blood pressure, fasting glucose, HBA1C, total cholesterol, HDL cholesterol, LDL cholesterol, and triglycerides.
- **Physical fitness.** Can you keep up the same level of activity you were doing when you were really in the swing of things? Have you noticed that you don't have the energy for brisk walks or your favorite physical activity?
- **Mood.** Reverting to old habits can be a sign of depression or anxiety; if you've been feeling down or worried, talk to your doctor or therapist.
- **Waist size.** Are you able to button your pants?
- **Energy level.** Healthier habits tend to lead to more energy—generally speaking, tiredness indicates that you need to take a little bit better care of yourself.
- **Your refrigerator and pantry.** At the beginning of any new eating plan, your fridge is probably overflowing with plant foods and your pantry is filled with cans of beans, nuts, seeds, and nutrient-dense alternative pastas. Is your fridge still bursting with colors of all the different plants, or do you only have some wilted kale from two weeks ago? When you open your pantry, do you see mostly chips and cookies?
- **Your "non-negotiables" frequency.** Everyone has foods they're not willing to give up for the rest of their lives—Kristin refers to them as "non-negotiables" with her clients. While you don't have

to avoid them forever, you do want to make sure they're not sneaking back into a heavy rotation. So ask yourself, How often are you having dessert? Eating out or ordering takeout? How many times a week are you eating junk food or high-carb foods like bread?

· **Your alcohol intake.** Has your consumption of alcoholic beverages crept up again?

If you notice any trends in a negative direction, you'll know it's time to recommit to one of the plans in this book and to do what it takes to start moving the needle in a positive direction again.

Expect the Unexpected

At some point, everyone's life goes a little sideways—you get sick or your loved ones get sick and you need to care for them, you move homes, or you go through an exceptionally busy time at work. It could even be great news that throws a kink in your dedication to taking better care of yourself—you could go on vacation, get married, have a baby, or become a grandparent.

It's not a question of *if* something will come along to knock you off your healthy habits; it's a question of *when.* And it could be something as small as the grocery store being out of the vegetable you planned to buy and use for that week's meals.

When you encounter a disruption in your routine, these strategies can help:

· **Admit that stumbling blocks will happen.** Researchers at Penn State found that when people faced setbacks, it lessened their commitment to pursuing a goal. The good news is that anticipating setbacks has the very real potential to help you not get sidetracked in your resolve. It takes away the element of surprise, which makes a challenge less of an emotional event. Then, you can remind yourself to find a substitution instead of taking it as a sign to quit.[3]

- **Find and accept support.** It may mean you sign up for a meal delivery service for a little while, or ask a friend to organize a meal train for you, or you think up something that would help when someone offers to assist you instead of saying, "No thanks, I'm OK."
- **Do what you can, even if it doesn't feel like much.** If you don't have the energy to go on runs or long walks, walk around the block instead. If you need the convenience of living on frozen foods for a while, remember to also buy some frozen vegetables that you can throw in the oven alongside your frozen dinner.
- **Don't be too hard on yourself.** It's OK to take a break. We're all going to face unplanned situations, and you're never going to be perfect all the time. Take it easy on yourself, and let go of any shame or guilt.
- **Get back to it as you can.** Most routine-altering situations are short-lived, and you can get back to healthy living in a couple of weeks or months. Just keep reminding yourself that the break you give yourself is temporary. Maybe you need to gradually get back to limiting your carbs, upping your nutrient density, and reducing your added sugars, but every step counts.
- **Revisit your why.** Remind yourself of why you wanted to take this journey in the first place. This will help you find your motivation again.

Choosing Meal Delivery Services and Frozen Meals

There are times in everyone's life when cooking can feel like one task too many. During those periods, frozen meals and meal delivery services can help you stay (mostly) true to your chosen plan.

When buying frozen meals, look for:

- Fewer than 450 milligrams of sodium
- At least three grams of fiber (more is better)
- Fewer than four grams of saturated fat
- Ingredients you can recognize and pronounce

When choosing a meal delivery service:

- Review a few weeks of sample menus, if possible (they generally make these available on their website and/or app). You want to make sure that they sound appealing to you and that they contain nutrient-dense ingredients.
- Check the prices before you sign up for anything and make sure they are in line with your budget.
- Read a few reviews to see how easy the meals are to prepare—will you be doing the cooking? Or will you be mostly reheating? Find one that's a match for your available time and energy.
- Read what the company has to say about the quality of their ingredients—do they use mostly or all organic ingredients?
- If you have any dietary restrictions, such as needing to eat gluten-free, low-sodium, vegan, or vegetarian foods, make sure the delivery service provides options suitable for your needs.

Taking Your Homemade Meals to Go

Whether you need to pack in a pinch to head to the office, or you need something practical that carries well throughout your day, try some of these meal ideas to help keep you on track with ease. A few supplies will make it easy: a bento box (segmented lunch box), a large Mason jar with a lid, and/or an insulated lunch box.

Bento Box Lunches

Keep your meal nutritionally balanced and think packable foods like fruits, chopped veggies, dips, nuts, seeds, wraps, sandwiches, salads, and sushi. The following meals lend themselves well to a bento box:

- Taco salad
- Greek salad and hard-boiled eggs
- Tuna salad sandwich and melon
- Low-carb wrap sandwich pinwheels, veggies, and dip
- Chicken, wild rice, veggies, and salsa

Mason Jar Meals

Preparing Mason jar meals is as simple as grabbing your favorite ingredients and layering!

- Layer 1: Salad dressing first, at the bottom
- Layer 2: Hard veggies (carrots, peppers, celery)
- Layer 3: Cooked fish or poultry
- Layer 4: Eggs, beans, and/or cheeses
- Layer 5: Soft veggies (cucumbers, roasted red peppers) and berries
- Layer 6: Greens (romaine, kale, spinach)
- Layer 7: Nuts, seeds, sprouts

Tips for Eating Out

Remember, a primary goal of ours when we developed these meal plans was to make them a doable and sustainable part of your life. For that reason, you can absolutely eat out at a restaurant or order takeout and still take good care of your liver, no matter which plan you are on.

In general, you'll want to keep these principles in mind:

- **Focus on lean protein and vegetables.** Sautéed chicken with a side of broccoli, or a piece of fish with the vegetable of the day, or a salad with grilled scallops, shrimp, or salmon on top are all ways to stay low carb and enjoy letting the professional do the work and perfect the flavors. You also probably want to steer clear of big plates of pasta, as there's really no way that's not going to turn into a carb fest. Nearly all restaurants these days provide ways to customize their meals to be healthier—you can get a burger on a bed of lettuce at Five Guys, for example.
- **Be sauce savvy.** For the most part, you want to either opt for something that's not doused in sauce (like the orange chicken at your favorite Chinese restaurant—it's loaded with sugar) or ask for the sauce on the side so that you can decide how much of it you'll eat.

- **Go easy on the other kind of sauce.** If you have a drink before dinner and wine with your meal, it will not only add more calories but also inhibit your ability to make healthy choices. Place your order for appetizers or entrees first, *before* ordering your drink; that way, you'll be able to put something in your stomach to counter the effects of alcohol. Restaurants want to get a drink in your hand as soon as possible because they know it means you'll be more likely to order more drinks—and more food—later.
- **Consider the preparation, not just the main ingredient.** Many restaurants have delicious Brussels sprouts or cauliflower appetizers. But if the cauliflower is breaded, deep-fried, and then smothered in a sticky (and therefore, sweet) sauce, it's really not doing you much good. If these types of appetizers are a once-a-week-or-less delicious indulgence for you, great—order them and enjoy them. But if you're thinking that you're sticking to your plan with these options, look for something roasted, sautéed, or grilled instead.
- **Choose colorful options.** For example, if you're picking up food from Chipotle, go easy on the rice, opt for a bowl instead of a burrito, and then focus on the foods that have the most color—the fajita vegetables, the guacamole, the salsa, and the black beans.
- **Order from the sides menu.** The list of appetizers or sides often has the most basic, yet still delicious, options in manageable portion sizes. For example, you might order a side of salmon with a side of broccoli.
- **Stay mindful.** You still want to take your time, chew your food well, and savor the experience of eating.

All that being said, if you only go out to dinner once or twice a month, enjoy yourself! One night out is not going to throw you into cirrhosis. What's problematic is when one big night out starts happening most nights.

Ibrahim's tip: I typically go out to dinner on Fridays as a way to honor the end of the workweek. Because I stick to a Modified Mediterranean plan throughout the week, I have wine and dessert when I'm out to eat. But as I'm sitting at the dinner table, I use my phone to sign up for a workout class the next day. (I do it when my girlfriend is using the restroom—no one wants to eat with someone who is on their phone!) That's a good rule of thumb: any time you mindfully choose to stray from your plan, put something on your schedule that will boost your physical activity the next day. It will help your liver burn up the extra glucose instead of storing it as fat.

Liver-Friendly Options at Different Types of Restaurants

Italian
Chicken marsala
Chicken or turkey meatballs with marinara sauce
Arugula salad with grilled protein of choice

Japanese
Brown-rice rolls
Rice-free rolls
Cucumber-wrapped rolls
Sashimi
Chicken yakitori
Miso soup
Seaweed salad

Mexican
Chicken fajitas
Ceviche
Guacamole
Grilled chicken, fish, or tofu with beans and salsa

Chinese
Stir-fry with vegetables and your protein of choice, with brown rice
(be mindful of portion size)
Soup (hot and sour, wonton)

Thai
Stir-fry with vegetables and your protein of choice, with brown rice
(be mindful of portion size)

Chicken satay
Green papaya salad
Soup (tom kha gai)

Vietnamese
Stir-fry with vegetables and your protein of choice, with brown rice
(be mindful of portion size)
Soup (pho)

One Year of Monthly Challenges

While, yes, we do want you to love your liver for life and establish new habits of moving, eating, and making time for relaxation for the long term, there is also something really motivating about a short-term goal. Inspired by the wellness committee at Minnesota Gastroenterology, where Ibrahim works, we've put together twelve different challenges that can help you systematically address the many areas that support your liver health.

You might find it easier to stick to new liver-friendly habits if you team up with a friend (or friends) to meet a challenge for one month and share results with each other. Or your community group, church group, or coworkers or neighbors might be interested in doing one of these monthlong challenges with you.

1. **Eat the rainbow challenge.** Aim to eat as many differently colored vegetables and fruits as you can each day—or even at each meal.
2. **Step challenge.** Get a little friendly competition going with a few others to see who can rack up the most steps in a month's time. Alternatively, you can use apps like The Conqueror or Challenge Hound, which let you see how far ahead or behind you are from your fellow challengers.
3. **Ditch the dining out challenge.** Can you go a full thirty days without visiting a restaurant or ordering takeout? Trying to do so can save you money, help you eat healthier, and force you to get better about preparing something at home, even when you really don't feel like it.

4. **Eat climate-friendly challenge.** In general, eating a plant-based diet is better for the Earth than eating animal-derived foods, such as meat and dairy. On the plant front, beans are some of the most climate-friendly and nutrient-dense (and cheap!) foods you can eat, followed closely by root vegetables (which keep for a longer time, reducing food waste), whole grains, seeds, and nuts that require little water to grow, such as pistachios, pecans, and hazelnuts. You can aim, for a month, to avoid beef and lamb, which require a lot of land to raise, and if you eat meat, stick to poultry and shellfish, which have a smaller carbon footprint than other forms of animal protein. Look for Fair Trade, shade-grown, or Rainforest Alliance certifications on your chocolate and coffee.

5. **Lose the booze challenge.** Give your liver a break by avoiding alcohol for a month—whether that's a dry January, dry July, sober October, or any thirty-day spread that makes sense for your schedule. It's a great opportunity to find new ways to take the edge off.

6. **Mindful eating challenge.** Aim to eat at least one meal a day while creating the conditions for being able to savor the experience of feeding yourself—actually sit down at a table (not in front of your computer), turn the TV off, keep the phone away, and put your fork down between each bite.

7. **Get more sleep challenge.** You can't necessarily will yourself to sleep more, but you can *allow* for at least seven hours of sleep a night by getting to bed earlier. Even twenty minutes earlier can make a big difference in how much sleep you get.

8. **Declutter your kitchen challenge.** Spend some time each week purging one area of your kitchen—your pantry, the fridge, your cabinets, and any places you store food.

9. **Reduce screen time challenge.** The average person spends four hours a day on their phones, which adds up to sixty days a year! The more time we spend looking at phones, tablets, and computers, the less time we are moving, talking to people, or giving our brains some much-needed quiet time. For guidance on doing a short-term screen-time challenge, visit screenlifebalance.com.

10. **No dessert challenge.** Having dessert after dinner can become an ingrained habit as your taste buds get trained to have

something sweet in order for you to feel full. You don't have to give up all sweet things for a month, but break the habit of ending your evening meal with dessert. (And if you truly need something sweet, opt for berries!)

11. **Relaxation challenge.** We understand that challenging yourself to relax is a bit of a paradox! But, the benefit of challenging yourself to do more of the things that reduce stress and promote relaxation is clear—you help yourself sleep better, digest better, and reduce your need to rely on things like comfort eating and drinking alcohol to take the edge off. For thirty days, aim to do one relaxation-promoting practice per day, whether that's meditating, a few yoga poses, journaling, or simply sitting still and doing nothing.

12. **The prep ahead challenge.** While meal planning can be a big undertaking, giving some forethought to what you're going to have for your meals makes it a lot easier to stick to healthy eating habits. For the next thirty days, find a twenty-minute slot in your week to jot down what you'll eat in the next seven days. Afterward, dedicate an hour or two to preparing some of that food in advance—roasting a few chicken breasts, cooking up a pot of quinoa or cauliflower rice, and prepping some fruit and veggies for easy snacking and future sautéing. Give yourself the experience of having most of your meals mostly cooked in advance so that each time you're hungry, it's a lot quicker and easier to put something delicious together than to order takeout.

Avoiding the Likely Outcomes

As we come to the end of the main part of the book, we want to circle back to the projections we shared in Chapter 1. If we, as individuals and collectively, don't change our eating patterns or behaviors, projections suggest that fatty liver disease could overtake cancer as a cause of death in the United States—and other countries are not far behind.

Modern medicine is great because it allows us to live longer than we ever have before. But the bad part of our longer life spans is that the body can now outlive the organs—the heart, the brain, and as you now understand, the liver.

The simple truth is, if you take care of your liver, you'll live longer than someone who does not. Not only will you live longer but you'll live better. You want your life to have vibrancy as you age and not just be racking up numbers with each passing birthday while also adding conditions, treatments, and medications that impede your quality of life, whether that's dementia, dialysis, or stroke.

A patient of Ibrahim's, Jerry, is an excellent example of how it is never too late to reap the benefits of taking care of your liver. At seventy-two, Jerry started experiencing mild pain in his upper right abdomen after eating and occasionally felt nauseated. Although his symptoms weren't glaring, he knew something wasn't right, so he went to his primary care doctor for a checkup.

When Jerry's liver enzymes came back elevated, he had an ultrasound and then a CAT scan, which revealed that he had cirrhosis and liver cancer. Jerry, who had never been much of a drinker, was shocked. Because he, like so many people, associated advanced liver disease with alcoholism, he was ashamed to even tell his family about his diagnosis.

When Ibrahim met with Jerry and reviewed his chart, he saw the risk factors that we've discussed in this book: type 2 diabetes, central obesity, and high blood pressure. Not paying attention to his diet and exercise over the decades had led to the silent progression of fatty liver to its most advanced stage.

All of this happened at a time when Jerry's daughter was pregnant with his first grandchild. Becoming a grandparent was Jerry's motivation to get healthier—he wanted to be part of that child's life for as long as possible.

Luckily, although Jerry's liver was riddled with scar tissue, it was still functioning. If the liver is like a car, Jerry's was dented and scratched on the outside, but the engine still worked, which is why he felt mostly OK except for the pain and nausea. The other piece of good news was that Jerry's cancer was limited to one very small tumor that had not spread.

There wasn't much Jerry could do on his end to treat the liver cancer—he needed medical intervention for that. And luckily, there is a very effective treatment for this type of liver cancer; Ibrahim was able to kill the tumor cells by applying heat to the tumor via a treatment that uses needles to convey microwaves directly to the affected area.

But there was something very impactful Jerry could do to keep his liver's engine running, and that was to change his diet and start moving more. He may not be able to erase the scratches and dents, but the car will continue to get him around. And by doing so, he is decreasing the chance of cancer coming back.

Jerry adopted a low-carb diet and started walking outside, limited his eating hours to a twelve-hour window (between 8:00 a.m. and 8:00 p.m.), worked with his doctor to take better care of his diabetes, and saw his metabolic risk factors greatly improve. He reduced his waist size, and both his blood sugar level and his blood pressure are down. When Ibrahim saw Jerry for his follow-up, he looked ten years younger. Jerry reports that he and his wife got a dog that helps keep him walking. And most importantly, he's had the energy to take his grandchild swimming in the community pool a few times a week.

Living in Minnesota, Jerry faces challenges in staying active during the winter, when it's not pleasant—or sometimes even possible—to walk outside. He uses a standing bike during the colder months but admits that he stays more focused on eating well during the winter because he knows he's not getting as much daily movement as he does during the warmer months.

We share Jerry's story because he is a prime example of how it is never too late to start taking better care of your liver—and that when you do, every aspect of your health improves. Even though he was in his seventies when he was diagnosed with the most advanced stage of fatty liver disease, with treatment and a solid food and exercise plan, Jerry was able to significantly improve his health. By doing so, he has extended his health span, the number of years in your life that are not impeded by disease, and probably his life span, the number of years that you are alive. And that is precisely what we hope this book will help you do, too.

Remember, while fatty liver is a highly prevalent disease, it is also a very slowly progressing disease. The key, then, is to start now so that whatever form of fatty liver disease you already have doesn't have a chance to progress any further—or so that it never has a chance to develop in the first place.

Fatty liver is reversible. Like Spider-Man, your liver can regenerate. It only needs you to partner with it.

meal suggestions for the renew your liver eating plans

Instead of giving you a scripted calendar of which meal to eat when, we put together lists of plan-compliant meals and snack options. Some are actual recipes (in **bold type** and included in the Recipes section of this book), while others are simple things you can pull together without instructions; a few are prepackaged products that we believe in.

You don't have to abide by these categories: lunch can be breakfast, breakfast can be dinner, and if you make an extra serving of dinner, the leftovers can be breakfast or lunch the next day.

You'll see in these lists that some meal ideas are small, while others are a more typical size—you can mix and match meals of different sizes to find the right approach for you. The goal is to make eating this way very doable, with lots of variety and not a lot of complicated cooking.

We also include snack suggestions for each of the plans starting on page 245.

Modified Mediterranean Plan Meal Suggestions

You can also choose meals from the Moderate-Carb and Low-Carb plans, since they won't nudge your carb intake out of the moderate range.

(Our Family plan isn't carb-restricted, so don't choose meals or snacks from it.)

Breakfast

1. Breakfast sandwich: Place 1 slice of cheese and 1 fried or scrambled egg (and maybe 1 turkey sausage patty or 1 piece of turkey bacon) on a toasted whole wheat English muffin.
2. Pancakes: Top 2 whole wheat or buckwheat pancakes with 1 tablespoon maple syrup and a handful of berries or chopped apples.

3. Breakfast burrito: To 1 or 2 scrambled or sliced hard-boiled eggs, add your favorite accompaniments, such as cooked turkey bacon, avocado, cilantro, green onion, or salsa, and roll everything up in a whole-grain or almond flour or chickpea flour tortilla (such as those by Siete).

4. Loaded toast: To 1 piece of 100 percent whole-grain or sprouted-grain (such as Ezekiel) toast, add toppings such as a small avocado smashed with salt and pepper, a little crumbled feta cheese, diced tomato, and diced raw onions, drizzled with extra virgin olive oil and balsamic vinegar. Or try ricotta cheese or cottage cheese with a dusting of cinnamon and a handful of berries. Or try your favorite nut butter with sliced banana or berries in lieu of jelly.

5. **Overnight Oats (page 254).**

Lunch

1. Quesadilla: Start with 1/2 cup shredded cheese and 1 whole-grain or almond flour or chickpea flour tortilla, and add protein as desired, such as turkey bacon, leftover chicken, or black beans. Serve with salsa, sour cream, avocado, and hot sauce to taste.

2. Corn salad: 1 ear corn, grilled and cut off the cob, mixed with 1/4 cup feta; 1/2 cup arugula, chopped; 6 cherry tomatoes, halved; 1/2 avocado, chopped; and 1/2 cup cooked whole wheat couscous, all drizzled with extra virgin olive oil and red wine vinegar.

3. Guacamole: Mix 1/2 cup smashed avocado; 1/4 cup tomato, diced; 1/4 cup red onion, diced, and top with cilantro, minced. Serve with corn tortilla chips.

4. **Feta Vegetable Couscous (page 291).**

Dinner

1. **Chicken Chili (page 303).** Top with 1/4 cup shredded cheese and serve with corn tortilla chips.

2. **Christmas Ravioli (page 292).** Serve with a side of steamed broccoli.

3. Tacos: Sauté 4 ounces (per person) crumbled tofu, ground chicken, or ground turkey with taco seasoning and serve in a whole-grain,

corn, chickpea flour, or almond flour tortilla with sliced avocado, shredded cheese, diced tomatoes, and salsa or hot sauce.

4. Burgers: Keep your patties to 4 ounces and choose from bison, turkey, chicken, or bean (such as those made by Dr. Praeger's or Amy's), and serve on a whole wheat or sprouted-grain bun (or if you're seeking a lower-carb option, use a cauliflower or keto bun) with a slice of cheese, lettuce, onion, and tomato, and a side of roasted sweet potato fries (such as from Alexia).

5. Stir-fry: Start with 2 cups total of a mix of vegetables (such as Brussels sprouts, mushrooms, zucchini, and broccoli), sauté in extra virgin olive oil and jazz up with fresh lemon juice, hot sauce, **Tahini Sauce (page 268)**, and/or soy sauce. Add a protein of choice, such as cooked chicken, salmon, or shrimp, and serve with 1/2 cup cooked brown rice.

6. Burrito bowl: Combine 4 ounces of your protein of choice (sautéed turkey, chicken, or tofu, or grilled chicken), 1/2 cup cooked brown rice, 1/2 cup black or pinto beans in a bowl and serve with salsa, guacamole, shredded cheese, sour cream, and/or hot sauce.

Moderate-Carbohydrate Plan Meal Suggestions

Remember, when you're on the Moderate-Carb plan, you can also eat any of the breakfasts, lunches, dinners, and snacks in the Low-Carb plan. Steer clear of the Family plan suggestions, as they aren't designed to be lower in carbs.

Breakfast

1. Breakfast burrito: To 1 or 2 scrambled or sliced hard-boiled eggs, add reasonable amounts of your favorite accompaniments, such as cooked turkey bacon, shredded cheese, raw or sautéed spinach, cream cheese, avocado, cilantro, green onion, or salsa, and roll everything up in a low-carb tortilla (such as those by Mission).

2. Loaded toast: To 1 piece sprouted-grain (such as Ezekiel) or low-carb (such as Carbonaut) toast, add toppings such as a small avocado smashed with salt and pepper, a little crumbled feta cheese, diced tomato, and diced raw onions; drizzle with extra virgin olive

oil and balsamic vinegar. Or try ricotta cheese or cottage cheese with a dusting of cinnamon and a handful of berries. Or try your favorite nut butter with sliced banana or berries in lieu of jelly.

3. Sweet potato hash: In a bowl toss together 1 serving (according to package) of Alexia Crispy Bite-Size Sweet Potato Puffs (cooked according to package instructions), 1 scrambled egg (cooked), and 1/4 cup shredded cheese.

4. Fruits and whey: Mix 1/2 cup cottage cheese with 1 small mandarin orange, peeled and divided into segments, or 1 small apple cut into small chunks, or a handful of berries, and a dusting of cinnamon or nutmeg. Serve in a bowl.

5. Granola and berries: Combine 1 serving (according to package) low-sugar, high-fiber granola (such as Purely Elizabeth) with 1/2 cup mixed berries and 1 cup of unsweetened nut milk or low-fat dairy milk.

6. Intact oatmeal: Combine 1 cup cooked, steel-cut oatmeal with 1/2 cup fresh-cut apple chunks or mixed berries and 1 teaspoon cinnamon, and sweeten with low-carb maple syrup (such as that made by Lakanto).

7. Matcha smoothie bowl: Blend 2 teaspoons matcha powder (found in the tea section of most grocery stores), 1/2 cup kale, 1/2 cup spinach, 6 mint leaves, a handful of ice, and 1 cup unsweetened almond milk. Pour into a bowl and top with a handful of walnuts; 1/2 banana, sliced; a handful of blackberries; and 1 tablespoon ground flaxseeds.

Lunch

1. **Heart-Healthy Hummus (page 261)**. Serve with **Whole Wheat Pita Fennel Chips (page 268)**, baby carrots, and celery sticks.

2. Quesadilla: Start with 1/2 cup shredded cheese and an almond flour or low-carb tortilla (such as those made by Mission), and add protein as desired, such as turkey bacon, leftover chicken, or pinto or black beans. Serve with salsa, sour cream, avocado, and hot sauce to taste.

3. Corn salad: 1 ear corn, grilled and cut off the cob, or 3/4 cup canned corn, mixed with 1/4 cup feta; 1/2 cup arugula, chopped; a

handful of cherry tomatoes, halved; 1/2 avocado, chopped; and 1/2 cup cooked quinoa. Drizzle with extra virgin olive oil and red wine vinegar.

4. Super-fast soup: Prepare 1 serving (according to package) canned lentil soup or split pea soup (such as Amy's), drizzle with extra virgin olive oil, and serve with **Keto-Friendly Crackers (page 265)** or your favorite low-carb crackers.

5. Chickpea salad: Mix 1/2 cup **Crunchy Chickpeas (page 256)**; 1-1/2 cups romaine lettuce, chopped; and 1/4 cup shredded Parmesan cheese. Drizzle with extra virgin olive oil and balsamic vinegar, add salt and pepper to taste. Serve with almond flour crackers, low-carb crackers, or **Keto-Friendly Crackers (page 265)**.

6. Caprese salad: In a bowl combine 8 cherry tomatoes, halved; 4 mozzarella pearls, halved; 4 leaves fresh basil, julienned; 1/2 cucumber, diced; 1/4 cup shallots, minced; and drizzle with balsamic vinegar and extra virgin olive oil, add salt and pepper to taste. Serve with almond flour crackers (such as those by Simple Mills), low-carb crackers, or **Keto-Friendly Crackers (page 265)**.

7. Kale salad: Mix 2 cups chopped, curly kale massaged with 1 tablespoon extra virgin olive oil and the juice of 1/4 of a lemon with 1/2 cup pre-cooked lentils; 1/4 cup shallots, minced; and 2 tablespoons grated Parmesan cheese.

8. Kale sweet potato salad: Combine 2 cups baby kale leaves with 1/2 of a roasted sweet potato, scooped out of the skin, and a handful of chopped pecans, with a drizzle of extra virgin olive oil and balsamic vinegar to taste.

9. **Buffalo Chicken Dip (page 264)**, 1/2 cup. Serve with carrot and celery sticks or a handful of corn tortilla chips.

10. Guacamole: Mix 1/2 cup smashed avocado; 1/4 cup tomato, diced; 1/4 cup red onion, diced; and top with cilantro, minced. Serve with jicama sticks and/or a handful of corn tortilla chips for dipping.

Dinner

1. **Chicken Chili (page 303)**, top with 1/4 cup shredded cheese and serve with low-carb corn tortilla chips (such as those by Quest).

2. **Butternut Squash Soup (page 282)**, serve with **Keto-Friendly Crackers (page 265)**.

3. **Stuffed Baked Sweet Potatoes (page 286)**, serve with a side of **Spicy Pulled Chicken (page 302)**.

4. **Lean, Green Pasta and Meatballs (page 296)**.

5. Burgers: Keep your patties to 4 ounces and choose from bison, turkey, chicken, or bean (such as those made by Dr. Praeger's or Amy's), and serve on a cauliflower or keto bun (such as those by Carbonaut) with a slice of cheese, lettuce, onion, and tomato. Serve with a green salad drizzled with extra virgin olive oil and your favorite vinegar or lemon juice.

6. Stir-fry: Start with 2 cups total of a mix of vegetables (such as Brussels sprouts, mushrooms, zucchini, and broccoli), sauté in extra virgin olive oil and jazz up with fresh lemon juice, hot sauce, **Tahini Sauce (page 268)**, and/or soy sauce. Add a protein of choice, such as cooked chicken, salmon, or shrimp, and serve on a bed of 1/2 cup pre-cooked lentils and 1/2 cup of either quinoa or cauliflower rice.

7. Burrito bowl: Combine 1/4 pound protein of choice (sautéed turkey, chicken, or tofu, or grilled chicken), 1/2 cup cauliflower rice or quinoa, and 1/2 cup black or pinto beans in a bowl and serve with salsa, guacamole, shredded cheese, sour cream, and/or hot sauce.

8. Tacos: Sauté 4 ounces (per person) crumbled tofu, ground chicken, or ground turkey with taco seasoning, and serve in almond flour or low-carb tortillas with sliced avocado, shredded cheese, and diced tomatoes.

9. **Grilled Chicken Breast, Baked Chicken Breast, Grilled Salmon**, or **Broiled Salmon (pages 278–281)**, season with your favorite marinade—such as low-carb teriyaki, low-carb BBQ sauce, pesto, za'atar, or Jamaican jerk seasoning—and serve with a side of roasted sweet potato, quinoa, or bean-based pasta.

10. Chicken fajitas: Sauté 4 ounces chicken chunks with 1/4 cup sliced onion and 1/2 cup sliced bell peppers. Serve with a side of 1/2 cup cooked quinoa or cauliflower rice, 1/2 cup cooked black or pinto beans, and no-sugar-added salsa and hot sauce to taste.

11. Watermelon salad: Combine 1/2 cup watermelon, cubed; 1 cup arugula; 1/4 cup feta or goat cheese; drizzle with balsamic

vinegar and extra virgin olive oil to taste, and serve with 1 **Grilled Chicken Breast (page 279)**.

12. No-cook bowl: Mix 1 cup pre-cooked lentils with 1 cup broccoli florets (raw, steamed, or roasted), 1/4 cup chopped pepper (red, green, orange, or yellow), and 2 tablespoons feta cheese; drizzle with extra virgin olive oil and red wine vinegar.

13. Easy tikka masala: Fill a sheet pan with chopped vegetables (zucchini, broccoli, bell peppers, onion, mushrooms, etc.), drizzle with extra virgin olive oil, add salt and pepper, and roast at 400°F until vegetables are starting to brown, about 20-25 minutes. Serve 2 cups of cooked vegetables with 1/2 cup of cooked quinoa and then mix in 1/4 cup of jarred tikka masala sauce. (Add 1 can of drained and rinsed chickpeas or 1 pound cooked chicken chunks for extra protein.)

14. Easy shrimp sauté: Sauté 4 ounces fresh or thawed, peeled, and deveined shrimp in extra virgin olive oil with 2 cloves minced garlic, then finish with a squeeze of lemon juice and the zest of 1/2 lemon. Serve over 1 cup of bean-based pasta or 1/2 cup of cooked quinoa. (To thaw shrimp from frozen, pour shrimp out of bag into a bowl of cold water for 10 to 20 minutes; drain shrimp thoroughly and then pat dry with paper towels before sautéing.)

15. Stuffed mushroom: Destem 1 portabella or 5 button mushrooms and stuff with a blend of chopped bell peppers, shredded mozzarella, and onion. Bake at 350°F for 25-30 minutes and serve with a side of bean-based pasta or quinoa.

16. Pesto gnocchi: Cook 1/2 package cauliflower or kale gnocchi (available at Trader Joe's) according to package instructions and serve with 1 or 2 tablespoons **Triple Herb Pesto (page 272)** or **Red Sauce (page 269)**.

Low-Carb Plan Meal Suggestions

Breakfast
1. **Peanut Butter Chocolate "Chaffles" (page 252)**.
2. Low-carb or keto-friendly protein shake (such as Atkins).

3. Two Birch Benders Keto Frozen Waffles with 1 tablespoon of Lakanto maple syrup.

4. One keto-friendly bagel, bun, or biscuit, spread with 1 tablespoon unsalted butter, with 1 slice of cheese and 1 scrambled egg sandwiched between the halves.

5. One cup keto-friendly cereal with 1/2 cup no-added-sugar nut milk.

6. Top 1 turkey or chicken sausage patty with 1 fried egg and 1/2 large avocado, sliced.

7. Combine 1 cup low-fat cottage cheese with 1/2 cup mixed berries and a handful of walnuts, chopped.

8. **Strawberry Chia Pudding (page 309).**

9. Avocado egg bake: Slice 1 avocado in half and remove the pit. Crack 1 egg into the hole left by the pit in each half of the avocado and bake at 350°F for 15 minutes. When done, garnish with chopped cilantro and hot sauce to taste.

10. Greek cottage cheese: Combine 1 cup low-fat cottage cheese with 1 teaspoon chopped fresh or dried dill; 1 mini cucumber, sliced into 1/4-inch coins; and a handful of cherry tomatoes, halved.

11. Spicy deviled eggs: Slice 2 hard-boiled eggs in half and put yolks in a bowl. Mash yolks with 1/2 avocado, 1 dollop sour cream, and add salt, pepper, and cayenne pepper to taste. Fill egg whites with yolk mixture.

12. **Chocolate Chia Pudding (page 309).**

13. Four **Parmesan Crisps (page 255)**, top each with 1/2 tablespoon cream cheese, 1 slice avocado, and 1/2 a cherry tomato.

14. Easy parfait: Combine 1 cup plain, low-fat Greek yogurt with 1/2 cup mixed berries, a handful of almonds or walnuts, and 1 tablespoon almond butter; top with 2 tablespoons unsweetened shredded coconut.

15. Eggs a hundred ways: Scramble, fry, poach, or hard-boil 1 or 2 eggs (or maybe 1 full egg and 1 egg white to cut down on saturated fat) and serve 1/2 an avocado, sliced; a handful of grape tomatoes, sliced; 1 or 2 pieces of smoked salmon, diced; 1 cup of spinach, sautéed; 1 cup of leftover cooked vegetables of any type; 1/4 cup roasted red peppers, diced; 2 tablespoons of any type of

cheese and/or salsa; garnish with a little sriracha or pesto, and/ or 1 green onion, sliced, or 1 tablespoon of cilantro, chopped. (If you want to have a little bacon or breakfast sausage with your egg, go for turkey or chicken options, and don't have it every day, as the nitrates in turkey bacon and sausage are still a concern. Of course, you can also have the "real" versions of bacon and sausage, but consider them the same way you would an ice cream sundae—as treats.)

Lunch

1. **Spinach Artichoke Dip** (page 263), serve with **Keto-Friendly Crackers (page 265)**.
2. **Warm Ricotta Dip** (without the raspberry swirl) **(page 260)**, serve with **Keto-Friendly Crackers (page 265)**.
3. Ricotta Caprese "salad": In a bowl, combine 1/2 cup ricotta cheese; a handful of cherry tomatoes, halved; and a few basil leaves, julienned; then drizzle with olive oil and add salt and pepper to taste. Serve with **Keto-Friendly Crackers (page 265)** or flaxseed crackers (such as Flackers).
4. Buffalo cauliflower: Toss 2 cups cauliflower florets in 1/4 cup buffalo sauce (such as the one by Primal Kitchen) and bake at 350°F for 30 minutes.
5. Un-breaded jalapeño poppers: Remove the top and seeds of 3 jalapeño peppers, stuff each with cheese of choice, and wrap each pepper with 1 piece of turkey bacon. Bake at 350°F for 30 minutes or until turkey bacon is crispy.
6. Quesadilla: Start with 1/2 cup shredded cheese and a keto tortilla (such as those made by Mission), and add protein as desired, such as 3 slices turkey bacon or a 1/2 cup leftover chicken. Serve with salsa, sour cream, avocado, and hot sauce to taste.
7. Chicken salad: Combine 1/2 cup **Baked Chicken Breast (page 278)**, chopped; 1/4 cup celery, diced; 1/4 cup red onion, diced; 1-2 tablespoons olive oil-based mayonnaise; 1 teaspoon Dijon mustard; 1 teaspoon fresh or dried dill; and add salt and pepper to taste. Serve on celery sticks, with **Keto-Friendly Crackers (page 265)** or flaxseed crackers (such as Flackers), or alone in a bowl.

8. Cauliflower "fried rice": Microwave a bag of frozen cauliflower rice according to directions on package; drain excess liquid; then sauté in extra virgin olive oil in a pan over medium heat with 1 cup mushrooms, sliced, and 1/4 cup shelled edamame. Season with soy sauce, salt, pepper, and sriracha to taste.

9. **Krissy's Keto Broccoli and Cheese Casserole (page 288).**

10. Tuna salad: Mix 1 can tuna with 1–2 tablespoons olive oil- or avocado oil-based mayonnaise; serve on 2 celery stalks.

11. Bell pepper sandwich: 1 bell pepper, cored, destemmed, and halved; fill one side of pepper with 2 slices of turkey breast, 1/4 cup spinach, 1 slice of cheese, and 1 slice of tomato. Then sandwich together with other half of pepper.

12. Lettuce wraps: Sauté 1/4 pound ground chicken with 1 tablespoon fresh ginger, peeled and chopped, and 1 tablespoon soy sauce. Serve wrapped in pieces of lettuce.

13. No-bagel everything wrap: Spread 2 tablespoons cream cheese on 2 ounces wild smoked salmon lox, sprinkle with everything bagel seasoning (sold at Costco and Trader Joe's), and roll up.

14. Egg salad: Combine 2 hard-boiled eggs, peeled and chopped; 1/2 cup spinach, chopped; and 1–2 tablespoons olive oil- or avocado oil-based mayonnaise. Garnish with fresh dill or cilantro, chopped.

15. Cucumber salad: In a bowl, toss together 2 mini cucumbers, sliced lengthwise and then into 1/4-inch coins; a handful of cherry tomatoes, halved; 1/4 cup onion, sliced; and 1/2 avocado, chunked. Sprinkle with salt and pepper and drizzle with extra virgin olive oil. Serve with **Keto-Friendly Crackers (page 265)** or flaxseed crackers (such as Flackers).

16. **Buffalo Chicken Dip (page 264)**, 1/2 cup, serve with celery sticks and/or low-carb crackers.

17. Turkey pinwheel roll-ups: Take 2 slices of fresh turkey breast, top each with a slice of cheese and a few baby spinach leaves, then roll up and slice into circles.

18. Spicy shrimp sauté: Sauté or grill 4 jumbo shrimp, drizzle with sriracha, and serve on top of 1 cup cauliflower rice, prepared according to package directions.

19. Arugula salad: Combine 2 cups baby arugula leaves with 1/2 cup mixed berries and 1/4 cup low-fat cottage cheese; drizzle with extra virgin olive oil.

Dinner

1. **Easy African Peanut Stew (page 289)**.
2. **Spicy Pulled Chicken (page 302)**, serve either in a bowl or with a keto tortilla, with no-sugar-added salsa, sour cream, shredded cheese, sliced black olives, and cubed avocado.
3. **Chicken Chili (page 303)**, serve with shredded cheese, sour cream, diced onion, and low-carb tortilla chips (such as those by Quest).
4. **Zingy Baked Salmon with Cauliflower Rice (page 298)**.
5. **Sautéed Shrimp on Curried Spaghetti Squash (page 300)**, serve with steamed broccoli florets.
6. **Vegetarian Lasagna (page 297)**.
7. **No-Carb Pizza ("The Friday Night Special") (page 295)**.
8. **Krissy's Keto Broccoli and Cheese Casserole (page 288)**.
9. **Roasted Cauliflower and Mushroom Soup (page 284)**, serve with **Keto-Friendly Crackers (page 265)**.
10. Stuffed mushroom: Fill 1 large, destemmed portabella mushroom with 1/4 cup bell pepper, diced; 1/4 cup onion, diced; 1 clove garlic, minced; and top with 2 tablespoons shredded cheese. Bake at 350°F for 30 minutes, garnish with fresh parsley, chopped.
11. Low-carb pasta bowl: Zoodles (zucchini noodles, which are often available in the refrigerator case of the produce section), cooked according to package instructions, or 1/2 spaghetti squash, sliced in half lengthwise, deseeded, and then roasted cut-side down on a cookie sheet in a 400°F oven until tender (30–40 minutes). Serve with Parmesan cheese and a drizzle of extra virgin olive oil, your favorite pesto, or **Red Sauce (page 269)**; add grilled or baked chicken or salmon if you like.
12. Tacos: Sauté crumbled tofu, ground chicken, or ground turkey with taco seasoning and serve in a whole-grain, corn, chickpea flour, or almond flour tortilla with sliced avocado, shredded cheese, diced tomatoes, and salsa or hot sauce.

13. Burgers: Keep your patties to 4 ounces and choose from bison, turkey, chicken, or bean (such as those made by Dr. Praeger's or Amy's), and serve on a cauliflower or keto bun (such as those by Outer Aisle or Carbonaut) with a slice of cheese, lettuce, onion, and tomato with a green salad on the side drizzled with extra virgin olive oil and your favorite vinegar or lemon juice.

14. Stir-fry: Start with 2 cups total of a mix of vegetables (such as Brussels sprouts, mushrooms, zucchini, and broccoli), sauté in extra virgin olive oil and jazz up with fresh lemon juice, hot sauce, **Tahini Sauce (page 268)**, and/or soy sauce. Add a protein of choice, such as cooked chicken, salmon, or shrimp, and serve on 1/2 cup cooked cauliflower rice.

15. Burrito bowl: Combine 1/4 pound protein of choice (sautéed turkey, chicken, or tofu, or grilled chicken), 1/2 cup cooked cauliflower rice, 1/4 cup black or pinto beans in a bowl and serve with salsa, guacamole, shredded cheese, sour cream, and/or hot sauce.

16. Either **Grilled Chicken Breast, Baked Chicken Breast,** or **Broiled Salmon (pages 278–281)**, season with your favorite marinade—such as low-carb teriyaki, low-carb BBQ sauce, pesto, or Jamaican jerk seasoning—and serve with a side of roasted Brussels sprouts, roasted cauliflower, sautéed peppers and onions, or steamed green beans.

17. Not-spaghetti: Bake 1/2 spaghetti squash, deseeded, at 450°F for 1 hour, then top with 1/4 cup ricotta, 1/4 cup **Red Sauce (page 269)**, and 1/4 cup combined grated Parmesan and shredded mozzarella cheese.

18. No-carb chicken parm: Bake 1 chicken breast in a casserole dish with 1 cup **Red Sauce (page 269)** at 400°F for 25 minutes. Remove from oven, top with 1 slice of fresh mozzarella, place back in oven, and cook for an additional 5–10 minutes.

19. **Baked Eggplant (page 292)**.

20. Buffalo chicken zucchini: Slice 1 zucchini into 1/4-inch coins and bake on a greased cookie sheet at 350°F for 25 minutes, then top with 1/2 cup **Buffalo Chicken Dip (page 264)**.

21. Chicken arugula salad: Combine 2 cups baby arugula leaves with 1/2 cup chopped **Grilled or Baked Chicken Breast (pages 278–279)**,

1/4 cup toasted pine nuts, and 1/4 cup grated Parmesan cheese; drizzle with extra virgin olive oil and balsamic vinegar.

22. Stuffed pepper: Remove top and core of bell pepper, stuff with 3 ounces parcooked ground turkey, 1/4 cup **Red Sauce (page 269)**, 1 tablespoon Italian seasoning, and bake at 350°F for 20 minutes. Top with 1/4 cup shredded mozzarella cheese and continue baking until cheese is melted.

Family Plan Meal Suggestions

These meal suggestions are for when you live with kids and/or extended family and you want to be able to cook one meal that (a) everyone will eat, and (b) will be more nutrient-dense than typical American family fare. That said, these meals aren't carb-restricted in any way, so if you're trying to follow any of the other plans that do seek to lower total carb levels, it's best to stick to the meal suggestions for your particular plan. Any of the suggestions for all of our other plans are also acceptable on the Family plan (while you don't want kids to be concerned with eating low carb at every meal, it's OK for them to have low-carb meals once in a while).

Note: As with all the other meal plans in this book, these meal suggestions are geared toward serving one person. Because this is the Family plan, you may need to double, triple, or quadruple your ingredients to prepare the correct amount of food for your family.

Breakfast

1. Fruit soup: In a bowl, combine 1/2 grapefruit, peeled and sectioned; 1 small banana, sliced; 1 kiwi, sliced; 6 grapes, halved; and squeeze remaining juice from grapefruit rind over the top.

2. Almond butter and banana bagel sandwich: Halve and toast 1 whole-grain bagel, until slightly browned; evenly spread 2 tablespoons almond butter, 1 tablespoon over each half; place 1 small banana, sliced, on one bagel half; sprinkle 1 tablespoon of ground flaxseeds evenly on the other half of bagel; then press the bagel halves together.

3. Stick-to-your-ribs oatmeal: Mix 1 cup cooked rolled oats with 1/2 banana, sliced; 1/4 cup blueberries; and 1 tablespoon almond butter, and drizzle 1 tablespoon honey over the top.

4. **Overnight Oats (see page 254 for instructions),** mix in 1/2 cup berries (strawberries, blueberries, blackberries, raspberries) and 1 tablespoon dark chocolate chips.

5. Healthy cereal: One serving (according to the nutrition label) high-fiber, low-sugar cereal (Nature's Path has great options for kids and adults) with 1 cup unsweetened nut milk or low-fat dairy milk.

6. Pancake sandwich: Two frozen protein pancakes or waffles (such as those by Birch Benders or Kodiak) prepared according to package instructions; drizzle 1 pancake with 1 tablespoon of maple syrup, and sandwich 1 turkey sausage patty between pancakes.

7. Prep-ahead egg muffins: Scramble 6 eggs in a bowl, then mix in 1/4 cup shredded cheese and 1/4 cup turkey bacon, chopped finely. Pour into greased six-count muffin tin pan and bake at 350°F for 20 minutes.

8. One apple, sliced and dipped in 2 tablespoons no-added-sugar peanut or other nut butter mixed with 2 tablespoons uncooked rolled oats, lightly drizzle with honey, and dust with cinnamon or nutmeg.

9. Protein toast: One piece 100% whole-grain toast, top with 1/2 cup cottage cheese, dust with cinnamon and drizzle with honey.

10. Turkey sausage pancake sticks: Using a protein pancake mix (such as Kodiak), prepare batter according to package instructions and pour into medium casserole dish. On stove top, partially cook 1 package of turkey sausage links. Submerge as many small turkey sausages links vertically into the pancake mix across the casserole as possible (two rows). Bake at 400°F for 10–15 minutes. Cut into sticks and serve.

Lunch

1. Grilled cheese and soup: Toast 2 pieces of 100% whole-grain bread (such as Dave's Killer Bread) with 2 slices of cheese melted

between them, and serve with 1 serving of canned or boxed roasted red pepper or tomato soup (such as Pacific Foods) according to package.

2. Higher-fiber sushi: Brown rice sushi roll from the grocery store sushi counter with a side of low-sodium soy sauce.

3. Pesto turkey panini: 2 slices 100% whole-grain bread, 1 tablespoon of your favorite pesto, 1 slice tomato, and 2 slices mozzarella cheese. Assemble sandwich, then cook over medium-low heat in a skillet, pressing the sandwich down with a spatula as it cooks, 1–2 minutes per side.

4. Red lentil pasta salad: Combine 2/3 cup red lentil pasta, cooked and drained; 1/4 cup celery, diced; 1/4 cup tomato, diced; 1/4 cup bell pepper; drizzle with extra virgin olive oil, add 1 tablespoon Italian seasoning, and salt and pepper to taste.

5. Chicken pocket: Stuff 1/2 of a 100% whole wheat pita with 2 slices roasted chicken, 1 slice mild cheddar cheese, and 2 tablespoons of hummus. Serve with carrot sticks.

6. Turkey mozzarella sticks: Wrap 1 mozzarella cheese stick with 1 slice of turkey and roll up in a romaine lettuce leaf. Serve 2 for lunch.

7. Classic nut butter sandwich: 2 slices 100% whole-grain bread and 2 tablespoons nut butter. (Option: Add 1/2 small banana, sliced.)

Dinner

1. "Walking tacos" (for nights you need to eat on the go): To a single-serving-sized bag of Quest Nutrition Tortilla chips, add 1/2 cup sautéed taco meat of choice (turkey, chicken, beef, plant-based, tofu), a small handful of shredded lettuce, 2 tablespoons of no-sugar-added salsa, 2 tablespoons of shredded cheese, and 1 tablespoon of guacamole.

2. Pizza: Choose a thin-crust pizza or cauliflower crust pizza, skip the pepperoni and sausage (although feel free to load up on vegetable toppings), keep it to 2 slices, and serve with your favorite salad green drizzled with extra virgin olive oil and lemon juice.

3. Chicken and rice: Grilled chicken strips with a side of baby carrots (with ranch dressing for dipping) and a side of brown rice.

4. Higher-fiber pizza: Whole wheat pizza shell topped with shredded mozzarella cheese, sauce, red pepper strips, and turkey pepperoni.

5. Healthier pasta and meatballs: Prepared chicken or turkey meatballs (from the frozen food section of the grocery store, prepared according to package directions), serve with **Red Sauce (page 269)**, whole wheat penne pasta, Parmesan cheese, and a drizzle of extra virgin olive oil.

recommended snacks for the renew your liver plans

Modified Mediterranean Plan Snacks

You can also have any of the snacks listed on the Moderate-Carb and Low-Carb plans.

1. Cheesy roll-up: Whole-grain tortilla with melted cheese inside dipped in salsa.
2. **Heart-Healthy Hummus (page 261)** or **Baba Ganoush (page 265)** with **Whole Wheat Pita Bread (page 266).**
3. One medium banana with 2 tablespoons nut butter.
4. Guacamole with diced tomatoes, onions, and cilantro with a squeeze of fresh lime. Serve with corn tortilla chips.
5. Two or 3 dates, pitted, with a shmear of goat cheese or your favorite nut butter and a sprinkle of sea salt.
6. Top 1 piece of whole-grain toast with ricotta, sliced tomato, salt, and pepper; drizzle with extra virgin olive oil and a splash of balsamic vinegar.

Moderate-Carb Plan Snacks

You can also have any of the snacks for the Low-Carb plan listed below.

1. **Crunchy Chickpeas (page 256).**
2. **Holiday Roasted Chickpeas (page 257).**
3. **Party-Pleasing Edamame Dip (page 261)**, serve with **Keto-Friendly Crackers (page 265)** or your favorite store-bought low-carb crackers.
4. Baked green pea snacks (such as Harvest Snaps or those sold at Trader Joe's).

5. Refried pinto beans topped with melted cheese with low-carb crackers.
6. Unsweetened apple sauce with cinnamon.
7. Ants on a log: Celery sticks topped with almond butter and raisins or dried cranberries.
8. Cottage cheese with cantaloupe chunks.
9. Cheesy roll-up: Almond or chickpea flour tortilla rolled up with melted cheese inside (make it dairy-free by choosing a plant-based cheese).
10. **Whole Wheat Pita Bread (page 266)** or **Whole Wheat Pita Fennel Chips (page 268)**, serve with **Roasted Red Pepper Dip (page 262)**.
11. **Whole Wheat Pita Fennel Chips (page 268)**.
12. Guacamole with diced tomatoes, onions, and cilantro with a squeeze of fresh lime. Serve with jicama sticks.
13. **Tabbouleh (page 282)**.
14. Two small figs sliced (without cutting all the way through) and stuffed with a walnut and a schmear of feta or goat cheese.
15. **Cheese and Fig Bites (page 259)**.
16. **Avocado Melon Smoothie (page 251)**.
17. One apple, sliced, and served with 2 tablespoons nut butter.

Low-Carb Plan Snacks

All of these fit the low-carb definition of 26 percent or less of carbohydrates. Any snack that you find at the grocery store marketed as keto will also fit within the parameters of the Low-Carb plan.

For the dips listed here, have them with crudités (red pepper, celery, snow peas, cucumbers, radishes, and carrots, although be careful with carrots as they can get higher in carbs if you eat a lot of them).

1. **Savory Rosemary Cashews (page 258)**.
2. Two pieces of smoked salmon with cream cheese and everything bagel seasoning (available at Costco and Trader Joe's), rolled up.
3. **Spinach Artichoke Dip (page 263)**.
4. **Buffalo Chicken Dip (page 264)**.

5. **Warm Ricotta Dip with Raspberry Swirl (page 260).**
6. Carrots, celery, or bell pepper sticks with ranch dressing for dipping.
7. Celery sticks topped with almond butter or cream cheese and blueberries.
8. **Crispy Brussels Sprout Chips (page 255).**
9. Cheesy zucchini chips: Slice 1 small zucchini into coins; lay flat on baking sheet, drizzle with extra virgin olive oil, and sprinkle with salt and pepper. Bake at 350°F for 15 minutes, then open oven and sprinkle evenly and generously with Parmesan cheese and bake for another 15 minutes.
10. A handful of olives
11. Cottage cheese with **Keto-Friendly Crackers (page 265)** or flax-seed crackers (such as Flackers).
12. Cheesy roll-up with keto tortilla and melted cheese inside.
13. Nuts: A handful of walnuts, pistachios, almonds, cashews, maca-damias, or pine nuts.
14. Seeds: A handful of pumpkin seeds or sunflower seeds.
15. Berries: A handful of strawberries, blackberries, raspberries, or blueberries (with a dollop of ricotta cheese if you like).
16. Stuffed olives: Stuff 3 large pitted green olives with feta, mozza-rella, or ricotta cheese.
17. Guacamole with crudités, keto crackers, or flaxseed crackers (such as Flackers).
18. **Parmesan Crisps (page 255).**
19. **Protein-Powered Cookie Cream (page 305).**
20. **Low-Carb Peanut Butter Cups (page 306).**
21. **Keto-Friendly Crackers (page 265).**
22. Cucumber slices topped with cottage cheese and everything but the bagel seasoning (sold at Costco and Trader Joe's).
23. Simple Mills almond flour crackers with cottage cheese.
24. Celery sticks with cream cheese and everything but the bagel seasoning.
25. Plain low-fat yogurt with a handful of keto granola and a handful of fresh berries (raspberries, blueberries, and blackberries).

26. Hard-boiled eggs.
27. Deviled eggs: Slice 2 hard-boiled eggs in half and put yolks in a bowl. Mash yolks with 1/2 avocado, 1 dollop sour cream, and add salt and pepper (and cayenne pepper or hot sauce if you like it spicy) to taste. Fill egg whites with yolk mixture.
28. String cheese.

Family Plan Snacks

All the snacks on all the meal plans are acceptable for the Family plan. Also keep in mind that kids want to be kids. You don't want to ban them from ever having their favorites, whether that's chips, cookies, or ice cream, but see if you can sell them on some of the healthier snacks we've listed for the other Renew Your Liver plans so that those beloved foods become more of a treat and less of a go-to option.

recipes

Breakfasts

Avocado Melon Smoothie
Peanut Butter Chocolate "Chaffles"
Breakfast of Champions: Five Ways to Prepare Oatmeal

Snacks and Sides

Crispy Brussels Sprout Chips
Parmesan Crisps
Crunchy Chickpeas
Holiday Roasted Chickpeas
Savory Rosemary Cashews
Cheese and Fig Bites
Warm Ricotta Dip with Raspberry Swirl
Party-Pleasing Edamame Dip
Heart-Healthy Hummus
Roasted Red Pepper Dip
Spinach Artichoke Dip
Buffalo Chicken Dip
Baba Ganoush
Keto-Friendly Crackers
Whole Wheat Pita Bread
Whole Wheat Pita Fennel Chips

Sauces

Tahini Sauce
Red Sauce
Traditional Basil Pesto
Triple Herb Pesto

Nutty Vegan Pesto
Spicy Vegan Cilantro Pesto
Cashew Spinach Pesto
Pumpkin Seed Pesto with Parsley
Dill and Lemon Pesto
High-Protein Green Pea Pesto

Basic Animal Proteins

Baked Chicken Breast
Grilled Chicken Breast
Broiled Salmon
Grilled Salmon

Main Meals, from Light to Hearty

Tabbouleh
Butternut Squash Soup
Roasted Cauliflower and Mushroom Soup
Stuffed Baked Sweet Potatoes
Sweet Potato Holiday Casserole
Krissy's Keto Broccoli and Cheese Casserole
Easy African Peanut Stew
Feta Vegetable Couscous
Baked Eggplant
Christmas Ravioli
No-Carb Pizza ("The Friday Night Special")
Lean, Green Pasta and Meatballs
Vegetarian Lasagna
Zingy Baked Salmon with Cauliflower Rice
Pan-Seared Salmon with a Ginger Turmeric Sauce and Cauliflower
Rice
Sautéed Shrimp on Curried Spaghetti Squash
Spicy Pulled Chicken
Chicken Chili

Desserts

Apple Crisp
Protein-Powered Cookie Cream
Low-Carb Peanut Butter Cups
Miraculous Chocolate Chip Cookies
Peanut Butter Mousse
Strawberry Chia Pudding
Chocolate Chia Pudding
Pumpkin Spice Chia Pudding

Key:

MM—Modified Mediterranean
MC—Moderate carb
LC—Low carb
KF—Keto friendly
GF—Gluten-free
V—Vegan
VGT—Vegetarian

Breakfasts

In addition to oatmeal, chia pudding, cereal, eggs and scrambles, and other breakfast ideas you've read about in this book, here are some breakfast recipes you might enjoy.

Avocado Melon Smoothie (MM, GF, VGT)

Many of Kristin's patients have requested variations on smoothie recipes. They were getting tired of mixed berries and yogurt and wanted a liver-friendly alternative. This option, with avocado as the base and melons as the fruit, is thick, delicious, and perfect on a hot summer day. In general, to keep smoothies liver friendly, you want to avoid relying on high-glycemic fruits, such as bananas and mangoes, and instead use small amounts of berries, apples, or melon to sweeten the mix. You can also add greens, such as kale or the more mildly flavored spinach, to up the nutrient content. And use no-sugar-added nut or seed milk, water, or low-fat cow's milk as the liquid base.

Prep time: 5 minutes
Total time: 5 minutes

SERVES 1

INGREDIENTS:
1 ripe avocado, pitted
1/2 cup cantaloupe chunks
1/2 cup honeydew chunks
1 scoop of plain Greek yogurt
Scoop of ice
Drizzle of honey

INSTRUCTIONS:
1. Place all ingredients into the blender.
2. Blend until smooth.

Peanut Butter Chocolate "Chaffles" (Cheesy Waffles) (MM, MC, LC, GF, VGT)

Kristin wanted to create low-carb waffles that were satisfying and kept low blood sugar at bay. One mini waffle maker and numerous waffles later, this sweet "chaffle" (cheesy waffle) recipe was born. The cheese and egg bind for a basic waffle batter; the peanut butter and chocolate complement the savory flavor with just enough sweet (you can use almond butter or your favorite nut or seed butter in place of the peanut butter if you like).

Prep time: 5 minutes
Cook time: 8-16 minutes
Total time: 13-21 minutes

SERVES 2

INGREDIENTS:
1 whole egg

1 egg white
1/2 cup mozzarella cheese (shredded preferred)
2 tablespoons cream cheese or ricotta cheese
2 tablespoons cocoa powder
2 tablespoons powdered peanut butter
2 tablespoons almond or coconut flour
1/4 cup sugar alternative (see pages 138–144)
Avocado oil spray
2 tablespoons natural peanut butter

INSTRUCTIONS:
1. Preheat mini waffle maker.
2. In a food processor or using an immersion blender, combine egg, egg white, mozzarella, and cream cheese or ricotta cheese. Blend until smooth.
3. Add cocoa powder, powdered peanut butter, almond or coconut flour, and sugar alternative to cheese and egg mixture. Blend again, until smooth and evenly mixed.
4. Spray waffle maker with avocado oil. Pour 1/4 of chaffle mixture into waffle maker, close top, and cook for 2–4 minutes. Move chaffle to a plate.
5. Repeat baking process until you have 4 chaffles.
6. Spread natural peanut butter on 2 of the chaffles, and then make 2 sandwiches with the remaining 2 chaffles.

Breakfast of Champions: Five Ways to Prepare Oatmeal

Microwaved Oatmeal. Mix 1/2 cup oats (steel-cut or rolled preferred) with 1 cup liquid (mix of water, milk, or unsweetened nondairy milk) and a pinch of salt and microwave for 2–3 minutes, keeping your eye on it after about a minute and a half so that it doesn't boil over. Remove and let the oatmeal sit for a few minutes so it can absorb more liquid, then add your topping of choice—such as a handful of blueberries and a tablespoon of ground flaxseeds.

Overnight Oats. These require even *less* prep time in the morning than microwaved oats—because you make them the night before! Combine 1/2 cup of your favorite oats and 1/2 cup of your favorite milk in a Mason jar with a lid. Mix in 1 tablespoon ground flaxseeds if you want extra fiber and beneficial fats, then cover and stick in the fridge overnight. You can add more flavorings in the morning, like cinnamon, berries, or walnuts.

Stove-Top Steel-Cut Oats. The basic ratio for steel-cut oats is 4 cups liquid (3 cups water and 1 cup of your favorite style of milk) to 1 cup of oats. For extra flavor, melt 1/2 tablespoon of butter or coconut oil in the pan first and then toast the oats over medium heat until they become fragrant. Then add the liquid and a pinch of salt, turn up to medium-high to bring to a boil, then turn down to a simmer until the oats reach the consistency you prefer, usually about 15–25 minutes, stirring occasionally.

Instant Pot Steel-Cut Oats. Pre-make your breakfast for the week with an Instant Pot or other pressure cooker. The ratio is 2 cups steel-cut oats to 5 cups liquid (a mix of water and your favorite milk, although using just water works fine, too). Program the Instant Pot to cook for 4 minutes, then let the pressure release naturally. Altogether, the cooking process will take about 20 minutes—resist the temptation to rush the steam release, as that's when the oats will really absorb the liquid.

To-Go Oats. Pour 1/2 cup rolled oats into an 8-ounce insulated container. Add a handful of roasted pecans and your favorite berry, 1/2 teaspoon of sweetener (see list that starts on page 138), and fill almost to the top with hot water. In an hour, it's ready to eat—whether you're at the office, a kid's soccer game, or on your commute to work.

SNACKS AND SIDES

Crispy Brussels Sprout Chips (MM, MC, LC, GF, KF, VGT)

Kristin loves Brussels sprouts, but her kids do not always share her enthusiasm. She says, "When my six-year-old told me he would eat them in chip form, I asked my intern, Olivia Dottore, to see if she could find a way to provide just that. She really delivered! Everyone in my family gobbles these down."

Prep time: 10 minutes
Cook time: 30 minutes
Total time: 40 minutes

SERVES 2

INGREDIENTS:
1 pound Brussels sprouts
Zest of 1 lemon
1–2 cups grated Parmesan cheese
Extra virgin olive oil or avocado oil
Salt

INSTRUCTIONS:
1. Preheat oven to 425°F.
2. Peel enough leaves off the sprouts to cover a baking sheet.
3. Sprinkle the leaves evenly with lemon zest, cheese, oil, and salt.
4. Bake until crispy, about 30 minutes.

Parmesan Crisps (MM, MC, LC, GF, KF, VGT)

This recipe works great on the Low-Carb eating plan. It's a wonderful substitute for carb-heavy crackers and provides just the right amount of flavor.

Prep time: 2 minutes
Cook time: 10 minutes
Total time: 12 minutes

SERVES 4

INGREDIENTS:
8-10 ounces fresh Parmesan cheese
Oil of choice, such as extra virgin olive oil or avocado oil

INSTRUCTIONS:
1. Grate Parmesan cheese on the medium-sized holes of a box grater.
2. Drizzle a small amount of oil on a sauté pan. Using a paper towel, spread the oil until it covers the pan.
3. Pile small circles of shredded cheese around the pan.
4. Cook on medium-high heat for about 5 minutes, or until cheese seems to be sticking to the pan.
5. Flip the cheese and cook until crispy, another 5 minutes.
6. Remove crisp from pan and place on paper towel to dry.

Crunchy Chickpeas (MM, MC, GF, V, VGT)

The roasted chickpeas were so popular in our first book, and chickpeas are such a great source of protein and fiber, we wanted to add them again with some suggestions for other herbs and spices. This blend has a great smoky flavor, thanks to the paprika. Consider saving the liquid from at least one of the cans of chickpeas to use to make Peanut Butter Breakfast Mousse—it will stay fresh, sealed in a glass jar, 2–3 days in the refrigerator.

Prep time: 5 minutes
Cook time: 30 minutes
Total time: 35 minutes

SERVES 10

INGREDIENTS:
2 15.5-ounce cans unsalted chickpeas
3 tablespoons extra virgin olive oil or avocado oil

1 teaspoon garlic powder
1/2 teaspoon salt
1/2 teaspoon cumin
1-1/2 teaspoons smoked paprika
1 teaspoon onion powder

INSTRUCTIONS:

1. Preheat oven to 425°F.
2. Drain the chickpeas in a colander, then transfer to a flat surface and dry thoroughly with a paper towel.
3. Pour the chickpeas into a medium-sized bowl and mix in all ingredients.
4. Transfer the chickpeas to a baking sheet lined with parchment paper.
5. Bake for approximately 30 minutes, mixing every 10 minutes. Most chickpeas should be crunchy when you take them out.

Holiday Roasted Chickpeas (MM, MC, GF, V, VGT)

We love holiday cookies as much as the next person, but not every holiday treat needs to be a dessert. These roasted chickpeas are a wonderful thing to give as a gift to a friend (put them in a Mason jar with a pretty ribbon) or to keep out on your counter during the busy end-of-year time for a healthy, grab-it snack. You could even leave them out for Santa, if that's a tradition in your household!

Prep time: 5 minutes
Cook time: 30 minutes
Total time: 35 minutes

SERVES 4

INGREDIENTS:
1 15.5-ounce can chickpeas
Extra virgin olive oil
1-1/2 teaspoons ginger
1 tablespoon cinnamon
1 tablespoon nutmeg

INSTRUCTIONS:

1. Preheat oven to 425°F.
2. Strain the can of chickpeas into a colander and allow to dry out for as long as possible. If there is no time for drying, use a dish towel to dab chickpeas dry.
3. Transfer chickpeas to a clean bowl and saturate in olive oil.
4. Add in ginger, cinnamon, and nutmeg. Mix until all chickpeas are fully covered. Amounts are suggestions; feel free to make this recipe your own with each amount of spice.
5. Spread chickpeas out on a baking sheet and place into the oven for about 30 minutes or until chickpeas are browned and look crispy.

Savory Rosemary Cashews (MM, MC, LC, GF, VGT)

The great news about this recipe is that it's highly versatile. You can swap cashews with almonds or pecans, or switch the savory herbs to something sweeter (by replacing the rosemary with cinnamon). Just keep the fat and the cooking time/temp the same and you are good to go.

Prep time: 5 minutes
Cook time: 8 minutes
Total time: 13 minutes

SERVES 10

INGREDIENTS:

3 cups raw cashews
2 tablespoons melted butter or extra virgin olive oil
3 tablespoons fresh or dried rosemary
1 teaspoon cayenne pepper
1/4 teaspoon cumin
1/4 teaspoon sea salt

INSTRUCTIONS:

1. Preheat oven to 350°F.
2. Mix cashews and melted butter or olive oil in bowl.
3. Add in remaining ingredients, mixing well.
4. Roast for 8 minutes, making sure not to overcook.

Cheese and Fig Bites (MM, MC, GF, VGT)

Having a party? This is the perfect recipe to satisfy your guests, without all the additives that store-bought puff pastries provide. You can use the dough in the recipe with your favorite combinations—roasted mushrooms and goat cheese, for example, or pesto and a cherry tomato. Have fun experimenting!

Prep time: 20 minutes
Cook time: 30 minutes
Total time: 50 minutes

SERVES 14

INGREDIENTS:
Extra virgin olive oil or avocado oil spray
2 cups almond flour
1 teaspoon salt
1/2 cup cold unsalted butter, cut into small cubes
1/2 cup cold water
1 package of 14 mini Babybel cheese rounds, peeled
4-1/2 tablespoons fig spread

INSTRUCTIONS:
1. Preheat oven to 400°F.
2. Grease mini muffin pan with olive oil or avocado oil spray and set aside.
3. Make the puff pastry dough: In the bowl of a food processor, combine almond flour, salt, and cold butter. Pulse a few times, just until butter is evenly dispersed. Add the cold water and pulse a few more times just until a rough dough forms.
4. Working on a floured surface (use a little extra almond flour to keep dough from sticking), roll the dough into a rectangle about 12 inches by 18 inches. Fold the dough in half, then in half again so that you have four layers of dough stacked on top of each other, and roll out dough one more time (using a little more almond flour so the dough doesn't stick to your rolling pin or rolling surface) so that it is again about 12 inches by 18 inches.

5. Wrap 1 Babybel cheese round with a piece of puff pastry dough that is approximately 3 inches square, leaving top slightly uncovered. In uncovered spot, spread 1 teaspoon fig spread.
6. Repeat until all Babybel cheese rounds are encased in dough and topped with fig spread.
7. Place on a greased cookie sheet and bake for 30 minutes or until browned.

Warm Ricotta Dip with Raspberry Swirl (MM, MC, GF, VGT)

We love dips because they are so versatile—you can use them as a dip or a spread or even alter slightly and make them into a sauce. This recipe combines the best of sweet and savory and is a good source of protein, thanks to the ricotta. Serve with Keto-Friendly Crackers, Whole Wheat Pita Bread, or your favorite low-carb cracker.

Prep time: 5 minutes
Cook time: 10-20 minutes
Total time: 15-25 minutes

SERVES 4

INGREDIENTS:
8 ounces ricotta cheese
Zest of 1 lemon
2 tablespoons fresh chopped mint
Extra virgin olive oil
Honey (optional)
1 6-ounce package fresh raspberries

INSTRUCTIONS:
1. Preheat oven to 400°F.
2. Mix ricotta, 1/2 of the lemon zest, 1/2 of the mint, drizzle of olive oil, and honey (optional) in bowl and transfer to oven-safe dish. Place in oven for 10-20 minutes until warm.
3. While mixture is in the oven, muddle (smash) freshly washed raspberries until smooth.

4. Remove ricotta mix from the oven and top with raspberry puree.
5. Using a fork, swirl raspberry puree throughout dip.
6. Top with remaining lemon zest and mint.

Party-Pleasing Edamame Dip (MM, MC, GF, V, VGT)

This is a favorite in Kristin's house for any occasion—light appetizers with friends, as a side, or as a sauce for roasted or grilled veggies. With a robust flavor, plenty of protein, and lots of fiber, this dip covers a lot of bases. She stores any leftovers in an airtight container in the fridge and uses the dip as a spread in place of mayonnaise.

Prep time: 10 minutes
Total time: 10 minutes

SERVES 12

INGREDIENTS:
1 12-ounce bag frozen shelled edamame, thawed
1/2 teaspoon salt
1/2 teaspoon soy sauce
Juice from 1 medium lemon
1/4 cup tahini
1 garlic clove, peeled
4 tablespoons extra virgin olive oil (reserve 1/2 tablespoon for drizzle)
1/2 teaspoon cumin

INSTRUCTIONS:
1. Combine all ingredients in a food processor and process until well combined.
2. Slowly add water, 1 tablespoon at a time, to reach desired consistency.

Heart-Healthy Hummus (MM, MC, GF, V, VGT)

Hummus is the black purse of the food world—it goes great with everything! It makes a great addition to any appetizer plate, can be a whole lunch (with some whole wheat pita and carrot and/or celery sticks), or is a perfect snack that, thanks to its high fiber content, will help you feel full until your next mealtime. It's also really easy to make—a bonus!

Prep time: 5 minutes
Total time: 5 minutes

SERVES 5

INGREDIENTS:
2 15.5-ounce cans unsalted chickpeas
3 garlic cloves, peeled
Juice from 1 lemon
4 tablespoons tahini
6 tablespoons extra virgin olive oil
1 teaspoon coriander
2 teaspoons cumin
1 teaspoon salt

INSTRUCTIONS:
In a blender or food processor, add all ingredients and mix until the consistency you want. If you want a smoother consistency, slowly add water until it reaches the desired texture.

Roasted Red Pepper Dip (MM, MC, LC, GF, VGT)

Creamy, nutty, tangy, and a little sweet, this roasted red pepper dip will be your new fave snack/appetizer/sauce.

Prep time: 5 minutes
Total time: 5 minutes

SERVES 6

INGREDIENTS:
1 12-ounce jar roasted red peppers, drained
1/2 cup extra virgin olive oil
1/4 cup walnuts
1/4 cup almonds
3 garlic cloves, peeled
Salt, to taste

Zest of 1 lemon

2 tablespoons Italian seasoning

2 tablespoons heavy whipping cream (optional)

INSTRUCTIONS:

1. Add all ingredients into blender (or bowl if using immersion blender). To make it creamy, add heavy whipping cream.
2. Blend until smooth.
3. Enjoy warm or cold.

Spinach Artichoke Dip (MM, MC, LC, GF, VGT)

Every once in a while, you might crave a comforting favorite. Because this dip has a high fat content, a little goes a long way. Instead of dipping crackers into the dip, serve it with raw pepper strips. You can also use it as a spread for a turkey sandwich, or swirl a spoonful into a bowl of warm bean-based pasta.

Prep time: 10 minutes

Cook time: 60 minutes

Total time: 1 hour, 10 minutes

SERVES 10

INGREDIENTS:

2 10-ounce boxes frozen chopped spinach, thawed

1 5.2-ounce package Boursin cheese, garlic and herb flavor

1 8-ounce package cream cheese

2 cups shredded white cheddar cheese

1/2 cup shredded mozzarella cheese

1-1/2 12-ounce jars artichoke hearts, drained

1 teaspoon garlic powder, or 2 cloves fresh garlic, minced

Salt and pepper, to taste

INSTRUCTIONS:

1. Preheat oven to 350°F.
2. Drain spinach, squeezing out excess water.
3. Add spinach, cheeses, and artichoke hearts into a bowl and mix thoroughly.
4. Add garlic powder (or fresh, if preferred) and salt and pepper to taste.

5. Place mixture in oven-safe dish and bake for 1 hour or until warm and cheese is fully melted.
6. Mix and serve!

Buffalo Chicken Dip (MM, MC, LC, GF)

One of the most challenging occasions for Kristin's and Ibrahim's patients when trying to stick to a lower-carb eating style is a party. This dip changes that. Serve it with corn tortilla chips if you're on the Modified Mediterranean or Family plans, and/or crudités or Keto-Friendly Crackers if you're on the Moderate-Carb or Low-Carb plans (provide a spoon since the crackers might break if you try to use them as a scoop). Either way, you can enjoy yourself—and the party—knowing that you're giving your liver a break from the high carbs found in most finger foods. One note of caution: The hot sauce really gives this a lot of zip! If your spice tolerance is lower, use half the bottle.

Prep time: 10 minutes
Cook time: 20 minutes
Total time: 30 minutes

SERVES 8

INGREDIENTS:
1 rotisserie chicken, skin removed, deboned and chopped fine
1 8-ounce package cream cheese, room temperature
1 8-ounce package Mexican blend shredded cheese
1 14-ounce bottle Bolthouse Farms Classic Ranch Yogurt dressing (available at Target and Walmart)
1 12-ounce bottle Frank's RedHot Original Cayenne Pepper Sauce

INSTRUCTIONS:
1. Preheat oven to 350°.
2. Place all ingredients in a large mixing bowl and mix thoroughly.
3. Transfer mixture to an oven-safe dish (such as a glass roasting pan or ceramic pie plate) and bake for 20 minutes until cheese is melted and dip is heated through.

Baba Ganoush (MM, MC, LC, GF, VGT)

Baba ganoush is Ibrahim's favorite Levantine appetizer. "Baba" is an Arabic word that means "father" and is also a term of endearment. "Ganoush" means "indulged" or "spoiled." The word combination "baba ganoush" is interpreted as "indulged or spoiled daddy." Ibrahim promises you the name matches the personality of this amazing dish, which is a silky eggplant dip with rich flavor.

Prep time: 10 minutes
Cook time: 20 minutes
Total time: 30 minutes (plus 10 minutes cooling time)

SERVES 4

INGREDIENTS:
3 medium eggplants, sliced in half lengthwise
2-3 garlic cloves, peeled and minced or run through a garlic press
3 tablespoons tahini
1/2 cup fresh lemon juice, from about 4 lemons
1 teaspoon salt
Extra virgin olive oil
1-2 tablespoons fresh pomegranate seeds, to taste

INSTRUCTIONS:
1. Preheat oven to 350°F and line a baking sheet with parchment paper; slice eggplants and place them, cut-side down, on the baking sheet. Roast in oven until soft, about 20 minutes, then let sit on the counter until cool enough to handle, about 10 minutes.
2. Peel the eggplants and puree the flesh, either in a food processor or using a potato masher in a medium-sized mixing bowl.
3. Add garlic, tahini, lemon juice, and salt, and mix well.
4. Drizzle olive oil on top and serve with a few fresh pomegranate seeds.

Keto-Friendly Crackers (MM, MC, LC, GF, VGT)

These crackers are amazing even if you are not looking for a low-carb approach. When Kristin serves these at parties, everyone asks her for the recipe. Spruce them up by making them sweet with cinnamon, exotic with cumin or turmeric, or tried and true with a little bit of salt and pepper.

Prep time: 5 minutes
Cook time: 30-35 minutes
Total time: 35-40 minutes (plus 10 minutes cooling time)

SERVES 4

INGREDIENTS:
4 cups easy-to-melt cheese (such as cheddar or mozzarella)
2 cups almond flour
2 tablespoons oregano or Italian seasoning
Salt, to taste

INSTRUCTIONS:
1. Preheat oven to 375°F.
2. Shred cheese and melt in a microwave-safe bowl in the microwave, for about 60 seconds, checking on it every 15-20 seconds to make sure it doesn't burn.
3. Add almond flour, seasoning, and salt to cheese.
4. Knead mixture until evenly textured.
5. Roll out dough to approximately 1/8 inch thick, and cut into triangles or preferred shape.
6. Place on baking sheet and put in oven.
7. Bake for about 15 minutes or until crispy on upward-facing side, and then flip.
8. Bake for another 15 to 20 minutes until brown and crispy.
9. Place pan on a wire rack and let cool for 10 minutes.

Whole Wheat Pita Bread (MM, V, VGT)

Kristin found this recipe in a newspaper and, over the course of many years, tweaked it to make it her own. Don't worry about the sugar—you need it to activate the yeast, and it's such a small amount that it won't impact total grams of carbs per pita. Kristin makes this bread to add as a whole-grain side to dishes or to serve as an awesome dipper for dips and hummus.

Prep time: 90 minutes
Cook time: 18–35 minutes × number of balls
Total time: about 2–3 hours

SERVES 2 TO 4

INGREDIENTS:
1 cup lukewarm water
1/2 teaspoon granulated sugar
2 teaspoons active dry yeast
1-1/2 cups whole wheat flour, divided
1-1/4 cups all-purpose flour, divided
1 teaspoon salt
2 tablespoons extra virgin olive oil

INSTRUCTIONS:
1. In a large mixing bowl, add water, sugar, and yeast. Mix until dissolved.
   Then add 1/4 cup whole wheat flour and 1/4 cup all-purpose flour and
   whisk together. Set aside, uncovered, for about 15 minutes or until frothy.
2. Preheat the oven to 475°F and place a baking sheet in the oven.
3. Add salt, olive oil, and the rest of both flours (1 cup of all-purpose
   flour and 1-1/4 cup of whole wheat flour). Mix thoroughly. In a
   standard mixer with a kneading attachment or using hands, knead
   for 1 minute (or until all dry pieces are gone).
4. Continue kneading until smooth. Cover the bowl and allow the
   dough to rest for 10 minutes. Knead again for 2–3 minutes.
5. Cover the bowl with plastic wrap as tightly as possible and allow
   dough to rise until it has doubled from original size. This will
   usually take about 1 hour.
6. Deflate dough using hands and create 12–15 3-inch dough balls. Place
   dough balls on a different (room temperature) baking pan and cover
   with a damp towel for 10 minutes.
7. Remove 2 dough balls while keeping others covered. Flatten each
   into a disk and place in the oven on the hot baking sheet. Once
   dough is puffy (about 2–3 minutes), flip dough disks over and bake
   for another 1–2 minutes. Remove to a platter on the counter and cover
   with a dish towel to keep warm while the other pitas cook.
8. Continue the same process with the rest of the dough balls.

Whole Wheat Pita Fennel Chips (MM, V, VGT)

Many of Kristin's patients have heard of fennel but have never used it in a recipe. This was her way to get fennel into the kitchens of her patients because, as a plant, it's a great source of fiber, vitamins, and minerals.

Prep time: 10 minutes
Cook time: 15–20 minutes
Total time: 25–30 minutes

SERVES 6 TO 8

INGREDIENTS:
2 tablespoons minced garlic
1/4 cup extra virgin olive oil
1 package whole wheat pitas (or 4 homemade pitas)
Ground fennel seeds, to taste
Salt, to taste

INSTRUCTIONS:
1. Preheat oven to 350°F.
2. Mix garlic and oil.
3. Cut pitas into triangles and open. Lay triangles on baking sheet.
4. Brush olive oil and garlic mixture onto triangles. Sprinkle fennel seeds and salt evenly on triangles.
5. Bake until crispy (about 15 to 20 minutes) or until browned.

SAUCES

Tahini Sauce (MM, MC, LC, GF, V, VGT)

Tahini, a smooth paste made of ground sesame seeds, is of Arabic origin. And since sesame seeds are rich in calcium, tahini is a great way to up the mineral content of your meals while also adding a delicious savory element. (Fun fact: the pronunciation of the word "tahini" is the same in English, Arabic, and Hebrew.)

Prep time: 3 minutes
Total time: 3 minutes

SERVES 2 TO 4

INGREDIENTS:
3/4 cup tahini
2 tablespoons extra virgin olive oil
Pinch of salt
3 garlic cloves, peeled
Juice of 1/2 lemon

INSTRUCTIONS:
1. Place ingredients into blender (or bowl if using immersion blender).
2. Blend together, slowly adding water until sauce is at desired thickness.

Red Sauce (MM, MC, GF, V, VGT)

This is Kristin's favorite Italian American red sauce recipe that uses diced/ crushed tomatoes as a shortcut. It's great on bean-based pasta, of course, but also perfect in Vegetarian Lasagna and on top of No-Carb Pizza (a.k.a. "The Friday Night Special").

Prep time: 15 minutes
Cook time: 2–3 hours
Total time: 2 hours, 15 minutes to 3 hours, 15 minutes

SERVES 10 TO 12

INGREDIENTS:
1 large yellow onion, diced
4 garlic cloves, minced
2 28-ounce cans tomato puree
1 28-ounce can tomato paste
1 28-ounce can diced/crushed tomatoes
2 tablespoons garlic powder
2 tablespoons Italian seasoning
2 tablespoons dried oregano
1 tablespoon dried basil
Granulated sugar, to taste

INSTRUCTIONS:

1. Sauté onion on medium heat until translucent, about 8 minutes. Add minced garlic and cook until fragrant, about 1 minute.
2. Add all cans of tomato (puree, paste, diced/crushed). Using the puree can, add 2 cans of water. Stir to combine, then bring contents to a boil and reduce to a simmer.
3. Add seasonings (garlic powder, Italian seasoning, dried oregano, and dried basil). Stir every 5 minutes or so until flavors meld and sauce develops a smooth consistency, about 2–3 hours.
4. Taste and determine if any sugar is needed. If so, slowly add up to 1 tablespoon of sugar, tasting after each addition to get the right level of sweetness.

PESTO CHANGE-O: A QUICK WAY TO ADD VARIETY AND NUTRIENT DENSITY TO YOUR MEALS

True pesto hails from Liguria, a region in the northwest of Italy. It's a fresh, fragrant, salty sauce traditionally made from pine nuts, sea salt, garlic, Parmigiano-Reggiano cheese, pecorino cheese, fresh basil, and extra virgin olive oil that can be used in a variety of ways in a variety of dishes—as a pasta sauce, or a dressing for grilled vegetables, or a condiment swirled into a bowl of soup. Today, pesto has ventured beyond Italy and become one of the world's most popular sauces. During its travels, pesto has morphed to incorporate many different cultures, tastes, and dishes.

We consider pesto a liver-friendly food because it helps deliver plenty of the polyphenol-rich extra virgin olive oil that is a staple of the Mediterranean diet, the many nutrients that are naturally abundant in fresh herbs, vitamin B12 from cheese, antibacterial properties from garlic, and protein and minerals from nuts. And it packages all these benefits in a heaping helping of flavor that can make even the simplest dishes something swoon-worthy.

When you riff on the basic formula of pesto to weave in other ingredients— including seeds, nutritional yeast (if you want to make it vegan), and tofu— you not only vary the flavor profile but also mix up the nutrients.

If you want to put some extra love—and elbow grease—into your pesto, you can use a mortar and pestle to pound the ingredients yourself. If you want to make less effort, a food processor or high-speed blender will do the job in a snap.

Traditional Basil Pesto (MM, MC, LC, GF, VGT)

This original pesto is like a great pair of shoes—it goes with everything. Of course, you know to add it to pasta, but it's also an excellent addition to scrambled eggs, as a marinade for chicken (along with a squeeze of lemon juice or douse of vinegar), a mix-in for quinoa and/or cooked lentils, or even thinned with a little more olive oil and a splash or two of your favorite vinegar to make a delicious vinaigrette! Keep some frozen in ice cubes (see note for instructions) and you always have an easy way to add freshness and nutrient density to a quick meal or snack.

Prep time: 5 minutes
Total time: 5 minutes

SERVES 6

INGREDIENTS:
2 cups fresh basil leaves
2 tablespoons pine nuts or walnuts
2 large garlic cloves
1/2 cup extra virgin olive oil
1/2 cup grated Parmesan cheese
Salt, to taste

INSTRUCTIONS:
1. Process basil, nuts, and garlic in a food processor until minced.
2. With the machine running on low, slowly pour in the olive oil until you get a smooth consistency.
3. Stop the food processor, add in half the cheese and salt, and pulse a few times just until combined.
4. Last, add in the rest of the cheese and process minimally until combined.

Note: Leftovers will keep for up to one week in a tightly sealed jar in the refrigerator. Kristin pours a thin layer of extra virgin olive oil to cover the surface of the mixture, which will keep the basil bright green. Or portion out into ice cube trays and put in freezer until frozen, then transfer to an airtight freezer-safe bag. Will keep up to three months in the freezer.

Triple Herb Pesto (MM, MC, LC, GF, VGT)

The trifecta of herbs that gives this pesto its name is basil, cilantro, and mint. When you mix those three, it creates a delightfully light and bright flavor that's a great accompaniment to grilled chicken and vegetables, a schmear of ricotta cheese on a piece of whole-grain toast, or even swirled into scrambled eggs.

Prep time: 2 minutes
Total time: 2 minutes

SERVES 6

INGREDIENTS:
2 cups fresh basil
1/2 cup mint
1/2 cup cilantro
4 garlic cloves, peeled
1-1/2 tablespoons diced shallot
1 cup pine nuts
1/2 cup grated Parmesan cheese
3/4 cup extra virgin olive oil
Salt, to taste

INSTRUCTIONS:
1. Place all ingredients except salt into blender. Blend until smooth.
2. Add salt to taste.

Note: Leftovers will keep for up to one week in the refrigerator.

Nutty Vegan Pesto (MM, MC, LC, GF, VGT)

According to the Climate Change 2022 Report from the United Nations, shifting your diet from animal- to plant-based food has a high potential for reducing carbon emissions and mitigating climate change, as well as improving human health.[1] With macadamia nuts taking the place of cheese, this yummy dairy-free pesto has a rich, creamy flavor and benefits that extend above and beyond deliciousness.

Prep time: 5 minutes
Total time: 5 minutes

SERVES 6

INGREDIENTS:
1/4 cup extra virgin garlic olive oil
1/4 cup walnuts
1/4 cup macadamia nuts
1/2 cup pecans
1 teaspoon sea salt
3 ounces fresh basil

INSTRUCTIONS:
1. Put all ingredients in a food processor or blender.
2. Blend to desired consistency.

Note: Leftovers will keep for up to one week in the refrigerator.

Spicy Vegan Cilantro Pesto (MM, MC, LC, GF, VGT)

Parmesan cheese is a hallmark pesto ingredient, but you can still make a delicious herby sauce without it by swapping it out for nutritional yeast—a good source of vitamin B12 with a cheesy, nutty flavor that's reminiscent of Parmesan cheese. The cilantro and jalapeño give this sauce a kick beyond the typical bite of raw garlic, and the tofu mellows things out while delivering a good amount of plant-based protein. Try a tablespoon of this with your favorite drained and rinsed canned beans (adzuki, black, and pinto are good matches) wrapped in a low-carb tortilla or on a bed of your favorite salad green.

Prep time: 5 minutes
Total time: 5 minutes

SERVES 6

INGREDIENTS:
2 cups cilantro leaves, packed
1/4 cup sunflower seeds, roasted, unsalted, and shelled

1 jalapeño pepper, destemmed, deseeded, and roughly chopped
4 garlic cloves, peeled
1 tablespoon lime juice (from 1 lime, if using fresh)
8 ounces firm tofu, drained
1/4 cup extra virgin olive oil
1/4 cup nutritional yeast (optional)
Salt, to taste

INSTRUCTIONS:
1. Put all ingredients in a food processor or blender.
2. Blend until smooth and creamy.

Note: Leftovers will keep for up to one week in the refrigerator.

Cashew Spinach Pesto (MM, MC, LC, GF, V [if using nutritional yeast], VGT)

You'll be surprised how creamy this sauce is, thanks to the soaked cashews. Use it to slather slices of grilled or roasted eggplant or zucchini. Or mix it into warm pasta—it will melt and coat your noodles while still delivering a pleasant zing thanks to the lemon juice.

Prep time: 5 minutes (plus 30 minutes soaking time)
Total time: 35 minutes

SERVES 6

INGREDIENTS:
1/4 cup cashews
4 cups fresh spinach
1 cup fresh basil
2-3 tablespoons grated Parmesan cheese or nutritional yeast
2 garlic cloves, peeled
1/4 cup low-sodium vegetable broth
2 tablespoons lemon juice (from about 1 large lemon, if using fresh)
Salt, to taste

INSTRUCTIONS:

1. Place cashews in a bowl and add enough boiling water to cover. Let them soak for 30 minutes, then drain.
2. In a high-speed blender or food processor, add all ingredients and blend until you get a smooth consistency.

Note: Leftovers will keep in a tightly sealed jar in the refrigerator up to two days.

Pumpkin Seed Pesto with Parsley (MM, MC, LC, GF, V [if omitting Parmesan cheese], VGT)

This is a great way to use up leftover herbs, with a hearty taste—thanks to the pumpkin seeds—that makes a standard sautéed chicken breast sing. It's also great as a dip with Whole Wheat Pita Chips or Keto-Friendly Crackers (or your favorite nutrient-dense cracker). The fiber and minerals from the pumpkin seeds make this pesto a delicious way to add extra nutrition to your meal or snack.

Prep time: 5 minutes
Total time: 5 minutes

SERVES 6

INGREDIENTS:
1/2 cup shelled pumpkin seeds
2 garlic cloves, peeled
2 tablespoons grated Parmesan cheese (optional)
3/4 cup fresh parsley leaves
3/4 cup fresh basil leaves
2 tablespoons fresh lemon juice
1/2 cup extra virgin olive oil
Salt, to taste

INSTRUCTIONS:

1. Combine the pumpkin seeds, garlic, and Parmesan cheese (if using) in a food processor and pulse for 20 seconds until ground.

2. Add in the parsley, basil, lemon juice, and oil and pulse again for 40 seconds to combine into a thick sauce.

Note: Leftovers will keep in a tightly sealed jar in the refrigerator up to two days.

Dill and Lemon Pesto (MM, MC, LC, GF, V, VGT)

This sauce just tastes like spring and makes a great accompaniment to grilled or roasted salmon and/or vegetables (especially asparagus if it's in season!) or as the dressing for a quick chickpea salad (combine a drained and rinsed can of chickpeas with a cup of halved cherry tomatoes and mix with this pesto to taste).

Prep time: 5 minutes
Total time: 5 minutes

SERVES 6

INGREDIENTS:
5 tablespoons walnuts
5 garlic cloves, peeled
Zest of 1 large lemon
6 ounces fresh dill
Salt, to taste
3/4–1 cup extra virgin olive oil

INSTRUCTIONS:
1. Place walnuts and garlic into a food processor and process until chopped.
2. Add in the lemon zest, dill, and salt, and process until a paste is formed.
3. Continue to pulse while slowly pouring in the olive oil until a thick sauce forms.

Note: Leftovers will keep in a tightly sealed jar in the refrigerator up to two days.

High-Protein Green Pea Pesto (MM, MC, LC, GF, V [if omitting Parmesan cheese], VGT)

This hearty sauce is almost a meal in itself—kind of a cross between pesto and hummus. Eat it smeared on a piece of whole-grain toast or in a low-carb tortilla with a couple of slices of avocado for more of a meal, or as a dip with red pepper strips or cucumber spears for a nutrient-dense snack.

Prep time: 5 minutes
Total time: 5 minutes

SERVES 6

INGREDIENTS:
1 cup frozen peas, thawed
3/4 cup packed basil leaves
2 garlic cloves, peeled
1/4 cup shredded Parmesan cheese (optional)
1/4 cup tahini
5 tablespoons extra virgin olive oil
Fresh ground black pepper and salt, to taste

INSTRUCTIONS:
1. In a food processor combine peas, basil, garlic, and cheese (if using), and pulse until finely chopped.
2. Run the processor on low while adding the tahini first, and then 1 tablespoon of the olive oil at a time until the mixture is well blended.
3. Add salt and pepper to taste.

Note: Leftovers will keep in a tightly sealed container in the refrigerator up to two days.

BASIC ANIMAL PROTEINS

When you know how to prepare a few different, basic versions of our two favorite animal proteins, you can customize them in multiple ways (we suggest a few of those ways in our Meal Suggestions for each of the Renew Your Liver eating plans). You can prep either a few chicken breasts or salmon filets on Sunday night and have a building block for multiple meals throughout the week.

Leftovers will keep in the refrigerator for three days or in the freezer for up to four months. To freeze, wrap in waxed paper and then store in a freezer-safe plastic bag that you've labeled and dated so that you don't forget what's in it. To thaw, place in the refrigerator overnight. You can reheat in the microwave, a toaster oven, or in a pan on the stove top with the other ingredients of whatever dish you're adding it to.

Baked Chicken Breast (MM, MC, LC, GF)

Baked chicken breast blends with so many different sauces, sides, and flavor profiles, which is why we included it in so many of our suggested meals. You can certainly bake one half of a breast at a time if you are cooking for one, but cooking several at once will save you cooking time on a future meal.

Prep time: 5 minutes
Cook time: 40-45 minutes
Total time: 45-50 minutes

SERVES 4

INGREDIENTS:
4 halves boneless, skinless chicken breasts
Extra virgin olive oil, to taste
Salt and pepper, to taste

INSTRUCTIONS:
1. Preheat oven to 375°F.
2. Place the chicken breasts in a 9-inch × 12-inch glass or ceramic baking dish. (For easier cleanup, line pan with foil.)
3. Drizzle with extra virgin olive oil and sprinkle of salt and pepper on both sides.
4. Place on center rack in the oven and bake until a thermometer (we love the Thermapen) reads 160°F in the thickest part of the breast, about 40-45 minutes. (Check it after 35 minutes as overcooked chicken breast will become dry.)

5. Serve immediately, or let cool to room temperature, about 15 minutes, before refrigerating or freezing.

Grilled Chicken Breast (MM, MC, LC, GF)

Grilled chicken breast is even more flavorful than baked chicken— especially if you have time to marinate it before you grill it, although it's still good if you only have time to drizzle with olive oil and add salt and pepper to taste before tossing on the grill. It can hold its own on top of a salad or with a side of your favorite vegetable (such as steamed green beans, roasted broccoli, sautéed spinach, or baked sweet potato). Top it with a tablespoon or two of your favorite pesto if you want to jazz it up further. Pounding the chicken breast before grilling will help it be more tender and cook more evenly. You can also slice it into equal-sized strips, and it will grill up even more quickly.

Prep time: 10 minutes
Cook time: 12 minutes
Total time: 22 minutes (plus 1 hour marinating time)

SERVES 4

INGREDIENTS:
4 halves boneless, skinless chicken breasts
1/2 cup of your favorite marinade (such as low-sugar teriyaki, low-sugar BBQ, or Italian dressing) or a drizzle of extra virgin olive oil
Salt and pepper, to taste

INSTRUCTIONS:
1. Place chicken breasts on a poultry-only cutting board and use a meat tenderizer to pound chicken to about 1/2-inch thickness.
2. If marinating in advance, place chicken breasts in a bowl and cover with your marinade of choice. Turn to coat, then cover bowl with plastic wrap and let sit in the fridge for at least 1 hour and as long as 12 hours. If not marinating in advance, place chicken breasts in a bowl and drizzle with extra virgin olive oil, add salt and pepper to taste, and toss to coat.

3. Preheat grill to medium-high (about 400°F). Once grill is hot, place chicken on grill and cook about 6 minutes per side, until chicken reads 160°F using a meat thermometer.
4. Serve immediately, or let cool to room temperature, about 15 minutes, before refrigerating or freezing.

Broiled Salmon (MM, MC, LC, GF)

Broiled salmon is about as easy as it gets—you don't even need to flip it. Jazz the filets up with your favorite seasoning and then have fun finding how many different things you can pair it with. Look for wild-caught salmon filets or sustainably farmed Atlantic salmon.

Prep time: 5 minutes
Cook time: 7-9 minutes (plus 5 minutes resting time)
Total time: 17-19 minutes

SERVES 3

INGREDIENTS:
1 pound salmon filets
Your choice of seasoning, such as lemon pepper, Old Bay seasoning, dried dill, and salt and pepper, to taste
Extra virgin olive oil, for drizzling
Fresh lemon wedges, optional, for serving

INSTRUCTIONS:
1. Position your top oven rack to about 6 inches from the top of your oven.
2. Turn broiler on high.
3. Place salmon pieces skin side down on a sheet pan that you've covered with foil.
4. Drizzle with extra virgin olive oil, then sprinkle with salt, pepper, and seasoning of choice.
5. Cook until internal temperature is at least 135°F (for medium rare) or 140°F (for well done) and fish flakes easily with a fork, about 7-9 minutes.
6. Let salmon rest 5 minutes before serving to let it continue cooking. Squeeze juice from lemon wedges over the salmon, if using.

7. Serve immediately, or let cool to room temperature, about 15 minutes, before refrigerating or freezing.

Grilled Salmon (MM, MC, LC, GF)

Grilled salmon is a restaurant-worthy treat that you can easily make at home. It pairs with so many things—drizzled with soy sauce and a little toasted sesame oil, served on a bed of brown rice, quinoa, or cauliflower rice, or served with grilled asparagus, or atop your favorite salad. As with broiled salmon, look for wild-caught salmon filets or sustainably farmed Atlantic salmon.

Prep time: 5 minutes
Cook time: 12-16 minutes
Total time: 17-21 minutes

SERVES 3

INGREDIENTS:
1 pound salmon filets
Your choice of seasoning, such as lemon pepper, Old Bay seasoning, dried dill, and salt and pepper, to taste
Extra virgin olive oil, for drizzling and for oiling grill grates
Fresh lemon wedges, optional

INSTRUCTIONS:
1. Sprinkle salmon flesh with your seasoning of choice and salt and pepper.
2. Make sure grill grates are clean before you turn grill on. Once cleaned, preheat grill to medium.
3. Use tongs and a paper towel to thoroughly oil grill grates so that salmon doesn't stick.
4. Put salmon directly on grill grates skin side down.
5. Cook salmon 6-8 minutes per side, until fish flakes easily with a fork.
6. Squeeze juice from lemon wedges over the salmon, if using.
7. Serve immediately, or let cool to room temperature, about 15 minutes, before refrigerating or freezing.

MAIN MEALS, FROM LIGHT TO HEARTY

Tabbouleh (MM, MC, LC, V, VGT)

This recipe is straight from Ibrahim's mother's kitchen. An immigrant from Syria, his mother influenced his life in many ways, especially in her approach to cooking and gathering around a table of delicious and healthy Mediterranean food. With fresh veggies and bulgur wheat, this is a dish that is both delicate and packed with nutrients. Ibrahim says, "When I eat this salad, I can feel the love! And I hope you will, too."

Prep time: 15 minutes
Total time: 15 minutes (plus 10-15 minutes soaking time)

SERVES 2

INGREDIENTS:
2 bunches fresh Italian parsley, coarsely chopped, about 4 cups
1/2 bunch fresh mint, coarsely chopped, about 3/4 cup
1 bunch green onions, finely chopped, white and light green parts only
1 tablespoon bulgur wheat, soaked in a small bowl of water until soft, 10-15 minutes
1/4-1/2 cup extra virgin olive oil
1/4-1/2 cup fresh lemon juice, from 3-4 lemons
1 teaspoon salt
1 medium tomato, coarsely chopped

INSTRUCTIONS:
Mix all ingredients in a bowl and enjoy.

Butternut Squash Soup (MM, MC, GF, V, VGT)

Kristin's first experience with butternut squash soup came courtesy of the chef at the Cleveland Clinic, who taught her how to choose a butternut squash and create a soup that was ultimately a meal. She added in some more onion and garlic and it became her family's go-to Friday-night dinner during the fall months.

Prep time: 20 minutes
Cook time: 70 minutes
Total time: 1 hour, 30 minutes

SERVES 6 TO 8

INGREDIENTS:
1-1/2 to 2 medium-sized butternut squash
Extra virgin olive oil
Salt and pepper, to taste
1 cup raw pepitas (optional)
1-2 tablespoons paprika (optional)
4 tablespoons unsalted butter
2 cups yellow onion, chopped (about 2)
1 cup celery, chopped (about 2 stalks)
1 cup carrots, chopped (about 3 large)
5-7 garlic cloves, minced
4-8 sprigs thyme
4 cups no-salt-added or low-sodium chicken or vegetable stock
1 teaspoon chili flakes
1 cup heavy whipping cream

INSTRUCTIONS:
1. Preheat oven to 350°F. Line a large baking sheet with parchment paper for easy cleaning.
2. Slice each butternut squash in half and set face up on a tray. Drizzle thoroughly with olive oil and dust with salt and pepper. Bake for 1 hour or until soft enough to easily scoop out with a spoon.
3. (Optional) On another baking sheet, spread out pepitas, saturate with olive oil, and dust with paprika. Roast in oven for about 15-20 minutes. Set aside.
4. In a large soup pot or Dutch oven, melt butter and add onions, celery, carrots, garlic, and thyme. Sauté on medium heat until onions are translucent, about 8 minutes.
5. Add chicken (or vegetable) stock and chili flakes to the pot and reduce heat to medium-low. Cook until carrots are tender.
6. Once carrots are tender, remove thyme sprigs from the pot and add in the roasted butternut squash.

7. Using an immersion blender (or regular blender), blend ingredients in pot together until texture is smooth. Note: If using a traditional blender, work in small batches and start the blender on a low speed setting before increasing. Hot liquids will create steam and expand when blended in a traditional blender, which could result in explosion.
8. Add heavy whipping cream to soup and blend (or mix) again until well combined. Season with salt and pepper to taste.
9. Serve in soup bowls and garnish with toasted paprika and roasted pepitas, if using.

Notes: You can make the recipe vegetarian by using vegetable stock. You can make the recipe vegan by using vegetable stock, using olive oil instead of butter, and skipping the heavy whipping cream or replacing it with a nondairy option.

Roasted Cauliflower and Mushroom Soup (MM, MC, LC, GF, V, VGT)

Bill Althoff provided this recipe. Chef Bill is a private chef who has cooked for numerous dignitaries, including President Ronald Reagan, President George H. W. Bush, and King Hussein and Queen Noor of Jordan. Chef Bill's most recent client read our first book, Skinny Liver, and asked him to modify some of his recipes to be more liver friendly. Kristin and Ibrahim are so happy to be able to share this recipe (as well as his recipes for Sautéed Shrimp on Curried Spaghetti Squash and Pan-Seared Salmon with a Ginger Turmeric Sauce and Cauliflower Rice) with you now, for those times you want to enjoy fine dining that is also low carb.

Yes, this soup takes a long time to prepare. But it is so silky and savory—and so good for your liver—that it is absolutely worth it. It also makes a lot, so you can have plenty of leftovers for the week ahead if you make it on a Sunday afternoon, or you can freeze your leftovers (in a plastic freezer bag) and have a meal at the ready for another day. (To thaw, place soup in the refrigerator overnight and then reheat over low heat in a pot on the stove top.)

Prep time: 15 minutes
Cook time: About 2 hours
Total time: 2 hours, 15 minutes

SERVES 8

INGREDIENTS:
1 cup garlic cloves, peeled (from 3–5 heads)
1 cup extra virgin olive oil
2 pounds cauliflower (about 2 small heads), stem removed and cut
into 1-inch pieces
Kosher salt and ground black pepper, to taste
12 ounces white button mushrooms, stems removed and sliced thin
(about 5 cups)
5 ounces baby Bella mushrooms, stems removed and sliced thin
(about 2 cups)
1/4 cup shallots, peeled and sliced thin (about 2 shallots)
2 quarts low-sodium vegetable stock
2–3 fresh chives, minced (optional)

INSTRUCTIONS:
1. Preheat oven to 350°F.
2. In a small, high-sided roasting pan or Pyrex dish, combine peeled
   garlic cloves and olive oil. Place in the oven for 25–30 minutes or
   until the garlic cloves are a light golden brown.
3. Remove and allow to cool slightly (15–20 minutes). (Garlic cloves will
   get darker during cooling, which is desired.)
4. Use a fine mesh strainer or slotted spoon to remove roasted garlic
   cloves from the oil and set both aside.
5. While garlic is cooling, increase oven temperature to 450°F.
6. Place cut cauliflower pieces in a mixing bowl or plastic container
   and drizzle reserved garlic oil over cauliflower pieces until lightly
   coated. Season coated cauliflower with salt and ground black pepper
   and mix thoroughly.
7. Transfer cauliflower pieces to a lined baking sheet and spread
   evenly. Roast for 40 minutes, stirring halfway through to ensure
   even browning.
8. Remove from the oven and set aside to cool.

9. While cauliflower is roasting, heat a large pot or Dutch oven over medium-high heat.
10. Add remaining garlic oil to completely coat the bottom of the pot. If the bottom of the pot is not completely coated, use more olive oil as needed.
11. Once oil is hot, add all sliced mushrooms and stir to coat with oil.
12. Cook mushrooms uncovered on medium-high heat until they are a light golden brown (approximately 30 minutes).
Note: mushrooms will release all their liquid and cook down at first; once the liquid evaporates, stir frequently to ensure even browning.
13. Once mushrooms are browned, reduce heat to low and add sliced shallots and all of the reserved roasted garlic cloves. Cook, stirring occasionally, until shallots are slightly translucent, about 5 minutes.
14. Once shallots are translucent, add roasted cauliflower pieces and all of the vegetable stock and stir.
15. Bring to a light simmer and cook for 30 minutes or until cauliflower begins to fall apart.
16. Remove from heat and blend soup using an immersion-stick blender or traditional blender until completely smooth. Season with salt and pepper to taste. Note: If using a traditional blender, work in small batches and start the blender on a low speed setting before increasing. Hot liquids will create steam and expand when blended in a traditional blender, which could result in explosion.
17. Serve immediately with minced chives or cool and freeze for later use.

Stuffed Baked Sweet Potatoes (MM, MC, GF, VGT)

We cannot think of a better dish for a family meal—whether it's a random Wednesday or a special occasion. Packed with kale, quinoa, cranberries, and fresh mozzarella, these baked sweet potatoes pack a lot of surprising flavor in one nutritious—and delicious—package.

Prep time: 10 minutes
Cook time: 50 minutes
Total time: 60 minutes

SERVES 4

Ingredients:
2 large sweet potatoes, halved
Extra virgin olive oil, to taste
Salt and pepper
4 cups fresh, curly kale
1-2 cloves fresh garlic, minced
1 cup tricolor quinoa, rinsed
1 8-ounce package fresh pearled mozzarella, drained
1/3 cup dried cranberries
Fig balsamic vinegar, to taste

INSTRUCTIONS:
1. Preheat oven to 425°F.
2. Line a baking sheet with parchment paper and place 2 halved large sweet potatoes face up. Drizzle with olive oil and sprinkle lightly with salt and pepper. Bake for 30 minutes or until soft.
3. While potatoes roast, sauté kale and garlic in olive oil in a large pan on the stove top over medium heat, until kale is darker green and slightly wilted.
4. In a medium saucepan, boil quinoa for about 10 minutes or as listed on package.
5. In a separate mixing bowl, mix quinoa, sautéed kale, pearled cheese, and cranberries.
6. Once potatoes are cooked, spoon a small crater out of the potato to create a bowl for stuffing. Spoon stuffing mixture onto the potato and top with a drizzle of fig balsamic vinegar.
7. Optional: top with walnuts, pecans, or nuts of your choice.

Sweet Potato Holiday Casserole (MM, MC, GF, VGT)

Kristin says, "My mom used to make this when I was a kid, and I referred to it as 'orange casserole' due to the bright and vibrant orange color. Today, I know that the orange color means that I can have my casserole and phytonutrients at the same time!"

Prep time: 10 minutes
Cook time: 2 hours
Total time: 2 hours, 10 minutes

SERVES 6 TO 8

INGREDIENTS:
5 medium-sized sweet potatoes (not yams)
3/4 cup granulated erythritol
1/2 cup low-fat milk or nondairy milk of choice (unsweetened/unflavored)
1/2 cup melted ghee
2 teaspoons vanilla extract
2 eggs, well beaten
1/2 cup erythritol-based brown sugar alternative
1-1/2 cups chopped pecans

INSTRUCTIONS:
1. Preheat oven to 425°F.
2. Using a fork, poke holes in each sweet potato. Place sweet potatoes in oven for 50 to 60 minutes or until tender. Remove potatoes from oven, then turn oven down to 350°F.
3. Allow potatoes to cool until OK to handle, about 15 minutes, then peel.
4. Mash potatoes in a large bowl.
5. Add granulated erythritol, low-fat milk or nondairy milk of choice, melted ghee, vanilla extract, and eggs to mashed sweet potatoes. Mix thoroughly.
6. Place contents from the bowl into a glass baking casserole dish. Evenly sprinkle pecans and 1/2 cup erythritol-based brown sugar alternative on top.
7. Bake at 350°F for 30 to 40 minutes until warm.

Krissy's Keto Broccoli and Cheese Casserole (MM, MC, LC, GF, VGT)

This nutty, cheesy casserole is a hit every time. Best of all, you can get this delightful dish on the table in only twenty-five minutes.

Prep time: 5 minutes
Cook time: 20 minutes
Total time: 25 minutes

SERVES 6

INGREDIENTS:
8 ounces cream cheese
1/2 cup half-and-half
2 cups mixed shredded cheese, such as a blend of cheddar,
Parmesan, and gruyere
1 tablespoon garlic powder
1 teaspoon salt
1 teaspoon pepper
2 pounds broccoli florets, steamed until al dente

INSTRUCTIONS:
1. Preheat oven to 400°F.
2. Mix all ingredients except broccoli.
3. Add broccoli to the cheese/seasoning mixture and mix until the broccoli is fully coated.
4. Bake for 15 minutes in an oven-safe casserole dish until cheese is fully melted.
5. Broil for 5 minutes until the top is crispy.
6. Serve hot.

Easy African Peanut Stew (MM, MC, LC, GF, V, VGT)

Ibrahim first learned this recipe when he hiked Mount Kilimanjaro. He says, "This was the favorite recipe of Chef Adam, the man who cooked for all the tourists and porters in the group. When we were at a high altitude with a low amount of oxygen after a strenuous, long day of hiking, this recipe stood out. I love it and hope you will, too!"

Prep time: 15 minutes
Cook time: 25 minutes
Total time: 40 minutes

SERVES 4

INGREDIENTS:
1 yellow onion, diced
5-9 garlic cloves, minced
2 sweet potatoes, peeled and cubed
4 quarts vegetable stock
1 cup no-added-sugar peanut butter
2-1/2 teaspoons ginger
1 teaspoon cayenne pepper
2 teaspoons cumin
1 teaspoon onion powder
1-1/2 teaspoons salt
1/4 teaspoon pepper
2 teaspoons curry powder
1 15-ounce can of crushed tomatoes
Cilantro, chopped; dry roasted peanuts or Crunchy Chickpeas, optional; for garnish

INSTRUCTIONS:
1. Dice the onion and put it in an Instant Pot on the sauté setting for about 6 minutes.
2. Add minced garlic to the onion and sauté for 2 more minutes, until fragrant.
3. While onion and garlic are cooking, peel and dice the sweet potatoes.
4. Turn off the sauté function on your Instant Pot and add in all other ingredients.
5. Mix all ingredients, then seal the Instant Pot and set for 4 minutes at high pressure. Once done, allow the Instant Pot to naturally release its steam for 10 minutes.
6. Remove pot from Instant Pot and use an immersion blender to mix into a thick stew.
7. Bowl up your soup and add toppings! I add a few tablespoons of chopped cilantro and a small handful of dry roasted peanuts or Crunchy Chickpeas to further enhance the flavor.

Feta Vegetable Couscous (MM, MC, VGT)

Ibrahim was first introduced to couscous, a type of North African pasta, in the beautiful city of Casablanca in Morocco. While it's a complete meal on its own, you may enjoy pairing it with some shrimp that you've sautéed with garlic in olive oil or perhaps a small piece of roasted salmon. Watching the movie Casablanca *while you eat it is an optional—but recommended!—enhancement.*

Prep time: 10 minutes
Cook time: 18 minutes
Total time: 28 minutes

SERVES 2

INGREDIENTS:
1 cup water
Extra virgin olive oil
1 cup whole wheat couscous
1 cup multicolored bell peppers, finely chopped
1/4 cup red or black olives, chopped
1 tablespoon oregano
1/2 cup feta cheese
1/2 cucumber, diced
Zest of 1 lemon
1/3 cup pine nuts
Salt and pepper, to taste

INSTRUCTIONS:
1. Bring 1 cup of water with a drizzle of olive oil to a boil on the stove.
2. Add couscous to water, cover pot, and remove from heat. Allow couscous to sit for 10-15 minutes.
3. Fluff with fork and transfer to serving bowl.
4. Add remaining ingredients and mix thoroughly. Add salt and pepper to taste.

Baked Eggplant (MM, MC, LC, GF, V, VGT)

This gooey dinner is like eggplant parmigiana without the carbs (or the frying). Serve it with your favorite bean-based pasta (good for Modified Mediterranean, Moderate-Carb, and Family plans), or with zoodles (for the Low-Carb plan) for a tasty meatless meal.

Prep time: 10 minutes
Cook time: 35-40 minutes
Total time: 45-50 minutes

SERVES 3

INGREDIENTS:
1 large or 2 medium eggplants
1 8-ounce ball fresh mozzarella
2 tablespoons extra virgin olive oil
1-2 teaspoons salt
1-2 teaspoons pepper
2 tablespoons Italian seasoning
1 25-ounce jar low-sugar tomato sauce or 3 cups Red Sauce

INSTRUCTIONS:
1. Preheat oven to 400°F.
2. Slice eggplant and mozzarella into 1/4-inch rounds.
3. On a large baking sheet, place eggplant rounds so that they are not touching each other, then drizzle with olive oil and sprinkle with salt, pepper, and Italian seasoning.
4. Bake for 30 minutes, flipping halfway through.
5. Remove pan from oven and top each eggplant round with 1 spoonful of tomato or Red Sauce and 1 mozzarella round.
6. Place back in oven for 5-10 minutes until mozzarella is melted and slightly browned.

Christmas Ravioli (MM, VGT [with plant-based meat])

This is a special occasion meal—both because it takes some time to prepare and because it uses white flour. But this is a treasured family recipe from

Ibrahim's good friend Federico Rossi—and sometimes you don't want to tinker with recipes that have been passed down through the generations! Born in Milan, Dr. Rossi has a family tradition of making ravioli for Christmas. He stuffs the ravioli with meat, with the exception of one ravioli that he leaves empty. Whoever gets the empty ravioli is the lucky host of Christmas dinner next year.

Prep time: 60-75 minutes
Cook time: 12-18 minutes
Total time: 72-93 minutes (plus 2-3 hours drying time)

SERVES 5 TO 6 (MAKES 100 RAVIOLI)

INGREDIENTS:
Stuffing
1 tablespoon extra virgin olive oil
1/4 cup each onion, celery, and carrot, diced small (you can often find this pre-made in the refrigerator case of the produce section, sometimes labeled "mirepoix")
Salt and pepper
12 ounces ground beef or plant-based substitute (such as Quorn crumbles)
2 eggs
1/3 cup grated Parmesan cheese
2 tablespoons grated Pecorino cheese

Pasta
3 cups white flour
1 cup semolina flour
4 large eggs
1 cup water
1 tablespoon extra virgin olive oil
1 tablespoon salt

INSTRUCTIONS:
Prepare the Stuffing:
1. Heat a sauté pan over medium heat with olive oil. Once pan is hot, sauté vegetables with a pinch of salt and pepper until vegetables

soften, 8–10 minutes. If mixture dries up you may add a splash of wine, water, or vegetable broth.

2. Add the ground beef or plant-based substitute to the pan and cook, stirring frequently, 8–10 minutes. If mixture dries up you may add a splash of wine or water.

3. Remove pan from heat and allow cooked meat and vegetable mixture to cool to room temperature.

4. Add eggs and grated cheeses and mix well, adding salt and pepper to taste, and a bit more grated cheese or water to achieve a consistency where the mixture holds together when you pinch a bit between your thumb and forefinger.

Make the Ravioli:

1. Place white flour and semolina in a large bowl. Make a well in the center about 2 inches deep and 3 inches across.

2. In a small separate bowl, beat eggs, water, and oil, then pour mixture into the well.

3. Stir flour and egg mixture together to form a ball. Turn onto a floured surface and knead until smooth and elastic (7–10 minutes) consistency. Add a little more flour if necessary to keep dough from sticking or water to keep dough from drying.

4. Cut pasta dough into 10 equal pieces. Working one at a time, roll each piece of dough to a 1/16-inch-thick sheet that is 3–4 inches wide and 10–12 inches long. (This is most easily done with a pasta-rolling machine.)

5. Place 1 teaspoon of filling, one after another, 1 inch apart along the left side of the pasta sheet. Fold the right half of the pasta sheet over the left half of the sheet, pressing down the outside edges, as well as pressing between each pile of filling, to seal the filling in.

6. Cut the now folded and pressed pasta sheets into squares with a pastry wheel to make 10–12 individual ravioli.

7. Carefully place each ravioli on a floured sheet pan, being careful to keep each ravioli separate so that they do not stick together.

8. Repeat with the remaining pieces of dough. (Remember to leave one empty!)

9. Allow ravioli to dry for 2–3 hours.

10. For any ravioli that you don't want to cook right away, you can store them in a freezer-safe plastic bag for up to 3 months.

Cook and Serve the Ravioli:

1. Bring a pot of salted water to a boil. Add ravioli, fresh or frozen. Return to a rolling boil, then reduce heat to a gentle simmer.
2. Cook until ravioli float to the top and are tender, 2-3 minutes if fresh and 6-8 minutes if frozen.
3. Drain the ravioli, then toss with melted butter or olive oil and grated Parmesan cheese, or your favorite pesto, or Red Sauce.

No-Carb Pizza ("The Friday Night Special") (MM, MC, LC, GF, VGT)

There's no denying how tempting it is to order a pizza on a Friday night—not only does it mean no cooking; it's also such a familiar, comforting taste. If you're trying to stick to low carb but want to enjoy a savory slice of pizza, try this nontraditional pizza, which Kristin calls the Friday Night Special. It has a great pizza flavor without the carbs. However, it does have a fair amount of saturated fat, so it's still more of an indulgence than an every-night-of-the-week type of thing.

Prep time: 10 minutes
Cook time: 10-12 minutes
Total time: 20-22 minutes

SERVES 1

INGREDIENTS:
2 eggs
2 tablespoons grated Parmesan cheese
1 tablespoon Italian seasoning
1/4 cup shredded mozzarella, plus more for sprinkling
1 tablespoon extra virgin olive oil
1-2 tablespoons no-sugar-added tomato sauce or Red Sauce
Sliced veggies or olives, to taste

INSTRUCTIONS:
1. Scramble the eggs in a bowl with Parmesan cheese, Italian seasoning, and mozzarella.

2. Put olive oil into a small, ovenproof sauté pan, heat it over medium-low heat, and pour in the egg and cheese mixture. Cook for about 5 minutes until the edges are set and starting to brown.
3. Using a spatula, carefully flip and finish cooking the other side for another minute or two.
4. Top with Red Sauce or no-sugar-added tomato sauce (and/or pesto), your favorite veggies (Kristin likes sliced red peppers, chopped sun-dried tomatoes, and a few torn pieces of fresh basil), and enough mozzarella cheese to cover your "pizza."
5. Pop the pan under the broiler until the cheese is melted and bubbly, 2–3 minutes (watch carefully to make sure it doesn't burn).

Lean, Green Pasta and Meatballs (MM, MC, GF)

This is one of our most popular recipes of all time. It is a simple but delightful weeknight meal that is absolutely packed with flavor. Using a jarred pesto makes this easy to make, but it also pairs well with our Traditional Basil Pesto, Nutty Vegan Pesto, or Triple Herb Pesto if you have leftovers of one of those recipes that you want to use up.

Prep time: 10 minutes
Cook time: 20–25 minutes
Total time: 30–35 minutes

SERVES 4

INGREDIENTS:
1 pound ground turkey
2 tablespoons extra virgin olive oil
1 tablespoon Worcestershire sauce
1 teaspoon garlic powder
1 teaspoon salt
1 teaspoon pepper
1 large egg
1/3 cup shredded Parmesan cheese
1 12-ounce bag frozen broccoli
1 8-ounce package edamame pasta
1/2 to 1 6.5-ounce jar kale pesto

INSTRUCTIONS:

1. Set oven to 350°F and line two baking sheets with parchment paper or cover with cooking oil.
2. In a mixing bowl, add ground turkey, extra virgin olive oil, Worcestershire sauce, garlic powder, salt, pepper, egg, and Parmesan cheese. Mix thoroughly.
3. Roll meat mixture into golf ball-sized balls and place on one baking sheet. Set in oven for 20-25 minutes, until lightly browned on the outside.
4. Place the broccoli (about 1/2 bag) onto a second baking sheet. Drizzle with olive oil and place in the oven with meatballs to roast.
5. While meatballs and broccoli are baking, place water for edamame pasta in a medium pan on the stove top. Once boiling, cook pasta until soft, drain water, and place back in the pot. Add 1/2 jar to 1 full jar of kale pesto sauce and mix thoroughly.
6. Plate pasta and add meatballs and broccoli on top.

Vegetarian Lasagna (MM, MC, LC, GF, VGT)

This recipe, with its plant-based protein and a moderate amount of carbohydrates, fits right in with what has come to be known as the "longevity diet"—a combination that has demonstrated a remarkable benefit on aging and disease risk factors. What's better than yummy foods that increase longevity?

Prep time: 5 minutes
Cook time: 37-45 minutes
Total time: 42-50 minutes

SERVES 6

INGREDIENTS:
1 24-ounce jar no-sugar-added tomato sauce or 3 cups Red Sauce
2 garlic cloves, chopped
1 12-ounce package meat alternative, such as Beyond Meat or Quorn crumbles
Extra virgin olive oil
1 box heart of palm lasagna "noodles"

1 15-ounce tub ricotta cheese
1 8-ounce container mozzarella pearls, drained
1/2 cup grated Parmesan cheese
Fresh basil

INSTRUCTIONS:
1. Preheat oven to 350°F.
2. Mix jar of tomato sauce or Red Sauce and minced garlic in a medium-sized bowl.
3. Sauté meat alternative in olive oil over medium heat until browned, 7–10 minutes.
4. Spread a thin layer of tomato sauce to cover the bottom of a glass or ceramic 9-inch × 12-inch baking dish, then create layers in the following order: noodles, tomato sauce, meat, ricotta. Repeat until there are two layers of each ingredient.
5. Top with pearled mozzarella and Parmesan cheese.
6. Place in oven for about 30–35 minutes, until cheese is browning on top.
7. Top with fresh basil and serve.

Zingy Baked Salmon with Cauliflower Rice (MM, MC, LC, GF)

This recipe has everything your liver loves—fiber, omega-3s, and even selenium (thanks to the garlic). Selenium is a mineral that helps cleanse your liver.

Prep time: 10 minutes
Cook time: 15–20 minutes
Total time: 25–30 minutes

SERVES 4

INGREDIENTS:
4 salmon filets, each 6–8 ounces
Extra virgin olive oil
Salt and pepper, to taste
Juice and zest of 1 lemon
2 garlic cloves, minced
1 8-ounce package cauliflower rice

INSTRUCTIONS:

1. Preheat oven to 350°F.
2. Place salmon filets on a baking sheet and drizzle with olive oil. Season with salt and pepper. Sprinkle lemon zest and garlic evenly over all filets.
3. Bake for 15–20 minutes, until salmon is baked through. Once cooked, squeeze fresh lemon juice over filets.
4. While salmon cooks, prepare riced cauliflower as directed on package.
5. Serve salmon on a bed of cauliflower rice and squeeze fresh lemon juice over filets.

Pan-Seared Salmon with a Ginger Turmeric Sauce and Cauliflower Rice (MM, MC, LC, GF)

This recipe is another of Chef Bill's (who also contributed the Roasted Cauliflower and Mushroom Soup and the Sautéed Shrimp on Curried Spaghetti Squash recipes). Bill says that when choosing salmon, look for wild Alaskan salmon, and if that's not available or affordable, opt for Atlantic salmon, but make sure that it is not artificially colored. He also suggests taking the skin off the salmon for consistency in cooking.

Prep time: 10 minutes
Cook time: 20 minutes
Total time: 30 minutes

SERVES 4

INGREDIENTS:
1 tablespoon avocado oil, divided
4 6-ounce filets of salmon, skin removed
Salt and pepper, to taste
1 tablespoon diced sweet onion
1 tablespoon fresh ginger, minced
2 teaspoons cornstarch
2 teaspoons water
1 cup vegetable stock
1/2 teaspoon ground turmeric

2 tablespoons virgin coconut oil

1 bulb fennel, tough outer leaves removed, diced

2 tablespoons shallot, minced

1 8-ounce package cauliflower rice

INSTRUCTIONS:

1. Preheat a sauté pan over medium-high heat until pan is warm, then pour in avocado oil.
2. Season salmon filets with salt and pepper and place salmon top down in hot pan. Sauté filets until light brown, typically about 6 minutes, then turn over for a few minutes until salmon is cooked through.
3. Remove from sauté pan, place in a glass baking dish pre-sprayed with nonstick spray, and set aside.
4. To the same pan, add a splash of avocado oil and turn down to medium heat. Add ginger and onions and sauté for 2 minutes.
5. Meanwhile, stir cornstarch into water.
6. Add vegetable stock to sauté pan, bring to boil. When boiling, stir in cornstarch until thickened to sauce consistency, about 2 minutes.
7. Add turmeric and salt and pepper to taste.
8. Preheat a large sauté pan over medium-high heat. Add coconut oil when hot, then add fennel and shallots and sauté 2 minutes.
9. Add cauliflower rice and stir until cauliflower is soft, about 5 minutes.
10. Add salt and pepper to taste.
11. Place a bed of cauliflower rice on each plate and place a salmon filet on top, then drizzle with a few tablespoons of sauce, to taste.

Sautéed Shrimp on Curried Spaghetti Squash (MM, MC, LC)

This recipe is also from Chef Bill. The spaghetti squash is a tasty and slightly crunchy alternative to pasta, and the curry powder delivers tons of flavor and great anti-inflammatory benefits thanks to the turmeric (which gives it its yellow color). To make this a super quick weeknight meal, precook the spaghetti squash—it will keep in an airtight glass container in your fridge for three days. You can reheat it in the microwave or in a separate sauté pan

with a little olive oil over medium-low heat until it reaches your desired
temperature (which takes about five to ten minutes).

Prep time: 10 minutes
Cook time: 55 minutes
Total time: 1 hour, 5 minutes

SERVES 2

INGREDIENTS:
1 medium spaghetti squash
Cooking spray
Salt and pepper, to taste
1 tablespoon curry powder
1 pound raw jumbo pink shrimp, peeled, deveined, and tails removed
2 tablespoons avocado oil, divided
2 teaspoons all-purpose flour
1/2 cup white wine
1 cup vegetable stock

INSTRUCTIONS:
1. For spaghetti squash, preheat oven to 350°F, carefully cut squash in
   half lengthwise and remove seeds. Line a sheet pan with aluminum
   foil and spray inside of squash with cooking spray or brush with oil.
   Shake salt, pepper, and curry powder over squash then place on
   sheet pan flesh down. Bake for 45 minutes, then remove from oven.
2. Let cool. Then, with a fork, scrape each half of squash out of skin
   and into a bowl. Add more seasoning as needed.
3. Meanwhile keep shrimp cool in fridge. Once squash is out of the
   oven and seasoned, heat 1 tablespoon oil in your favorite sauté pan.
4. Add shrimp to pan, right from refrigerator. Sauté until shrimp is
   bright pink on both sides, about 3 minutes, then remove from pan.
5. For sauce, add 1 more tablespoon of oil and, when heated, sprinkle in
   flour.
6. When flour is incorporated into oil and bubbling quickly, 1-2
   minutes, add white wine and half the vegetable stock. Continue
   stirring until thickened, about 3 minutes. You may need to add
   additional vegetable stock until desired consistency.
7. Add salt and pepper to taste.

Spicy Pulled Chicken (MM, MC, LC, GF)

This low-maintenance recipe yields chicken that is absolutely brimming with flavor—think tender, falling-apart chicken with taco flavors. You can use this chicken in many of the no-recipe dinners we included in the lists of suggested dinners in each of our plans.

Prep time: 5 minutes
Cook time: 30 minutes
Total time: 35 minutes

SERVES 5

INGREDIENTS:
3 cups unsalted chicken stock
1/2 teaspoon turmeric
1 teaspoon cayenne pepper
1 tablespoon cumin
2 teaspoons garlic powder
1 teaspoon smoked paprika
1 teaspoon dried oregano
1 tablespoon chili powder
1 tablespoon Old Bay Seasoning
1/2 teaspoon salt
1/2 teaspoon pepper
2 to 3 pounds boneless chicken—a mix of breasts and thighs
Salt and pepper to season chicken

INSTRUCTIONS:
1. Pour chicken stock into Instant Pot or pot on the stove. Add all spices, including salt and pepper, and stir to combine.
2. Season chicken with additional salt and pepper and place in Instant Pot or pot.
3. Close top to Instant Pot and cook on high pressure for 13-16 minutes. Allow steam to naturally release for 10 minutes. (If using a pot, boil in chicken stock until cooked all the way through—a meat thermometer should read 165°F—about 10-12 minutes.)

4. Remove chicken from the Instant Pot (or pot) and allow to cool about 5 minutes.
5. Once cool, use two forks to shred the chicken by pulling forks in opposite directions through the chicken.

Chicken Chili (MM, MC)

This recipe is dangerously good—spicy, smoky, and (thanks to the barley) hearty. Make this once, and you'll want to add it to your regular dinner rotation. With plenty of fiber from the beans and the barley and phytonutrients from the peppers, your liver will be as happy as your taste buds. (If you'd like to keep this recipe grain- or gluten-free, omit the barley and serve over brown rice or cauliflower rice.)

Prep time: 20 minutes
Cook time: 1 hour
Total time: 1 hour, 20 minutes

SERVES 6

INGREDIENTS:
2 split chicken breasts
Extra virgin olive oil or avocado oil
3 garlic cloves, minced
1 yellow onion, diced
4 bell peppers (any color), cubed
1 28-ounce can tomato puree
1 28-ounce can crushed tomatoes
1 15-ounce can black beans, drained
1 cup barley
1 tablespoon garlic powder
1 tablespoon cumin
1 teaspoon cayenne pepper
1 tablespoon chili powder
Salt to taste
Shredded Mexican blend cheese
1 avocado, sliced
Fresh cilantro, chopped

INSTRUCTIONS:
1. Preheat oven to 400°F.
2. Pat chicken dry, drizzle with olive oil or avocado oil, and bake in a glass baking dish until golden brown (30 minutes).
3. Remove chicken from oven and allow to cool while working on the next four steps.
4. While the chicken cools, sauté garlic and onion on medium heat in a large pot or Dutch oven until fragrant, about 8 minutes. Add bell peppers and sauté for 5 minutes.
5. Add tomato puree, crushed tomatoes, beans, barley, and spices. Bring contents to a boil, and then reduce heat to low.
6. Once cool enough to handle, remove bones from chicken and chop or shred to desired size and add to pot.
7. Cover and simmer, stirring every few minutes, until barley is cooked, about 25 to 30 minutes.
8. Season with salt to taste. Top with shredded cheese, sliced avocado, and cilantro.

DESSERTS

Apple Crisp (MM, VGT)

This one is fun to put together and offers a great way for kids to get involved in meal prep. It is an elegant, but essentially simple, dish.

Prep time: 15 minutes
Cook time: 35 minutes
Total time: 50 minutes

SERVES 6

INGREDIENTS:
1/4 cup butter
6-8 small apples, peeled, cored, and cut into slices (Kristin uses honeycrisp)
1/4 cup maple syrup (or Lakanto maple syrup to keep carbs lower)
1/4 cup whole wheat flour or almond flour

1/4 teaspoon baking powder
1/4 teaspoon baking soda
1/2 teaspoon cinnamon
1 tablespoon salted butter, divided
Canola oil blend
1/2 cup old-fashioned oats
1 tablespoon brown sugar

INSTRUCTIONS:

1. Preheat oven to 400°F.
2. Melt butter.
3. Reserving 1 teaspoon melted butter for topping, combine all ingredients except oats, brown sugar, and oil in a medium-sized bowl and mix well.
4. Spray a 9-inch × 9-inch glass baking dish with canola oil blend. Add apple mixture to pan. Top with oats and brown sugar, then drizzle with the remaining butter.
5. Bake for at least 30 minutes, allowing the mixture to bubble, then increase temperature to 425°F to brown the top. Bake for another 5 minutes.

Protein-Powered Cookie Cream (MM, MC, LC, VGT)

You have to try this homemade cookie cream recipe. It is more than the sum of its parts! A big hit with young children, but people of all ages enjoy this delightful dish. Kristin loves Quest cookies because they are high in protein and relatively low in carbs, their ingredient list is good, and they're available most everywhere (even in gas stations!).

Prep time: 5 minute
Total time: 5 minutes

SERVES 1

INGREDIENTS:
2 Quest peanut butter chocolate chip cookies
1 pint organic heavy whipping cream

1 tablespoon pure vanilla extract
1-2 tablespoons powdered erythritol

INSTRUCTIONS:
1. Cut cookies into small chunks.
2. Add whipping cream to a bowl and mix with either a hand mixer or stand mixer.
3. Once peaks are formed, add in vanilla extract, erythritol, and half the cookie chunks, reserving the other half as a topping.
4. Enjoy on pretty much anything you want to taste awesome—we love it on strawberries, or even straight from the spoon.

Low-Carb Peanut Butter Cups (MM, MC, LC, GF, V, VGT)

This is a super fun, quick, and healthy dessert. You won't believe how good these cups taste.

Prep time: 2 minutes
Cook time: 35 minutes
Total time: 37 minutes (plus 15 minutes to harden)

SERVES 12

INGREDIENTS:
1 cup stevia-sweetened chocolate chips (such as those made by Lily's)
1/2 cup no-sugar peanut butter
2 tablespoons erythritol-based confectioners' sugar
Peanuts (optional)

INSTRUCTIONS:
1. Melt half of chocolate chips either in the microwave or using a double boiler.
2. When liquid, divide the melted chocolate evenly among 12 cupcake liners or a silicone candy mold designed for peanut butter cups. Spread the chocolate evenly to cover the bottom of the liner or cups, then allow to cool enough to harden slightly, about 10 minutes.

3. Microwave the peanut butter in a microwave-safe bowl just enough to make it easy to pour, then mix in the sugar alternative.
4. Divide the sweetened peanut butter among the cupcake liners or candy mold, pouring in a smooth layer on top of the now-hardened chocolate layer you created in step 2.
5. Repeat step 1 with remaining 1/2 cup chocolate chips, covering peanut butter layer completely.
6. Refrigerate to allow the cups to harden completely, about 15 minutes.
7. Optional: Add chopped peanuts on top before the top layer hardens.

Miraculous Chocolate Chip Cookies (MM, MC, LC, GF, V, VGT)

Here we've given everyone's favorite—chocolate chip cookies—a healthy makeover. You won't believe this dessert is sugar-free!

Prep time: 10 minutes
Cook time: 10-15 minutes
Total time: 20-25 minutes

SERVES 12

INGREDIENTS:
3 cups almond flour
1-1/2 teaspoons baking powder
1 teaspoon baking soda
1 teaspoon salt
2 teaspoons vanilla extract
1/2 cup melted coconut oil
1/2 cup tahini
6 tablespoons water
3/4 cup erythritol-based brown sugar
1/4 cup granulated erythritol
1 cup Lily's stevia-sweetened chocolate chips

INSTRUCTIONS:
1. Preheat oven to 375°F (or 400°F if baking at high altitude).
2. Mix flour, baking powder, baking soda, and salt in a bowl and set aside.

3. Using a mixer, combine vanilla, coconut oil, tahini, and water until smooth.
4. Add the sugars to the wet mixture and mix for 2 minutes.
5. Add dry ingredients to the wet mixture, mix for 2 minutes until a dough forms.
6. Fold in the chocolate chips with a spoon or spatula.
7. Place on a baking sheet lined with parchment paper and bake for 8 minutes.
8. Flatten with a flat spatula and continue to bake until corners are brown, 3-5 minutes.

Note: Leftovers can be stored in an airtight container for up to a week.

Peanut Butter Mousse (MM, MC, LC, GF, V, VGT)

Did you know you could use the liquid from your chickpea can and turn it into a protein-packed mousse? Add in some cocoa, berries, or in this case, peanut butter (or your favorite nut or seed butter), and you have a whole new way to get your mousse fix.

Prep time: 2 minutes
Total time: 2 minutes

SERVES 4

INGREDIENTS:
1/4 cup drained chickpea liquid (from 1 can chickpeas)
1/2 teaspoon cream of tartar
2 tablespoons natural powdered peanut butter
3 tablespoons confectioners' sugar replacement
1 tablespoon pistachios, crushed

INSTRUCTIONS:
1. Drain aquafaba (liquid) from a can of chickpeas into a bowl. Add cream of tartar to liquid.
2. Using a hand or stand mixer, mix on low to medium speed for about 1 minute until the mixture is frothy.

3. Increase speed to high, add peanut butter and sugar replacement to the mixture, and mix until it forms a peak (about 6–8 minutes). Do not overmix or the mousse will deflate.
4. Place on a plate and top with crushed pistachios.

Strawberry Chia Pudding (MM, MC, LC, GF, V [if using alternative milk], VGT)

If you like strawberries, this recipe is for you! It is delightful and packed with flavor.

Prep time: 5 minutes (plus 1 hour wait time)
Total time: 1 hour, 5 minutes

SERVES 2

INGREDIENTS:
1/4 cup chia seeds
1/2 teaspoon pure vanilla extract
2 tablespoons maple syrup (or use Lakanto maple syrup if you are on the Low-Carb plan)
1 cup low-fat milk or unsweetened almond, oat, or cashew milk
1/2 teaspoon ground cinnamon
1 cup sliced fresh strawberries

INSTRUCTIONS:
1. Blend all ingredients except strawberries in a food processor or high-speed blender for 1 minute.
2. Pour mixture into small mixing bowl, cover, and refrigerate for at least 1 hour or as long as overnight. Once ready to serve, stir the pudding mixture and top with sliced strawberries.

Chocolate Chia Pudding (MM, GF, V [if using alternative milk], VGT)

This recipe is Ibrahim's grandmother's favorite. It's creamy and chocolatey yet packed with nutrients.

Prep time: 5 minutes (plus 1 hour wait time)
Total time: 1 hour, 5 minutes

SERVES 2

INGREDIENTS:
1 cup low-fat milk or unsweetened almond, oat, or cashew milk
3 tablespoons chia seeds
1/2 cup dates, pitted
1/8 teaspoon salt
1/2 teaspoon pure vanilla extract
1-1/2 tablespoons cocoa powder
2-3 tablespoons shredded coconut (optional)
2 tablespoons mini chocolate chips—regular or nondairy (optional, but not really!)

INSTRUCTIONS:
1. In a high-speed blender, add in milk, chia seeds, dates, salt, vanilla, and cocoa powder. Puree the mixture for at least 1 minute, until the seeds are pulverized and mixed.
2. Transfer mixture into a bowl and stir in optional toppings.
3. Cover and refrigerate for at least 1 hour or as long as overnight.
4. To serve, add shredded coconut, mini chocolate chips, and extra toppings or additional berries if you desire.

Pumpkin Spice Chia Pudding (MM, GF, V [if using alternative milk], VGT)

This savory autumnal treat warms you from the inside out and is a lot better for you than a traditional pumpkin spice latte that is typically packed with sugar.

Prep time: 10 minutes (plus 4 hours wait time)
Total time: 4 hours, 10 minutes

SERVES 4

INGREDIENTS:
1/4 cup chia seeds
2 cups low-fat milk or unsweetened almond, oat, or cashew milk
1 teaspoon ground cinnamon
1/4 teaspoon nutmeg
1/2 teaspoon ginger
1/4 teaspoon ground cloves
Pinch of black pepper (optional)
Pinch of chili powder (optional)
2 cups pumpkin puree
2 tablespoons maple syrup (or use Lakanto maple syrup if you are on the Low-Carb plan)
1 teaspoon vanilla extract

INSTRUCTIONS:
1. Combine chia seeds and milk in a bowl, cup, or jar, and let stand for 5 minutes.
2. Stir mixture rapidly, cover, and refrigerate at least 4 hours or overnight.
3. When ready to serve, whisk cinnamon, nutmeg, ginger, cloves, and optional black pepper and chili powder in a bowl.
4. Remove the chia mixture from the refrigerator, stir in pumpkin puree, spice mixture, maple syrup, and vanilla.

frequently asked questions

Should I be concerned about tracking ketones or glucose through a monitor?
Some of our patients who choose to do keto find valuable insight from using a ketone monitor. However, none of the Renew Your Liver plans are keto (even the Low-Carb plan allows more carbs than a keto diet does). A continuous glucose monitor can provide helpful insights into which foods cause your blood sugar to spike, but it's definitely an investment—of money, in the device itself, and of time and energy—in monitoring your results and perhaps becoming preoccupied with them. If you still want to track either ketones or glucose, we suggest working with a health care provider who can help you make sense of your results.

Do I have to cut all grains?
None of our plans require you to cut out all grains. We only counsel you to keep grain intake moderate (exactly how moderate depends on which plan you're following—refer back to page 130 for a breakdown of how many carbs—and therefore grains—are part of each plan) and to upgrade the grains you do eat to being as close to intact as you can. (Refer back to page 132 for information on intact grains.)

Will going gluten-free or dairy-free help with reversing liver damage?
If you have been diagnosed with a sensitivity to gluten—or you have good reason to suspect that you don't digest it well, such as bloating, gas, constipation, or diarrhea after eating it—it could be triggering inflammation that is making your whole body work harder, including your liver. An intolerance for the lactose in dairy has not been found to increase inflammation, however. If you're interested in trying a gluten-free or dairy-free diet, do it with a spirit of experimentation and pay close attention to how you feel. If you end up cutting out or

significantly reducing dairy, consider adding more nuts and seeds to replace the lost calcium.

If I'm going to have a burger, should I go with the real thing or a plant-based version?

It really depends on how often you're going to have one. If we're talking once a month, go for a beef burger and don't worry too much about the quality of the beef. If you'd like to have a burger once a week, aim to use grass-finished beef or bison. If you're following the Modified Mediterranean or Family plans, use a sprouted or whole wheat bun. If you're on the Moderate-Carb plan, use a low-carb bun, and if you're following the Low-Carb plan, use a broccoli or cauliflower bun (such as those made by the company Outer Aisle, located in the freezer section)—or skip the bun entirely.

The plant-based burger alternatives, such as Beyond Meat and Impossible, are still high in saturated fat and have long, complicated ingredient lists. They also have more carbs than a meat burger—six net carbs for an Impossible Burger versus zero carbs in a grass-fed beef burger. Ultimately, they haven't been around long enough for us to see studies verifying that they are better for your lipid profiles than meat-based burgers. If you really want to have a burger twice a week, try a veggie burger made with beans and quinoa, or a burger that you make out of ground chicken or turkey breast.

Is diet cola really better?

While you might assume that the fact that artificial sweeteners have no calories might mean they have no metabolic consequences, the data suggests otherwise. Kristin's patients come to her because they are addicted to sugar. They love it in *all* forms, and that includes artificial versions. Diet cola consumption has been linked with an increased risk of cardiovascular disease as well as belly fat. While both aren't good, what matters most is that the uber sweet taste is still hitting your taste buds, making it harder for you to ever really get off sugar.

Like anything, if you can enjoy a diet soda once in a while (let's say once a week or less), then have it and enjoy every sip. If it's something that you crave more of as soon as you finish a can or that you have a habit of drinking every day or most days, there are sodas made with stevia (such as those made by Zevia) that don't contain sugar or artificial sugar and that taste pretty good. Although different than the "real things," these sodas are also more expensive than traditional soft drinks, whether diet or regular. They are a better option for your liver health and your whole body health.

Are natural sugars—like agave, honey, and maple syrup—better for you?
Natural sugars still have a large impact on both insulin and blood sugar. Therefore, they should be viewed the same as white sugar and brown sugar and consumed in moderation. It's not that you can never have them; it's just that they should not be viewed as everyday options. See our rundown of alternative sweeteners starting on page 142.

What about all the new candy out there made with stevia and/or sugar alcohols?
Since stevia and sugar alcohols such as erythritol have not been found to have an impact on insulin or blood sugar, these treats can be a nice substitution for full-sugar candy. Again, everything in moderation— just because it's made with sugar alcohol, it still may be (depending on brand) low in nutrient density and not something you want to eat a lot of regularly. Look for brands with protein and/or fiber to obtain higher nutrient density.

Are sucralose and aspartame as bad as everyone says?
In small enough amounts, artificial sugars are fine—such as in the one diet soda that you have as an afternoon pick-me-up once or twice a week or the sugar-free gum or mints you have on occasion. Most of the studies that show adverse effects of artificial sugar consumption evaluated very high amounts. That being said, if you're drinking one or more diet sodas per day, or stirring sucralose into multiple cups of coffee per day, it can become problematic. Better to use an alternative sweetener, such as stevia (refer back to page 142 for our list of sugar alternatives), that doesn't impact your blood sugar, your microbiome, or your liver.

What medicine can I take for pain or headache if I have fatty liver?
You've likely heard somewhere that if you have liver disease, you should not be taking acetaminophen (Tylenol). Well, that is false! Believe it or not, acetaminophen is safe in moderation, even for patients with fatty liver. You can take up to two or three tablets/capsules of Tylenol 500 mg daily.

The one caution is that Tylenol has a synergistic effect with alcohol. In other words, limit your Tylenol intake if you plan on drinking alcohol later that day or if you had alcohol the night before.

In terms of other pain medicine, less is more. Nonsteroidal anti-inflammatory drugs (NSAIDs) such as ibuprofen (Advil and Motrin) are associated with increased risk of stomach ulcers and kidney injuries in the general population, and individuals with fatty liver are no exception. For day-to-day pain relief, stick with Tylenol, but if you had something to drink recently, go with ibuprofen.

The liver does not like narcotics (such as tramadol, codeine, and oxycodone), as it has to work to metabolize them. If you have any stage of liver disease, you will likely have higher levels of side effects from these medications—such as foggy memory and drowsiness—than the general population. Because clearance of these drugs in patients with fatty liver can be decreased, talk to your doctor about the correct dosage and timing between doses.

If you have recurring pain, it's important to look for the cause. While it's OK to treat occasional pain, unless you identify the cause of chronic pain and fix it, the pain is likely to come back once the medicine wears off.

Should I take milk thistle supplements?
Ibrahim can barely make it through a day of seeing patients without someone asking him about milk thistle, an herb that has been shown to reverse liver damage as a result of mushroom poisoning. (There is a type of mushroom that amateur mushroom foragers can easily misidentify and that can cause severe liver damage, even liver failure.) For this reason, many people assume that milk thistle is protective against other forms of liver disease, including NAFLD, and that it is generally supportive of the liver. But the science does not support

this. While milk thistle isn't harmful to your liver, it's not particularly helpful either. Ibrahim would rather see you take the money you might spend on milk thistle every month and reallocate it toward liver-supportive foods that have more evidence behind them, such as deeply hued produce, coffee, and green tea.

What about turmeric?

Turmeric, the bright yellow spice that gives curry powder its telltale color, is a perfect example of the benefit of eating deeply hued fruits, vegetables, grains, and spices. Its main active component, curcumin, is a strong antioxidant that can lower inflammation. Like most things in life, however, too much turmeric can be harmful. There have been isolated case reports of liver injury during use of turmeric dietary supplements.[1]

Rather than take turmeric as a supplement, we recommend that you add it to food—a teaspoon in cottage cheese, or added to scrambled eggs, or sprinkled over nuts that you then roast, or even in a delicious beverage known as golden milk that you drink. Eating turmeric means that you're getting culinary-grade spice and minimizes the chance of ordering a potentially contaminated supplement of questionable quality.

net carb chart of recommended foods

Here we've created a list of foods, arranged according to category and in ascending order of number of net carbs, so that if you are on the Moderate-Carb or Low-Carb plan, you can choose your fruits, vegetables, and nuts with care, and avoid inadvertently consuming more carbs than you intend to.

Food	Serving Size	Net Carbs
Fruit		
Blackberries	1 cup	6.2
Raspberries	1 cup	6.6
Plum	1 plum	7.5
Kiwi	1 kiwi	8.25
Watermelon	1 cup, chunked	11.1
Cantaloupe	1 cup, chunked	11.4
Strawberries	1 cup	11.5
Granny Smith apple	1 medium apple	11.6
Red delicious apple	1 medium apple	12.8
Peach	1 peach	13
Honeycrisp apple	1 medium apple	13
Orange	1 medium orange	14.5
Pineapple	1 cup, diced	19.7
Cherries	1 cup	21
Pear	1 pear	22
Bananas	1 banana	24.4
Grapes	1 cup	26
Vegetables		
Kale	1 cup	0.1
Spinach	1 cup	0.4

Food	Serving Size	Net Carbs
Green onion	1 medium onion	0.7
Romaine lettuce	1-3/4 cups, chopped	1
Asparagus	1/2 cup, chopped	1.2
Celery	2 medium stalks	1.5
Iceberg lettuce	1-1/2 cups, chopped	1.6
Cucumber	1/2 cup, sliced	1.6
White mushroom	1 cup, sliced or chopped	1.6
Portabella mushroom	1 whole mushroom	2.2
Shiitake mushroom	3 mushrooms	2.4
Green bell pepper	1 pepper	2.9
Avocado	1 avocado	3
Cauliflower	1 cup	3.3
Broccoli	1 cup	3.6
Orange bell pepper	1 pepper	4
Red bell pepper	1 pepper	4
Green beans	1 cup	4.3
Brussels sprouts	1 cup	4.6
Carrot	1 large carrot	4.9
Tomato	1 cup, chopped	4.9
Yellow bell pepper	1 pepper	5.4
Peas	1/2 cup	6.3
White onion	1/4 onion	1.2
Yellow onion	1 onion	2.4
Red onion	1/4 onion	2.9
Sweet yellow corn	1 medium ear	17
Sweet potato	1 medium potato	22
Sweet white corn	1 large ear	23

Nuts

Food	Serving Size	Net Carbs
Brazil nuts	6 nuts	1.2
Pecans	19 pecan halves	1.2

Food	Serving Size	Net Carbs
Macadamia nuts	10–12 nuts	1.5
Hazelnuts	21 whole nuts	2
Walnuts	7 walnuts	2
Almonds	23 almonds	2.6
Pine nuts	167 pine nuts	2.7
Pistachios	49 pistachios	4.7
Cashews	18 cashews	7.6

health risk assessment

Here is the assessment we shared in Chapter 1; keep a copy of this on your computer or in your Regenerative Health journal and periodically check in to gauge your progress. Remember, the more checks progressing toward Column D, the more you are taking steps toward loving your liver and regenerating your health.

Liver Health Risk Assessment

	Column A	*Column B*	*Column C*	*Column D*
Diet				
I eat red meat (beef or pork) or red processed meat (sausages, hot dogs, pepperoni, etc.)	Pretty much every day _____	A few times a week _____	Once a week or so _____	Rarely _____
I eat more than 25 grams of added sugar in a day (the amount in 1/2 a can of soda, 1–2 scoops of ice cream, 2 cookies, or a slice of cake)	Pretty much every day _____	A few times a week _____	Once a week or so _____	Rarely _____
I eat more than 50 grams of low-fiber carbs in a day (from an assortment of white bread, wraps/ tortillas, pasta, white rice, crackers, pretzels, standard breakfast cereals)	Pretty much every day _____	A few times a week _____	Once a week or so _____	Rarely _____
I eat fast food	Pretty much every day _____	A few times a week _____	Once a week or so _____	Rarely _____
I eat at least three servings of fruits and vegetables of different colors	Rarely _____	Once a week or so _____	A few days per week _____	Every day _____
I have a total of at least seven servings of fruits and/or vegetables in a day (a serving equals a large handful of fruit and colorful vegetables and two handfuls of fresh raw greens)	Rarely _____	Once a week or so _____	A few days per week _____	Every day _____
I eat at least 20 grams of fiber in a day (for example, from a blend of beans, oats, vegetables, nuts, seeds, berries, avocados, quinoa)	Rarely _____	Once a week or so _____	A few days per week _____	Every day _____

	Column A	Column B	Column C	Column D
Exercise				
The average number of hours I spend sitting in a day are	10 or more	8–10	5–8	Less than 5
	____	____	____	____
I get some light exercise—such as an easy walk, light yoga, or anything that doesn't make me out of breath, for at least 30 minutes	Rarely	Once a week or so	A few times a week	Most days
	____	____	____	____
I work out to the point of being able to notice my breathing	Rarely	Once a week or so	A few times a week	Most days
	____	____	____	____
In general, I spend this much of my day either standing or moving around (i.e., not sitting)	An hour or less	1–2 hours	3–4 hours	4 hours or more
	____	____	____	____
Alcohol				
I drink alcohol	5 or more days per week	3–4 days per week	1–2 days per week	Less than once per week
	____	____	____	____
When I drink alcohol, I have this many servings (one serving equals one drink—5 ounces of wine or 1 ounce of hard alcohol—for women, or two drinks for men)	4 or more	3–4	2–3	1
	____	____	____	____
Smoking or Vaping				
My relationship with smoking or vaping is	I currently smoke cigarettes or vape multiple times per day	I currently smoke cigarettes or vape 1–2 times per day	I used to smoke cigarettes or vape, and I quit less than five years ago	I used to smoke cigarettes or vape, and I quit more than five years ago, or I have never smoked or vaped
	____	____	____	____
Coffee				
I drink unsweetened coffee	Rarely or never	Once or twice a week	2 or more cups per day	1–2 cups per day
	____	____	____	____

	Column A	*Column B*	*Column C*	*Column D*
Sleep				
Most nights I sleep	Less than 5 hours	5–6 hours	6–7 hours	7 hours or more
	_____	_____	_____	_____
I have been diagnosed with sleep apnea	I have been diagnosed with sleep apnea and am not treating it	I don't know if I have sleep apnea but am told I snore loudly with periods of not breathing	I have sleep apnea and I am treating it	I do not have sleep apnea
	_____	_____	_____	_____
Stress Management				
I do practice something to reduce my experience of stress (for example, meditate, stretch, garden, journal, talk to a counselor, do yoga)	Rarely _____	Once a week or so _____	A couple times per week _____	Most days _____
Waist Size The circumference of my waist is (see page 45 for measuring instructions)	40 or higher (for men) or 35 or higher (for women) _____			39 or lower (for men) or 34 or lower (for women) _____
Type 2 Diabetes	I have been diagnosed with type 2 diabetes	My doctor has told me I'm prediabetic	I have not consulted with a doctor about my blood sugar levels	I've had my blood sugar levels tested and my doctor tells me they are in a healthy range
	_____	_____	_____	_____

resources

Websites

LiverTox: Clinical and Research Information on Drug-Induced Liver Injury

This website is run by the National Institutes of Health. It allows you to look up any drug, including herbs and supplements, and it will link you to any clinical research that has examined the potential for liver injury from using that drug, herb, or supplement.

https://pubmed.ncbi.nlm.nih.gov/31643176

NASH Knowledge

This website was started by a family whose father was diagnosed with non-alcoholic cirrhosis despite getting regular checkups every year (he wasn't aware that he had fatty liver until it had gotten to "the ugly" phase). The site hosts a liver disease support group, provides education for families who are trying to prevent or reverse NAFLD, and has a podcast called "Love Your Liver."

www.nash-now.org

Associations for the Study of Liver Disease

There are multiple professional organizations that collate and disseminate best practices and latest research on fatty liver from around the world. Although geared toward professionals, they are written in lay-friendly language—and the international organizations also offer their information in multiple languages.

American Association for the Study of Liver Diseases (AASLD)

www.aasld.org

European Association for the Study of the Liver (EASL)

https://easl.eu

The Asian Pacific Association for the Study of the Liver (APASL)
  http://apasl.info

Additional Recipes

Cleveland Clinic Health Library
The Cleveland Clinic has a large archive of recipes and health information on their website—Kristin often visits it for her own education and inspiration and recommends it to her patients for more recipe ideas and information on how to address their particular health challenges.
  https://my.clevelandclinic.org/health
  https://my.clevelandclinic.org/departments/wellness/patient-resources/recipes

Resources for Additional Support

The Academy of Nutrition and Dietetics
If you'd like to work with a registered dietitian to help you implement diet and lifestyle changes that are customized to you, your liver, and your life, the Academy of Nutrition and Dietetics has a feature on their website to help you find a registered dietitian near you.
  www.eatright.org/find-a-nutrition-expert

Tracking with Terah
Terah Becker is a registered nurse in Ibrahim's practice who is a certified coach in macro tracking—approaching diet with a specific ratio of protein, fats, and carbs that is tailored to you and your health goals. Terah always motivates the staff in Ibrahim's practice to eat better and move more and offers both group programs and one-on-one coaching.
  www.instagram.com/trackingwithterah

Nutrigenomics Testing
Nutrigenomics testing can help determine if there are certain foods you are less likely to tolerate, or nutrient deficiencies you're more

prone to, as well as insights into how much and what kinds of physical activity your body needs to feel its best. Kristin has been offering this service to her patients for years—if it's something you're interested in exploring, contact her via her website.

www.kristinkirkpatrick.com

Books

The Longevity Diet by Valter Longo, PhD (Avery, 2018)
This highly researched approach to promoting both health span (the number of years you are well) and life span (the number of years you live) aligns well with the Renew Your Liver plans. It also includes guidance on doing a five-day fasting mimicking diet, where you gain the majority of the benefits of fasting while still eating enough well-chosen calories to not *feel* like you're fasting.

The Great Age Reboot by Michael F. Roizen, MD (National Geographic, 2022)
Dr. Roizen is the chief wellness officer at the Cleveland Clinic and a mentor to Kristin. His book unpacks the latest research on what practices will help us avoid the chronic diseases of aging—including fatty liver disease—and enjoy our unprecedented longer life spans.

Skinny Liver by Kristin Kirkpatrick and Ibrahim Hanouneh (DaCapo Lifelong Books, 2017)
Of course, we have to recommend our first book, too. While our understanding of metabolic health has evolved, and some of our dietary recommendations have changed as a result, the book is still a great overview of liver health.

acknowledgments

I was nearly eighteen years old when I arrived in this country as an immigrant from Syria. I was born in Latakia, a small town on the Mediterranean coast. I'll always be grateful to America for giving me, along with so many others, a chance. I try in my current work to repay you—to contribute to society by promoting a robust nutrition plan, so crucial to the health and well-being of our country.

I would like to express my sincere gratitude to my friend and coauthor Kristin Kirkpatrick for her continuous support, motivation, enthusiasm, and immense knowledge. I could not have imagined a better teammate to work with.

I also owe a great debt of gratitude to the many members of the *Regenerative Health* project. Special thanks to our writer, Kate Hanley, for her patience and continued support; and to our editor, Renée Sedliar, and literary agent, Bonnie Solow, for their encouragement, insightful comments, and stimulating discussions. This project would not have been possible without you, all of you.

To my mentor, Dr. Nizar Zein, who inspired me to work hard and dream big. I am truly lucky to have a genius mentor like you.

To my uncle in Heaven, Dr. Hadi Hanouneh! I will forever be grateful for your love and guidance.

To my caring, loving, and supportive parents, siblings Dima and Mo, and significant other Stephanie: my heartfelt thanks for your love and prayers and for all the joy you have given me.

And finally, to my patients, who remind me every day how to cherish a life and savor every blessing.

—Ibrahim

To my sons, Jake and Boden. You both are the center of my universe, the loves of my life, and my reason for being on this Earth. I am insanely proud of you both. You inspire me every day.

To my husband, Andy—thank you for being my best friend and partner in this journey of life. I wouldn't want to be on it with anyone else.

To my parents, Mrs. Arlene Franco (registered nurse) and Dr. Irving Franco (Cleveland Clinic cardiologist). You instilled a love of medicine and health care services in me from a very young age. You not only supported me in finding my best health but also instilled in me a desire to help others.

I also want to acknowledge the contributions, guidance, and support of our amazing liver team.

To Dr. Ibrahim Hanouneh—you are not only one of the best physicians I have ever known; you are one of the best humans as well. I continue to be in awe of you and am honored to be creating this book with you. This project could never happen without you. Thank you for being my guide, my medical mind, and most importantly, my dear friend.

To Kate Hanley—you are amazing. You did what so many people cannot: take detailed medical information and put it on paper so everyone can understand and benefit from it. I am overwhelmed by your talent.

To my agent, Bonnie Solow. You supported me, you guided me, and you always told me what I needed to hear to be successful. Most importantly, you had my back every step of the way. Thank you for taking me on so many years ago and staying with me for this book.

To my editor, Renée Sedliar, and the entire team at Hachette. Thank you for taking everything we threw at you and putting it into a form that made it even better.

To Olivia Dottore. Your enthusiasm and nutrition knowledge are unparalleled. I am grateful for your role in helping transform science into easy yet delicious recipes. You will shine in this world no matter what you do.

Writing a book takes time and patience. I want to express my sincere love and appreciation for everyone who played a role in allowing me to do it. To my siblings and my siblings-in-law, Jeff, Brian, Courtney, and Carter, and to my godparents, Wanda and Sam Pluzaric, I am grateful to call you all family. A special shout-out to Jeff—I never "hired" him to do my marketing, but he does it anyway.

To my colleagues at the Cleveland Clinic: Dr. Michael Roizen, Dr. Mladen Golubic, and Dr. Richard Lang. You remain my greatest medical mentors. To Mary Pipino, Dr. Mehmet Oz, Dr. Joseph Antoun, Audrey Zona, Dr. Jonathan Clinthorne, Colette Heimowitz, Ashley Koff, Jennifer Livingston, Grace Niu, Alyssa Nimedez, and Cynthia Sass, thank you for allowing me to be part of your amazing teams.

To my NBC and *Today Show* colleagues, especially Susan Wagner and Margaret O'Malley—thank you for allowing me an incredible platform to educate others on good health.

To my friends and colleagues at the Meadows—you changed me. I see the world with different eyes because of you all, and the important work you do. I am grateful to each and every one of you, especially Sean Walsh, Carrie Steffensen, Patty Evans, Scott Evans, Cindy Warren, Brandon Braley, Jim Corrington Jr., Jean Collins-Stuckert, Josh Ulrich, and Elizabeth Brown.

To my friends—you are the family I chose, and life is better with you in it. To my best friend Mia, I love you. You are my sister. I walk beside you always, on the good days and the bad. To the people who I call home—especially Carlynn Schlissberg, Olivia Dottore, Joe and Toya Gorley, Lisa Fritz, and Stephanie Olson. And to my friends who support me in love and laughter, Lisa Dottore, Mark Dottore, Jen Young, Rylie Ward, Anne Maria Nuno, Rita Petti, Julia Zumpano, Faye Ambler, Danielle Riedel, Heidi Silk, Kirsten and Jarod Pate, Angie and Tim Lombardi, and Lisa and Brian Thompson.

To Chef Bill Althoff—thank you for taking our liver-loving nutritional principles to the next level with your exquisite recipes and for sharing a few of them in these pages. And to the ultimate chefs, Charles Dottore and Jim Perko—you inspire me to be better in the kitchen.

To Kathy Kenny—my first teacher, who taught me how to write not just well but using correct grammar.

Finally—to my patients, who challenge me every day to be better.

—Kristin

notes

Chapter 1

1. Neda Sarafrazi, Edwina A. Wambogo, and John A. Shepherd, "Osteoporosis or Low Bone Mass in Older Adults: United States, 2017-2018," *NCHS Data Brief* (Hyattsville, MD), no. 405 (March 2021): 1-8, https://doi.org/10.15620/cdc:103477.

2. Ji Min Choi, Goh Eun Chung, Seung Joo Kang, Min-Sun Kwah, Jong In Yang, Boram Park, and Jeong Yoon Yim, "Association Between Anxiety and Depression and Nonalcoholic Fatty Liver Disease," *Frontiers in Medicine* 7 (January 18, 2021): 585618, https://doi.org/10.3389/fmed.2020.585618.

3. Samarth S. Patel and Mohammad S. Siddiqui, "The Interplay Between Nonalcoholic Fatty Liver Disease and Atherosclerotic Heart Disease," *Hepatology* 69, no. 4 (2019): 1372-1374, https://doi.org/10.1002/hep.30410.

4. Zobair M. Younossi, Maria Stepanova, Mariam Afendy, Youssef Younossi, Hesham Mir, and Manirath Srishord, "Changes in the Prevalence of the Most Common Causes of Chronic Liver Diseases in the United States from 1988 to 2008," *Clinical Gastroenterology and Hepatology: The Official Clinical Practice Journal of the American Gastroenterological Association* 9, no. 6 (2011): 524-530. e1; quiz e60, https://doi.org/10.1016/j.cgh.2011.03.020.

5. Stephen A. Harrison, Samer Gawrieh, Katharine Rober, Céline Fournier, Angelo H. Paredes, and Naim Alkhouri, "Prospective Evaluation of the Prevalence of Non-alcoholic Fatty Liver Disease and Steatohepatitis in a Large Middle-Aged US Cohort," *Journal of Hepatology* 75, no. 2 (2021): 284-291, https://doi.org/10.1016/j.jhep.2021.02.034.

6. Christopher D. Williams, Joel Stengel, Michael I. Asike, Dawn M. Torres, Janet Shaw, Maricela Contreras, Cristy L. Landt, and Stephen A. Harrison, "Prevalence of Nonalcoholic Fatty Liver Disease and Nonalcoholic Steatohepatitis Among a Largely Middle-Aged Population Utilizing Ultrasound and Liver Biopsy: A Prospective Study," *Gastroenterology* 140, no. 1 (January 2011):124-131, https://doi.org/10.1053/j.gastro.2010.09.038.

7. Mohammad Nasser Kabbany, Praveen Kumar Conjeevaram Selvakumar, Kymberly Watt, Rocio Lopez, Zade Akras, Nizar Zein, William Carey, and Naim Alkhouri, "Prevalence of Nonalcoholic Steatohepatitis-Associated Cirrhosis in the United States: An Analysis of National Health and Nutrition Examination Survey Data," *American Journal of Gastroenterology* 112, no. 4 (2017): 581-587, https://doi.org/10.1038/ajg.2017.5.

8. David Goldberg, Ivo C. Ditah, Kia Saeian, Mona Lalehzari, Andrew Aronsohn, Emmanuel C. Gorospe, and Michael Charlton, "Changes in the Prevalence of Hepatitis C Virus Infection, Nonalcoholic Steatohepatitis, and Alcoholic Liver Disease Among Patients with Cirrhosis or Liver Failure on the Waitlist for Liver Transplantation," *Gastroenterology* 152, no. 5 (2017): 1090–1099.e1, https://doi.org/10.1053/j.gastro.2017.01.003.

9. Centers for Disease Control and Prevention, "A Snapshot: Diabetes in the United States," CDC, page last reviewed February 18, 2020, https://www.cdc.gov/diabetes/library/socialmedia/infographics/diabetes.html.

10. International Diabetes Foundation, "IDF Diabetes Atlas," IDF, accessed February 17, 2022, https://diabetesatlas.org/.

11. Centers for Disease Control and Prevention, "Nearly One in Five American Adults Who Have Had COVID-19 Still Have 'Long COVID.'" CDC National Center for Health Statistics, last modified June 22, 2022, https://www.cdc.gov/nchs/pressroom/nchs_press_releases/2022/20220622.htm.

12. Yngve Falck-Ytter, Zobair M. Younossi, Giulio Marchesini, and Arthur J. McCullough, "Clinical Features and Natural History of Nonalcoholic Steatosis Syndromes," *Seminars in Liver Disease* 21, no. 1 (2001): 17–26, https://doi.org/10.1055/s-2001-12926.

13. Tracey G. Simon, Bjorn Roelstraete, Kayla Hartjes, Hamed Khalili, Henrik Arnell, and Jonas F. Ludvigsson, "Non-alcoholic Fatty Liver Disease in Children and Young Adults Is Associated with Increased Long-Term Mortality," *Journal of Hepatology* 75, no. 5 (2021): 1034–1041, https://doi.org/10.1016/j.jhep.2021.06.034.

Chapter 2

1. Max Roser, Hannah Ritchie, and Pablo Rosado, "Food Supply," *Our World in Data*, accessed October 5, 2022, https://ourworldindata.org/food-supply.

2. Roberto A. Ferdman, "Where People Around the World Eat the Most Sugar and Fat," *Washington Post*, February 5, 2015, https://www.washingtonpost.com/news/wonk/wp/2015/02/05/where-people-around-the-world-eat-the-most-sugar-and-fat/.

3. J. Nicholas Betley, "Eliminating the 'Hanger' from Hunger," *New England Journal of Medicine* 385, no. 21 (2021): 2005–2007, https://doi.org/10.1056/NEJMcibr2111841.

4. Filippa Juul, Niyati Parekh, Euridice Martinez-Steele, Carlos Augusto Monteiro, and Virginia W. Chang, "Ultra-processed Food Consumption Among US Adults from 2001 to 2018," *American Journal of Clinical Nutrition* 11, no. 115(1) (2022): 211–221, https://doi.org/10.1093/ajcn/nqab305.

5. Lu Wang, Euridice Martínez Steele, Mengzi Du, Jennifer L. Pomeranc, Lauren E. O'Connor, Kirsten A. Herric, Hanqui Luo, Zuehong Zhang, Dariush

Mozaffarian, and Fang Fang Zhang, "Trends in Consumption of Ultraprocessed Foods Among US Youths Aged 2-19 Years, 1999-2018," *JAMA* 326, no. 6 (2021): 519-530, https://doi.org/10.1001/jama.2021.10238.

6. Seung Hee Lee, Latetia V. Moore, Sohyun Park, Diane M. Harris, and Heidi M. Blanck, "Adults Meeting Fruit and Vegetable Intake Recommendations– United States, 2019," *MMWR Morbidity and Mortality Weekly Report* 71, no. 1 (2022): 1-9, https://doi.org/10.15585/mmwr.mm7101a1.

7. Kelly B. Scribner, Dorota B. Pawlak, and David S. Ludwig, "Hepatic Steatosis and Increased Adiposity in Mice Consuming Rapidly vs. Slowly Absorbed Carbohydrate," *Obesity* 15, no. 9 (2007): 2190-2199; Silvia Valtueña, Nicoletta Pellegrini, Diego Ardigo, Daniele Del Rio, Filippo Numeroso, Francesca Scazzina, Lucilla Monti, Ivana Zavaroni, and Furio Brighenti, "Dietary Glycemic Index and Liver Steatosis," *American Journal of Clinical Nutrition* 84, no. 1 (2006): 136-142.

8. Simin Liu, Walter C. Willett, Meir J. Stampfer, Frank B. Hu, Mary Franz, Laura Sampson, Charles H. Hennekens, and JoAnn E. Manson, "A Prospective Study of Dietary Glycemic Load, Carbohydrate Intake, and Risk of Coronary Heart Disease in US Women," *American Journal of Clinical Nutrition* 71, no. 6 (2000): 1455-1461.

9. Ali Aminian, Abbas Al-Kurd, Rickesha Wilson, James Bena, Hana Fayazzadeh, Tavankit Singh, Vance L. Albaugh, Faiz U. Shariff, Noe A. Rodrigues, Jian Jin, Stacy A. Brethauer, Srinivasan Dasarthy, Naim Alkhouri, Philip R. Schauer, Arthur J. McCullough, and Steven E. Nissen, "Association of Bariatric Surgery with Major Adverse Liver and Cardiovascular Outcomes in Patients with Biopsy-Proven Nonalcoholic Steatohepatitis," *JAMA* 326, no. 20 (2021): 2031-2042, https://doi.org/10.1001/jama.2021.19569.

10. Giovanni Cerón-Solano, Rossana C. Zepeda, Jose Gilberto Romero Lozano, Gabriel Roldán-Roldán, and Jean-Pascal Morin, "Bariatric Surgery and Alcohol and Substance Abuse Disorder: A Systematic Review" [Cirugía bariátrica y trastorno por abuso de alcohol y otras sustancias: una revisión sistemática], *Cirugia espanola* 99, no. 9 (2021): 635-647. S0009-739X(21)00109-3, advance online publication, https://doi.org/10.1016/j.ciresp.2021.03.006.

11. Wendy C. King, Jia-Yuh Chen, Anita P. Courcoulas, Gregory F. Dakin, Scott G. Engel, David R. Flum, Marcelo W. Hinojosa, et al., "Alcohol and Other Substance Use After Bariatric Surgery: Prospective Evidence from a US Multicenter Cohort Study," *Surgery for Obesity and Related Diseases: Official Journal of the American Society for Bariatric Surgery* 13, no. 8 (2017): 1392-1402, https://doi.org/10.1016/j.soard.2017.03.021.

12. Kenneth Blum, Ernest P. Noble, and Peter J. Sheridan, "Allelic Association of Human Dopamine D2 Receptor Gene in Alcoholism," *JAMA* 263, no. 15 (1990): 2055-2060, https://doi.org/10.1001/jama.1990.03440150063027.

13. "Metabolic and Bariatric Surgery," American Society for Metabolic and Bariatric Surgery, July 2021, accessed February 25, 2023, https://asmbs.org/resources/metabolic-and-bariatric-surgery.

14. Eduardo Vilar-Gomez, Yadina Martinez-Perez, Luis Calzadilla-Bertot, Ana Torres-Gonzalez, Bienvenido Gra-Oramas, Licet Gonzalez-Fabian, Scott L. Friedman, Moises Diago, and Manuel Romero-Gomez, "Weight Loss Through Lifestyle Modification Significantly Reduces Features of Nonalcoholic Steatohepatitis," *Gastroenterology* 149, no. 2 (2015): 367-e15, https://doi.org/10.1053/j.gastro.2015.04.005.

Chapter 3

1. Joana Araújo, Jianwen Cai, and June Stevens, "Prevalence of Optimal Metabolic Health in American Adults: National Health and Nutrition Examination Survey 2009-2016," *Metabolic Syndrome and Related Disorders* 17, no. 1 (2019): 46-52, https://doi.org/10.1089/met/2018/0105.

2. Ayana K. April-Sander and Carlos J. Rodriguez, "Metabolically Healthy Obesity Redefined," *JAMA Network Open* 4, no. 5 (2021): e218860, https://doi.org/10.1001/jamanetworkopen.2021.8860; Gordon I. Smith, Bettina Mittendorfer, and Samuel Klein, "Metabolically Healthy Obesity: Facts and Fantasies," *Journal of Clinical Investigation* 129, no. 10 (2019): 3978-3989, https://doi.org/10.1172/JCI129186.

3. Norbert Stefan, Fritz Schick, and Hans-Ulrich Häring, "Causes, Characteristics, and Consequences of Metabolically Unhealthy Normal Weight in Humans," *Cell Metabolism* 26, no. 2 (2017): 292-300, https://doi.org/10.1016/j.cmet.2017.07.008.

Chapter 4

1. Jeffrey B. Schwimmer, Manuel A. Celedon, Joel E. Lavine, Alyssa Chavez, Michael S. Middleton, and Claude B. Sirlin, "Heritability of Nonalcoholic Fatty Liver Disease," *Gastroenterology* 136, no. 5 (2009): 1585-1592, https://doi.org/10.1053/j.gastro.2009.01.050.

2. Stefano Romeo, Julia Kozlitina, Chao Xing, Alexander Pertsemlidis, David Cox, Len A. Pennacchio, Eric Boerwinkle, Jonathan C. Cohen, and Helen H. Hobbs, "Genetic Variation in PNPLA3 Confers Susceptibility to Nonalcoholic Fatty Liver Disease," *Nature Genetics* 40, no. 12 (2008): 1461-1465, https://doi.org/10.1038/ng.257.

3. Noura S. Abul-Husn, Xiping Cheng, Alexander H. Li, Yurong Xin, Claudia Schurmann, Panayiotiz Stevis, Yashi Liu, et al., "A Protein-Truncating HSD17B13

Variant and Protection from Chronic Liver Disease," *New England Journal of Medicine* 378, no. 12 (2018): 1096–1106, https://doi.org/10.1056/NEJMoa1712191.

4. Bo-Tao Li, Ming Sun, Yun-Feng Li, Ju-Qiong Wang, Zi-Mu Zhao, Bao-Liang Song, and Jie Luo, "Disruption of the ERLIN-TM6SF2-APOB Complex Destabilizes APOB and Contributes to Non-alcoholic Fatty Liver Disease," *PLoS Genetics* 16, no. 8 (August 2020): e1008955, https://doi.org/10.1371/journal.pgen.1008955.

5. Hui Gao, Shouseng Liu, Zhenzhen Zhao, Xinjuan Yu, Qun Liu, Yongnin Xin, and Shiying Xuan, "Association of GCKR Gene Polymorphisms with the Risk of Nonalcoholic Fatty Liver Disease and Coronary Artery Disease in a Chinese Northern Han Population," *Journal of Clinical and Translational Hepatology* 7, no. 4 (2019): 297–303, https://doi.org/10.14218/JCTH.2019.00030.

6. Hai-bo Zhang, Wen Su, Hu Xu, Xiao-yan Zhang, and You-fei Guan, "HSD17B13: A Potential Therapeutic Target for NAFLD," *Frontiers in Molecular Biosciences*, no. 8 (2022): 824776, https://doi.org/10.3389/fmolb.2021.824776.

7. Mohammed Eslam and Jacob George, "Genetic Contributions to NAFLD: Leveraging Shared Genetics to Uncover Systems Biology," *Nature Reviews Gastroenterology and Hepatology* 17 (2020): 40–52, https://doi.org/10.1038/s41575-019-0212-0.

8. José Ignacio Martínez-Montoro, Isabel Cornejo-Pareja, Ana María Gómez-Pérez, and Francisco J. Tinahones, "Impact of Genetic Polymorphism on Response to Therapy in Non-Alcoholic Fatty Liver Disease," *Nutrients* 13, no. 11 (November 15, 2021): 4077, https://doi.org/10.3390/nu13114077.

9. Michael Roerecke, Afshin Vafaei, Omer S. N. Hasan, Bethany R. Chrystoja, Marcus Cruz, Roy Lee, Manuela G. Neuman, and Jürgen Rehm, "Alcohol Consumption and Risk of Liver Cirrhosis: A Systematic Review and Meta-Analysis," *American Journal of Gastroenterology* 114, no. 10 (2019): 1574–1586, https://doi.org/10.14309/ajg.0000000000000340.

10. John J. Shelmet, George A. Reichard, Charles L. Skutches, Robert D. Hoeldtke, Oliver E. Owen, and Guenther Boden, "Ethanol Causes Acute Inhibition of Carbohydrate, Fat, and Protein Oxidation and Insulin Resistance," *Journal of Clinical Investigation* 81, no. 4 (1988): 1137–1145, https://doi.org/10.1172/JCI113428.

11. Jérôme Boursier, Olaf Mueller, Matthieu Barret, Mariana Machado, Lionel Fizanne, Felix Araujo-Perez, Cynthia D. Guy, et al., "The Severity of Nonalcoholic Fatty Liver Disease Is Associated with Gut Dysbiosis and Shift in the Metabolic Function of the Gut Microbiota," *Hepatology* 63, no. 3 (2016): 764–775, https://doi.org/10.1002/hep.28356; Cyrielle Caussy, Anupriya Tripathi, Greg Humphrey, Shirin Bassirian, Seema Singh, Claire Faulkner, Ricki Bettencourt, et al., "A Gut Microbiome Signature for Cirrhosis Due to Nonalcoholic Fatty Liver Disease," *Nature Communications* 10, no. 1 (2019): 1406, https://doi.org/10.1038/s41467-019-09455-9.

12. Steven Zhao, Cholsoon Jang, Joyce Liu, Kahealani Uehara, Michael Gilbert, Luke Izzo, Xianfeng Zeng, et al., "Dietary Fructose Feeds Hepatic Lipogenesis via Microbiota-Derived Acetate," *Nature*, no. 579 (2020): 586-591, https://doi.org/10.1038/s41586-020-2101-7.

13. Lixin Zhu, Susan S. Baker, Chelsea Gill, Wensheng Liu, Razan Alkhouri, Robert D. Baker, and Steven R. Gill, "Characterization of Gut Microbiomes in Nonalcoholic Steatohepatitis (NASH) Patients: A Connection Between Endogenous Alcohol and NASH," *Hepatology* 57, no. 2 (2013): 601-609, https://doi.org/10.1002/hep.26093.

14. Rohit Loomba, Victor Seguritan, Weizhong Li, Tao Long, Niels Klitgord, Archana Bhatt, Parambir Singh Dulai, et al., "Gut Microbiome-Based Metagenomic Signature for Non-invasive Detection of Advanced Fibrosis in Human Nonalcoholic Fatty Liver Disease," *Cell Metabolism* 25, no. 5 (2017): 1054-1062.e5, https://doi.org/10.1016/j.cmet.2017.04.001.

15. Peter J. Turnbaugh, Ruth E. Ley, Michael A. Mahowal, Vincent Magrini, Elaine R. Mardis, and Jeffrey I. Gordon, "An Obesity-Associated Gut Microbiome with Increased Capacity for Energy Harvest," *Nature*, no. 444 (2006): 1027-1031, https://doi.org/10.1038/nature05414.

16. Julia J. Witjes, Loek P. Smits, Ceyda T. Pekmez, Andrei Prodan, Abraham S. Meijnikman, Marian A. Troelstra, Kristien E. C. Bouter, et al., "Donor Fecal Microbiota Transplantation Alters Gut Microbiota and Metabolites in Obese Individuals with Steatohepatitis," *Hepatology Communications* 4, no. 11 (2020): 1578-1590, https://doi.org/10.1002/hep4.1601.

17. Laura Craven, Adam Rahman, Seema Nair Parvathy, Melanie Beaton, Justin Silverman, Karim Qumosani, Irene Hramiak, et al., "Allogenic Fecal Microbiota Transplantation in Patients with Nonalcoholic Fatty Liver Disease Improves Abnormal Small Intestinal Permeability: A Randomized Control Trial," *American Journal of Gastroenterology* 115, no. 7 (2020): 1055-1065, https://doi.org/10.14309/ajg.0000000000000661.

18. Mingfei Yao, Lingling Qv, Yanmeng Lu, Baohong Wang, Björn Berglund, and Lanjuan Li, "An Update on the Efficacy and Functionality of Probiotics for the Treatment of Non-alcoholic Fatty Liver Disease," *Engineering* 7, no. 5 (2021): 679-686, https://doi.org/10.1016/j.eng.2020.01.017.

19. Kathleen E. Corey, Joseph Misdraji, Lou Gelrud, Lindsay Y. King, Hui Zheng, Atul Malhotra, and Raymond T. Chung, "Obstructive Sleep Apnea Is Associated with Nonalcoholic Liver Disease and Advanced Liver Histology," *Digestive Diseases and Sciences* 60, no. 8 (August 2015): 2523-2528, https://doi.org/10.1007/s10620-015-3650-8; Tzu-Chieh Chou, Wen-Miin Liang, Chang-Bi Wang, Trong-Neng Wu, and Liang-Wen Hang, "Obstructive Sleep Apnea Is Associated with Liver Disease: A Population-Based Cohort Study," *Sleep Medicine* 16, no. 8 (2015): 955-960, https://doi.org/10.1016/j.sleep.2015.02.542.

20. Eric M. Matheson, Dana E. King, and Charles J. Everett, "Healthy Lifestyle Habits and Mortality in Overweight and Obese Individuals," *Journal of the American Board of Family Medicine: JABFM* 25, no. 1 (2012): 9-15, https://doi.org/10.3122/jabfm.2012.01.110164.

21. Hiromichi Imaizumi, Atsushi Takahashi, Nobuo Tanji, Kazumichi Abe, Yuji Sato, Yukio Anzai, Hiroshi Watanabe, and Hiromasa Ohira, "The Association Between Sleep Duration and Non-alcoholic Fatty Liver Disease Among Japanese Men and Women," *Obesity Facts* 8, no. 4 (2015): 234-242, https://doi.org/10.1159/000436997.

22. Gi-Ae Kim, Han Chu Lee, Jaewon Choe, Min-Ju Kim, Min Jung Lee, Hye-Sook Chang, In Young Bae, et al., "Association Between Non-alcoholic Fatty Liver Disease and Cancer Incidence Rate," *Journal of Hepatology* 68, no. 1 (January 2018): 140-146, https://doi.org/10.1016/j.jhep.2017.09.012.

23. Tracey G. Simon, Bjorn Roelstraete, Kayla Hartjes, Uzma Shah, Hamed Khalili, Henrik Arnell, and Jonas F. Ludvigsson, "Non-alcoholic Fatty Liver Disease in Children and Young Adults Is Associated with Increased Long-Term Mortality," *Journal of Hepatology* 75, no. 5 (2021): 1034-1041, https://doi.org/10.1016/j.jhep.2021.06.034.

24. Susan A. Carlson, E. Kathleen Adams, Zhou Yang, and Janet E. Fulton, "Percentage of Deaths Associated with Inadequate Physical Activity in the United States," *Preventing Chronic Disease* 15 (2018): 170354, http://dx.doi.org/10.5888/pcd18.170354.

25. Gretchen Reynolds, "Walking Just 10 Minutes a Day May Lead to a Longer Life," *New York Times*, January 26, 2022, https://www.nytimes.com/2022/01/26/well/10-minutes-walking-exercise.html.

26. Nathan A. Johnson and Jacob George, "Fitness Versus Fatness: Moving Beyond Weight Loss in Nonalcoholic Fatty Liver Disease," *Hepatology* 52, no. 1 (2010): 370-381, https://doi.org/10.1002/hep.23711.

27. Shelley E. Keating, Daniel A. Hackett, Helen M. Parker, Helen T. O'Connor, James A. Gerofi, Amanda Sainsbury, Michael K. Baker, et al., "Effect of Aerobic Exercise Training Dose on Liver Fat and Visceral Adiposity," *Journal of Hepatology* 63, no. 1 (2015): 174-182, https://doi.org/10.1016/j.jhep.2015.02.022.

28. Elin Ekblom-Bak, Björn Ekblom, Max Vikström, Ulf de Faire, and Mai-Lis Hellénius, "The Importance of Non-exercise Physical Activity for Cardiovascular Health and Longevity," *British Journal of Sports Medicine* 48, no. 3 (2014): 233-238, https://doi.org/10.1136/bjsports-2012-092038.

29. Christopher M. Depner, Edward L. Melanson, Robert H. Eckel, Janet K. Snell-Bergeon, Leigh Perreault, Bryan C. Bergman, Janine A. Higgins, et al., "Ad Libitum Weekend Recovery Sleep Fails to Prevent Metabolic Dysregulation During a Repeating Pattern of Insufficient Sleep and Weekend Recovery Sleep," *Current Biology* 29, no. 6 (2019): 957-967.e4, https://doi.org/10.1016/j.cub.2019.01.069.

30. Esra Tasali, Kristen Wroblewski, Eva Kahn, Jennifer Kilkus, and Dale A. Schoeller, "Effect of Sleep Extension on Objectively Assessed Energy Intake Among Adults with Overweight in Real-Life Settings: A Randomized Clinical Trial," *JAMA Internal Medicine* (February 2022): e218098. Advance online publication, https://doi.org/10.1001/jamainternmed.2021.8098.

31. Sarosh J. Motivala, A. Janet Tomiyama, Michael Ziegler, Srikrishna Khandrika, and Michael R. Irwin, "Nocturnal Levels of Ghrelin and Leptin and Sleep in Chronic Insomnia," *Psychoneuroendocrinology* 34, no. 4 (2009): 540–545, https://doi.org/10.1016/j.psyneuen.2008.10.016.

32. "Sleep Statistics," National Sleep Foundation. Updated November 21, 2021, https://www.sleepfoundation.org/how-sleep-works/sleep-facts-statistics.

33. Danbee Kang, Di Zhao, Seungho Ryu, Eliseo Guallar, Juhee Cho, Mariana Lazo, Hocheol Shin, Yoosoo Chang, and Eunju Sung, "Perceived Stress and Nonalcoholic Fatty Liver Disease in Apparently Healthy Men and Women," *Scientific Reports* 10, no. 38 (2020): 21978, https://doi.org/10.1038/s41598-019-57036-z.

34. Rachael A. Heckenberg, Pennie Eddy, Stephen Kent, and Bradley J. Wright, "Do Workplace-Based Mindfulness Meditation Programs Improve Physiological Indices of Stress? A Systematic Review and Meta-analysis," *Journal of Psychosomatic Research*, no. 114 (2018): 62–71, https://doi.org/10.1016/j.jpsychores.2018.09.010.

35. Sara B. Seidelmann, Brian Claggett, Susan Cheng, Mir Henglin, Amil Shah, Lyn M. Steffen, Aaron R. Folsom, Eric B. Rimm, Walter C. Willett, and Scott D. Solomon, "Dietary Carbohydrate Intake and Mortality: A Prospective Cohort Study and Meta-analysis," *Lancet Public Health* 3, no. 9 (2018): e419–e428, https://doi.org/10.1016/S2468-2667(18)30135-X.

36. Lee Crosby, Brenda Davis, Shivam Joshi, Meghan Jardine, Jennifer Paul, Maggie Neola, and Neal D. Barnard, "Ketogenic Diets and Chronic Disease: Weighing the Benefits Against the Risks," *Frontiers in Nutrition*, no. 8 (2021): 702802, https://doi.org/10.3389/fnut.2021.702802.

37. Zeneng Wang, Nathalie Bergeron, Bruce S. Levison, Xinmin S. Li, Sally Chiu, Xun Jia, Robert A. Koeth, et al., "Impact of Chronic Dietary Red Meat, White Meat, or Non-meat Protein on Trimethylamine N-oxide Metabolism and Renal Excretion in Healthy Men and Women," *European Heart Journal* 40, no. 7 (2019): 583–594, https://doi.org/10.1093/eurheartj/ehy799.

38. Vikas Menon, Sujita Kumar Kar, Navratan Suthar, and Naresh Nebhinani, "Vitamin D and Depression: A Critical Appraisal of the Evidence and Future Directions," *Indian Journal of Psychological Medicine* 42, no. 1 (2020): 11–21, https://doi.org/10.4103/IJPSYM.IJPSYM_160_19.

39. Melinda H. Spooner and Donald B. Jump, "Omega-3 Fatty Acids and Nonalcoholic Fatty Liver Disease in Adults and Children: Where Do We Stand?" *Current Opinion in Clinical Nutrition and Metabolic Care* 22, no. 2 (2019): 103–110, https://doi.org/10.1097/MCO.0000000000000539.

40. Rafael de Cabo and Mark P. Mattson, "Effects of Intermittent Fasting on Health, Aging, and Disease," *New England Journal of Medicine* 381, no. 26 (2019): 2541-2551, https://doi.org/10.1056/NEJMra1905136.

41. Rona Antoni, Tracey Robertson, M. D. Robertson, and Jonathan D. Johnston, "A Pilot Feasibility Study Exploring the Effects of a Moderate Time-Restricted Feeding Intervention on Energy Intake, Adiposity, and Metabolic Physiology in Free-Living Human Subjects," *Journal of Nutritional Science,* no. 7 (2018): E22, https://doi.org/10.1017/jns.2018.13.

42. Jenna B. Gillen, Brian J. Martin, Martin J. MacInnis, Lauren E. Skelly, Mark A. Tarnopolsky, and Martin J. Gibala,"Twelve Weeks of Sprint Interval Training Improves Indices of Cardiometabolic Health Similar to Traditional Endurance Training Despite a Five-Fold Lower Exercise Volume and Time Commitment," *PloS One* 11, no. 4 (2016): e0154075, https://doi.org/10.1371/journal.pone.0154075.

43. Yuki Hamada and Naoyuki Hayashi, "Chewing Increases Postprandial Diet-Induced Thermogenesis," *Scientific Reports* 11, no. 1 (2021): 23714, https://doi.org/10.1038/s41598-021-03109-x.

44. Lan Lam, "Can Baking Soda Remove Pesticides from Produce?," *Cook's Illustrated*, December 3, 2019, https://www.americastestkitchen.com/cooks illustrated/articles/2075-can-baking-soda-remove-pesticides-from-produce.

Chapter 5

1. Ming Ding, Ambika Satija, Shilpa N. Bhupathiraju, Yang Hu, Qi Sun, Jiali Han, Esther Lopez-Garcia, Walter Willett, Rob M. van Dam, and Frank B. Hu, "Association of Coffee Consumption with Total and Cause-Specific Mortality in 3 Large Prospective Cohorts," *Circulation* 132, no. 24 (2015): 2305-2315, https://doi.org/10.1161/CIRCULATIONAHA.115.017341.

2. Louise J. M. Alferink, Juliana Fittipaldi, Jessica C. Kiefte-deJong, Harry L. A. Janssen, Oscar H. Franco, and Sarwa Darwish Murad, "Coffee and Herbal Tea Consumption Is Associated with Lower Liver Stiffness in the General Population: The Rotterdam Study," *Journal of Hepatology* 67, no. 2 (August 2017): 339-348, https://doi.org/10.1016/j.jhep.2017.03.013.

3. Shaohua Chen, Narci C. Teoh, Shiv Chitturi, and Geoffrey C. Farrell, "Coffee and Non-alcoholic Fatty Liver Disease: Brewing Evidence for Hepatoprotection?" *Journal of Gastroenterology and Hepatology* 29, no. 3, 435-441, https://doi.org/10.1111/jgh.12422.

4. Qian Xiao, Rashmi Sinha, Barry I. Graubard, and Neal D. Freedman, "Inverse Associations of Total and Decaffeinated Coffee with Liver Enzyme Levels in National Health and Nutrition Examination Survey 1999-2010," *Hepatology* 60, no. 6 (2014): 2091-2098, https://doi.org/10.1002/hep.27367.

5. Eating more nutrient-dense foods will help kids feel their fullness, as the packaged junk foods so many kids love are designed to taste so good that they drown out the cues their bodies send that it's time to stop eating.

6. Xiao Chen, Zheng Zhang, Huan Li, Jiangtao Zhao, Xiao Wei, Weishi Lin, Xiangna Zhao, Aimin Jiang, and Jing Yuan, "Endogenous Ethanol Produced by Intestinal Bacteria Induces Mitochondrial Dysfunction in Non-alcoholic Fatty Liver Disease," *Journal of Gastroenterology and Hepatology* 35, no. 11 (2020): 2009-2019, https://doi.org/ 10.1111/jgh.15027.

7. Nimer Assy, Gattas Nasser, Iad Kamayse, William Nseir, Zaza Beniashvili, Agness Djibre, and Maria Grosovski, "Soft Drink Consumption Linked with Fatty Liver in the Absence of Traditional Risk Factors," *Canadian Journal of Gastroenterology [Journal canadien de gastroenterologie]* 22, no. 10 (2008): 811-816, https://doi.org/10.1155/2008/810961.

8. Karen R. Jonscher, Michael S. Stewart, Alba Alfonso-Garcia, Brian C. DeFelice, Xiaoxin X. Wang, Yuhuan Luo, Moshe Levi, et al., "Early PQQ Supplementation Has Persistent Long-Term Protective Effects on Developmental Programming of Hepatic Lipotoxicity and Inflammation in Obese Mice," *FASEB Journal* 31, no. 4 (April 2017): 1434-1448, https://doi.org/10.1096/fj.201600906R.

9. Shunming Zhang, Shubham Kumari, Yeqing Gu, Xiaohui Wu, Xiaoyue Li, Ge Meng, Qing Zhang, et al., "Soy Food Intake Is Inversely Associated with Newly Diagnosed Nonalcoholic Fatty Liver Disease in the TCLSIH Cohort Study," *Journal of Nutrition* 150, no. 12 (2020): 3280-3287, https://doi.org/10.1093/jn /nxaa297.

10. American Society for Biochemistry and Molecular Biology, "Soy Protein Alleviates Symptoms of Fatty Liver Disease, Study Suggests," *ScienceDaily*, April 22, 2012, https://www.sciencedaily.com/releases/2012/04/120422162417.htm.

11. Mingyao Sun, Yeyi Gu, Shannon L. Gilsan, and Joshua D. Lambert, "Dietary Cocoa Ameliorates Non-alcoholic Fatty Liver Disease and Increases Markers of Antioxidant Response and Mitochondrial Biogenesis in High Fat-Fed Mice," *Journal of Nutritional Biochemistry*, no. 92 (2021): 108618, https://doi.org /10.1016/j.jnutbio.2021.108618.

12. Alireza Bahrami, Farshad Teymoori, Tannaz Eslamparast, Golbon Sohrab, Ehsan Hejazi, Hossein Poustchi, and Azita Hekmatdoost, "Legume Intake and Risk of Nonalcoholic Fatty Liver Disease," *Indian Journal of Gastroenterology: Official Journal of the Indian Society of Gastroenterology* 38, no. 1 (2019): 55-60, https://doi.org/ 10.1007/s12664-019-00937-8.

13. Fei Yue, Wenjiao Li, Jing Zou, Xianhan Jiang, Gulbin Xu, Hai Huang, and Leyuan Liu, "Spermidine Prolongs Lifespan and Prevents Liver Fibrosis and Hepatocellular Carcinoma by Activating MAP1S-mediated Autophagy," *Cancer Research* 77, no. 11 (June 2017): 2938-2951, https://doi.org/10.1158/0008-5472 .CAN-16-3462.

14. Davood Soleimani, Zamzam Paknahad, Gholamreza Askari, Bijan Iraj, and Awat Feizi, "Effect of Garlic Powder Consumption on Body Composition in Patients with Nonalcoholic Fatty Liver Disease: A Randomized, Double-Blind, Placebo-Controlled Trial," *Advanced Biomedical Research* 5, no. 2 (2016): eCollection 2016, https://doi.org/10.4103/2277-9175.174962.

15. Penn State, "Green Tea Extract Combined with Exercise Reduces Fatty Liver Disease in Mice: Although Untested in Human Trials, Results Suggest a Potential Health Strategy," *ScienceDaily*, February 14, 2020, https://www.sciencedaily.com/releases/2020/02/200214134655.htm; Weslie Y. Khoo, Benjamin J. Chrisfield, Sudathip Sae-tan, and Joshua D. Lambert, "Mitigation of Nonalcoholic Fatty Liver Disease in High-Fat-Fed Mice by the Combination of Decaffeinated Green Tea Extract and Voluntary Exercise," *Journal of Nutritional Biochemistry*, no. 76 (2020): 108262, https://doi.org/10.1016/j.jnutbio.2019.108262.

16. Masanobu Hibi, Hideto Takase, Masaki Iwasaki, Noriko Osaki, and Yoshihisa Katsuragi, "Efficacy of Tea Catechin-Rich Beverages to Reduce Abdominal Adiposity and Metabolic Syndrome Risks in Obese and Overweight Subjects: A Pooled Analysis of 6 Human Trials," *Nutrition Research*, no. 55 (2018): 1-10, https://doi.org/10.1016/j.nutres.2018.03.012.

17. Gal Tsaban, Anat Yaskolka Meir, Ehud Rinott, Hila Zelicha, Alon Kaplan, Aryeh Shalev, Amos Katz, et al., "The Effect of Green Mediterranean Diet on Cardiometabolic Risk: A Randomised Controlled Trial," *Heart* 107, no. 13 (2021): 1054-1061, https://doi.org/10.1136/heartjnl-2020-317802.

18. Marta Guasch-Ferre, Yanping Li, Walter Willett, Qi Sun, Laura Sampson, Jordi Salas-Salvado, Miguel Ángel Martinez-Gonzale, Meir Stampfer, and Frank Hu, "Consumption of Total Olive Oil and Risk of Total and Cause-Specific Mortality in US Adults," *Current Developments in Nutrition* 5, no. S2 (2021): 1036, https://doi.org/10.1093/cdn/nzab053_029.

19. Nimer Assy, Faris Nassar, Gattas Nasser, and Maria Grosovski, "Olive Oil Consumption and Non-alcoholic Fatty Liver Disease," *World Journal of Gastroenterology* 15, no. 15 (2009): 1809-1815, https://doi.org/10.3748/wjg.15.1809.

20. Christine C. Hsu, Erik Ness, Kris V. Kowdley, "Nutritional Approaches to Achieve Weight Loss in Nonalcoholic Fatty Liver Disease," *Advances in Nutrition*, no. 8 (2017): 253-265, https://doi.org/10.3945/an.116.013730.

21. Constantine E. Kosmas, Ian Martinez, Andreas Sourlas, Kyriaki V. Bouza, Frederick N. Campos, Verenisse Torres, Peter D. Montan, and Eliscer Guman, "High-Density Lipoprotein (HDL) Functionality and Its Relevance to Atherosclerotic Cardiovascular Disease," *Drugs Context*, no. 7 (2018): 212525, https://doi.org/10.7573/dic.212525.

22. Elena S. George, Adrienne Forsyth, Catherine Itsiopoulos, Amanda J. Nicoll, Marno Ryan, Siddharth Sood, Stuart K. Roberts, and Audrey C. Tierney,

"Practical Dietary Recommendations for the Prevention and Management of Nonalcoholic Fatty Liver Disease in Adults," *Advances in Nutrition* 9, no. 1 (2018): 30-40, https://doi.org/10.1093/advances/nmx007.

23. Amel Nakbi, Wafa Tayeb, Abir Grissa, Manel Issaoui, Samia Dabbou, Issam Chargui, Meriem Ellouz, Abdelhedi Miled, and Mohamed Hammami, "Effects of Olive Oil and Its Fractions on Oxidative Stress and the Liver's Fatty Acid Composition in 2,4-Dichlorophenoxyacetic Acid-Treated Rats," *Nutrition and Metabolism*, no. 7 (2010): 80.

24. Linqiang Ma, Honggui Li, Jinbo Hu, Juan Zheng, Jing Zhou, Rachel Botchlett, Destiny Matthews, et al., "Indole Alleviates Diet-Induced Hepatic Steatosis and Inflammation in a Manner Involving Myeloid Cell 6-Phosphofructo-2-Kinase/Fructose-2,6-Biphosphatase 3," *Hepatology* 72, no. 4 (2020): 1191-1203, https://doi.org/10.1002/hep.31115.

25. Chenchen Xu, Mariya Markova, Nicole Seebeck, Anne Loft, Silke Hornemann, Thomas Gantert, Stefan Kabsich, et al., "High-Protein Diet More Effectively Reduces Hepatic Fat than Low-Protein Diet Despite Lower Autophagy and FGF21 Levels," *Liver International* 40, no. 12 (2020): 2982-2997, https://doi.org/10.1111/liv.14596.

26. Denisa Margină, Anca Ungurianu, Carmen Purdel, George Mihai Nitulescu, Dimitris Tsoukalas, Evangelia Sarandi, Mari Thanasoula, et al., "Analysis of the Intricate Effects of Polyunsaturated Fatty Acids and Polyphenols on Inflammatory Pathways in Health and Disease," *Food and Chemical Toxicology*, no. 143 (2020): 111558, https://doi.org/10.1016/j.fct.2020.111558; Kátia Cansanção, Marta Citelli, Nathalie Carvalho Leite, María-Carmen López de Las Hazas, Alberto Dávalos, Maria das Graças Tavares do Carmo, and Wilza Arantes Ferreira Peres, "Impact of Long-Term Supplementation with Fish Oil in Individuals with Non-alcoholic Fatty Liver Disease: A Double Blind Randomized Placebo Controlled Clinical Trial," *Nutrients* 12, no. 11 (2020): 3372, https://doi.org/10.3390/nu12113372.

27. Shunming Zhang, Jingzhu Fu, Qing Zhang, Li Liu, Ge Meng, Zhankin Yao, Hongmei Wu, et al., "Association Between Nut Consumption and Non-alcoholic Fatty Liver Disease in Adults," *Liver International: Official Journal of the International Association for the Study of the Liver* 39, no. 9 (2019): 1732-1741, https://doi.org/10.1111/liv.14164.

28. Shawn N. Katterman, Brighid M. Kleinman, Megan M. Hood, Lisa M. Nackers, and Joyce A. Corsica, "Mindfulness Meditation as an Intervention for Binge Eating, Emotional Eating, and Weight Loss: A Systematic Review," *Eating Behaviors* 15, no. 2 (2014): 197-204, https://doi.org/10.1016/j.eatbeh.2014.01.005.

29. Carolyn Dunn, Megan Haubenreiser, Madison Johnson, Kelly Nordby, Surabhi Aggarwal, Sarah Myer, and Cathy Thomas, "Mindfulness Approaches and Weight Loss, Weight Maintenance, and Weight Regain," *Current Obesity Reports* 7, no. 1 (2018): 37-49, https://doi.org/10.1007/s13679-018-0299-6.

30. Hugo J. Alberts, Roy Thewissen, and L. Raes, "Dealing with Problematic Eating Behaviour: The Effects of a Mindfulness-Based Intervention on Eating Behaviour, Food Cravings, Dichotomous Thinking and Body Image Concern," *Appetite* 58, no. 3 (2012): 847-851, https://doi.org/10.1016/j.appet.2012.01.009.

Chapter 6

1. Denisa Margină, Anca Ungurianu, Carmen Purdel, George Mihai Nitulescu, Dimitris Tsoukalas, Evangelia Sarandia, Maria Thanasoula, et al., "Analysis of the Intricate Effects of Polyunsaturated Fatty Acids and Polyphenols on Inflammatory Pathways in Health and Disease," *Food and Chemical Toxicology*, no. 143 (2020): 111558, https://doi.org/10.1016/j.fct.2020.111558.

Chapter 7

1. Masoumeh Akhlaghi, Maryam Ghasemi-Nasab, and Maryamsadat Riasatian, "Mediterranean Diet for Patients with Non-alcoholic Fatty Liver Disease, a Systematic Review and Meta-analysis of Observational and Clinical Investigations," *Journal of Diabetes and Metabolic Disorders* 19, no. 1 (2020): 575-584, https://doi.oeg/10.1007/s40200-019-00475-2.

2. Harpreet Gosal, Harsimran Kaur, Hyginus Chakwop Ngassa, Khaled A. Elmenawi, Vishwanath Anil, and Lubna Mohammed, "The Significance of the Mediterranean Diet in the Management of Non-alcoholic Fatty Liver Disease: A Systematic Review," *Cureus* 13, no. 6 (2021): e15618, https://doi.org/10.7759/cureus.15618.

3. Ludovico Abenavoli, Luigi Boccuto, Alessandro Federico, Marcello Dallio, Carmelina Loguercio, Laura Di Renzo, and Antonino De Lorenzo, "Diet and Non-alcoholic Fatty Liver Disease: The Mediterranean Way," *International Journal of Environmental Research and Public Health* 16, no. 17 (2019): 3011, https:/doi.org/10.3390/ijerph16173011.

Chapter 8

1. Sara B. Seidelmann, Brian Claggett, Susan Cheng, Mir Henglin, Amil Shah, Lyn M. Steffen, Aaron R. Folsom, Eric B. Rimm, Walter C. Willett, and Scott D. Solomon, "Dietary Carbohydrate Intake and Mortality: A Prospective Cohort Study and Meta-analysis," *Lancet Public Health* 3, no. 9 (2018): e419-e428, https://doi.org/10.1016/S2468-2667(18)30135-X.

2. Mohsen Mazidi, Niki Katsiki, Dimitri P. Mikhailidis, Naveed Sattar, and Maciej Banach, "Lower Carbohydrate Diets and All-Cause and Cause-Specific Mortality: A Population-Based Cohort Study and Pooling of Prospective

Studies," *European Heart Journal* 40, no. 34 (2019): 2870-2879, https://doi
.org/10.1093/eurheartj/ehz174; Russell J. de Souza, Mahshid Dehghan, and
Sonia S. Anand, "Low Carb or High Carb? Everything in Moderation . . . Until
Further Notice," *European Heart Journal* 40, no. 34 (2019): 2880-2882, https://
doi.org/10.1093/eurheartj/ehz269.

3. Sarah Gribbin, Joanne Enticott, Allison M. Hodge, Lisa Moran, Eleanor
Thong, Anju Joham, and Sarah Zaman, "Association of Carbohydrate and Saturated Fat Intake with Cardiovascular Disease and Mortality in Australian
Women," *Heart* 108, no. 12 (2022): 932-939, https://doi.org/10.1136/heartjnl
-2021-319654.

4. Kyungho Ha, Kisun Nam, and YoonJu Song, "A Moderate-Carbohydrate Diet
with Plant Protein Is Inversely Associated with Cardiovascular Risk Factors: The
Korea National Health and Nutrition Examination Survey 2013-2017," *Nutrition
Journal* 19, no. 1 (2020): 84, https://doi.org/10.1186/s12937-020-00603-2.

5. de Souza, Dehghan, and Anand, "Low Carb or High Carb?" 2880-2882.

6. Celeste E. Naude, Amanda Brand, Anel Schoonees, Kim A. Nguyen, Marty
Chaplin, and Jimmy Volmink, "Low-Carbohydrate Versus Balanced-Carbohydrate
Diets for Reducing Weight and Cardiovascular Risk," *Cochrane Database of
Systematic Reviews* 1, no. 1 (2022): CD013334, https://doi.org/10.1002/14651858
.CD013334.pub2.

7. de Souza, Dehghan, and Anand, "Low Carb or High Carb?" 2880-2882.

Chapter 9

1. Cara B. Ebbeling, Amy Knapp, Ann Johnson, Julia M. W. Wong, Kimberly F.
Greco, Clement Ma, Samia Mora, and David S. Ludwig, "Effects of a Low-
Carbohydrate on Insulin-Resistant Dyslipoproteinemia—a Randomized Controlled Feeding Trial," *American Journal of Clinical Nutrition* 115, no. 1 (2022):
154-162, https://doi.org/ 10.1093/ajcn/nqab287.

2. Jeannie Tay, Natalie D. Luscombe-Marsh, Campbell H. Thompson, Manny
Noakes, Jonathan D. Buckley, Gary A. Wittert, William S. Yancy Jr., and Grant D.
Brinkworth, "Comparison of Low- and High-Carbohydrate Diets for Type 2 Diabetes Management: A Randomized Trial," *American Journal of Clinical Nutrition*
102, no. 4 (2015): 780-790, https://doi.org/10.3945/ajcn.115.112581.

3. Tay et al., "Comparison of Low- and High-Carbohydrate Diets for Type 2 Diabetes Management," 780-790.

4. Cara B. Ebbeling, Henry A. Feldman, Gloria L. Klein, Julia M. W. Wong, Lisa
Bielak, Sarah K. Steltz, Patricia K. Luoto, Robert R. Wolfe, William W. Wong, and
David S. Ludwig, "Effects of a Low Carbohydrate Diet on Energy Expenditure
During Weight Loss Maintenance: Randomized Trial," *BMJ (Clinical Research
Ed.)* 363 (2018): k4583, https://doi.org/10.1136/bmj.k4583.

5. Kate Hallsworth and Leon A. Adams, "Lifestyle Modification in NAFLD/ NASH: Facts and Figures," *JHEP Reports: Innovation in Hepatology* 1, no. 6 (2019): 468-479, https://doi.org/10.1016/j.jhepr.2019.10.008.

Chapter 10

1. Juan Hernandez, Soufien Rhimi, Aicha Kriaa, Vincent Mariaule, Houda Boudaya, Amandine Drut, Amin Jablaoui, et al., "Domestic Environment and Gut Microbiota: Lessons from Pet Dogs," *Microorganisms* 10, no. 5 (2022): 949, https://doi.org/10.3390/microorganisms10050949.

2. Truls Østbye, Rahul Malhotra, Marissa Stroo, Cheryl Lovelady, Rebecca Brouwer, Nancy Zucker, and Bernard Fuemmeler, "The Effect of the Home Environment on Physical Activity and Dietary Intake in Preschool Children," *International Journal of Obesity* 37, no. 10 (2013): 1314-1321, https://doi.org/10.1038/ijo.2013.76.

3. Gisela Nyberg, Åsa Norman, Elinor Sundblom, Zangin Zeebari, and Liselotte Schäfer Elinder, "Effectiveness of a Universal Parental Support Programme to Promote Health Behaviours and Prevent Overweight and Obesity in 6-Year-Old Children in Disadvantaged Areas, the Healthy School Start Study II, a Cluster-Randomised Controlled Trial," *International Journal of Behavioral Nutrition and Physical Activity* 13, no. 4 (2016), https://doi.org/10.1186/s12966-016-0327-4.

4. Eric A. Klein, Ian M. Thompson Jr., Catherine M. Tangen, John J. Crowley, M. Scott Lucia, Phyllis J. Goodman, Lori Minasian, et al., "Vitamin E and the Risk of Prostate Cancer: The Selenium and Vitamin E Cancer Prevention Trial (SELECT)," *JAMA* 306, no. 14 (2011): 1549-1556, https://doi.org/10.1001/jama.2011.1437.

5. Kathryn T. Hall, Julie E. Buring, Kenneth J. Mukamal, M. Vinayaga Moorthy, Peter M. Wayne, Ted J. Kaptchuk, Elisabeth M. Battinelli, et al., "COMT and Alpha-Tocopherol Effects in Cancer Prevention: Gene-Supplement Interactions in Two Randomized Clinical Trials," *Journal of the National Cancer Institute* 111, no. 7 (2019): 684-694, https://doi.org/10.1093/jnci/djy204.

6. Megan E. Harrison, Mark L. Norris, Nicole Obeid, Maeghan Fu, Hannah Weinstangel, and Margaret Sampson, "Systematic Review of the Effects of Family Meal Frequency on Psychosocial Outcomes in Youth," *Canadian Family Physician [Médecin de famille canadien]* 61, no. 2 (2015): e96-e106.

7. Keeley J. Pratt, Joseph A. Skelton, Kristina H. Lewis, Christopher A. Taylor, Colleen K. Spees, and Callie L Brown, "Family Meal Practices and Weight Talk Between Adult Weight Management and Weight Loss Surgery Patients and Their Children," *Journal of Nutrition Education and Behavior* 52, no. 6 (2020): 579-587, https://doi.org/10.1016/j.jneb.2020.04.001.

Chapter 11

1. Suzanne Phelan, Tate Halfman, Angela Marinilli Pinto, and Gary D. Foster, "Behavioral and Psychological Strategies of Long-Term Weight Loss Maintainers in a Widely Available Weight Management Program," *Obesity* 28, no. 2 (2020): 421–428, https://doi.org/10.1002/oby.22685; Suzanne Phelan, James Roake, Noemi Alarcon, Sarah M. Ng, Hunter Glanz, Michelle I. Cardel, and Gary D. Foster, "In Their Own Words: Topic Analysis of the Motivations and Strategies of over 6,000 Long-Term Weight-Loss Maintainers," *Obesity*, no. 30 (2022): 751–761, https://doi.org/10.1002/oby.23372.

2. Olya Bullard and Rajesh V. Manchanda, "How Goal Progress Influences Regulatory Focus in Goal Pursuit," *Journal of Consumer Psychology* 27, no. 3 (2017): 302–317, https://doi.org/10.1016/j.jcps.2017.01.003.

3. Richard J. Vann, José Antonio Rosa, and Sean M. McCrea, "When Consumers Struggle: Action Crisis and Its Effects on Problematic Goal Pursuit," *Psychology and Marketing*, no. 35 (2018): 696–709, https://doi.org/10.1002/mar.21116.

Recipes

1. Priyadarshi R. Shukla, Jim Skea, Andy Reisinger, Raphael Slade, Roger Fradera, Minal Pathak, Alaa Al Khourdajie, et al., ed., "Climate Change 2022: Mitigation of Climate Change." Intergovernmental Panel on Climate Change, Working Group III Contribution to the Sixth Assessment Report of the Intergovernmental Panel on Climate Change, 2022, https://www.ipcc.ch/report/ar6/wg3/downloads/report/IPCC_AR6_WGIII_FullReport.pdf.

Frequently Asked Questions

1. Dina Halegoua-DeMarzio, Victor Navarro, Jawad Ahmad, Bharathi Avula, Huiman Barnhart, A. Sidney Barritt, Herbert L. Bonkovsky, et al., "Liver Injury Associated with Turmeric—A Growing Problem: Ten Cases from the Drug-Induced Liver Injury Network [DILIN]," *American Journal of Medicine* 136, no. 2 (February 2023): 200–206. Advance online publication, https://doi.org/10.1016/j.amjmed.2022.09.026.

Index

Page numbers in italics refer to figures. Page numbers followed by a *t* indicate in item in a table. Recipes appear in bold face.